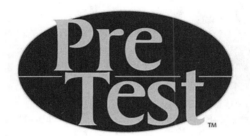

Pediatrics

PreTest™ Self-Assessment and Review

Notice

Medicine is an ever-changing science. As new research and clinical experience broaden our knowledge, changes in treatment and drug therapy are required. The authors and the publisher of this work have checked with sources believed to be reliable in their efforts to provide information that is complete and generally in accord with the standards accepted at the time of publication. However, in view of the possibility of human error or changes in medical sciences, neither the authors nor the publisher nor any other party who has been involved in the preparation or publication of this work warrants that the information contained herein is in every respect accurate or complete, and they disclaim all responsibility for any errors or omissions or for the results obtained from use of the information contained in this work. Readers are encouraged to confirm the information contained herein with other sources. For example and in particular, readers are advised to check the product information sheet included in the package of each drug they plan to administer to be certain that the information contained in this work is accurate and that changes have not been made in the recommended dose or in the contraindications for administration. This recommendation is of particular importance in connection with new or infrequently used drugs.

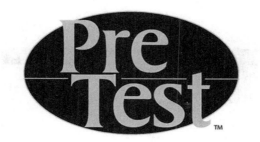

Pediatrics

PreTest™ Self-Assessment and Review
Twelfth Edition

Robert J. Yetman, MD
Professor of Pediatrics
Director, Division of Community and General Pediatrics
Department of Pediatrics
The University of Texas Medical School at Houston
Houston, Texas

Mark D. Hormann, MD
Associate Professor of Pediatrics
Director, Medical Student Education
Division of Community and General Pediatrics
Department of Pediatrics
The University of Texas Medical School at Houston
Houston, Texas

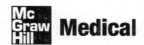

New York   Chicago   San Francisco   Lisbon   London   Madrid   Mexico City
Milan   New Delhi   San Juan   Seoul   Singapore   Sydney   Toronto

Pediatrics: PreTest™; Self-Assessment and Review, Twelfth Edition

Copyright © 2009, 2006, 2003, 2001, 1998, 1995, 1992, 1989, 1987, 1985, 1982, 1978 by The McGraw-Hill Companies, Inc. All rights reserved. Printed in the United States of America. Except as permitted under the United States Copyright Act of 1976, no part of this publication may be reproduced or distributed in any form or by any means, or stored in a database or retrieval system, without the prior written permission of the publisher.

PreTest™ is a trademark of The McGraw-Hill Companies, Inc.

2 3 4 5 6 7 8 9 0   DOC/DOC   14 13 12 11 10

ISBN 978-0-07-159790-6
MHID 0-07-159790-5

This book was set in Berkeley by International Typesetting and Composition.
The editors were Kirsten Funk and Peter J. Boyle.
The production supervisor was Sherri Souffrance.
Project management was provided by Arushi Chawla, International Typesetting and Composition.
RR Donnelley was printer and binder.

This book is printed on acid-free paper.

Library of Congress Cataloging-in-Publication Data

Pediatrics : PreTest self-assessment and review. — 12th ed. / [edited by]
   Robert J. Yetman, Mark D. Hormann.
       p. ; cm.
   Includes bibliographical references and index.
   ISBN-13: 978-0-07-159790-6 (pbk. : alk. paper)
   ISBN-10: 0-07-159790-5 (pbk. : alk. paper) 1. Pediatrics—Examinations,
questions, etc. I. Yetman, Robert. II. Hormann, Mark.
   [DNLM: 1. Pediatrics—Examination Questions. WS 18.2 P371   2009]
RJ48.2.P42   2009
618.9200076—dc22

                                                    2008052985

Student Reviewers

Fatima Cody-Stanford, MD, MPH
University of South Carolina
PGY-2

Stacy Cooper
SUNY Upstate Medical University
Class of 2008

Ilana Harwayne-Gidansky
SUNY Downstate College of Medicine
Class of 2009

Erica Katz
Stony Brook University School of Medicine
Class of 2008

Tina A. Nguyen
SUNY Upstate Medical University
Class of 2008

Contents

Introduction

Pediatrics: PreTest™ Self-Assessment and Review, Twelfth Edition, provides comprehensive self-assessment and review within the field of pediatrics. The 500 questions in the book have been designed to be similar in format and degree of difficulty to the questions in Step 2 of the United States Medical Licensing Examination (USMLE). They may also be a useful study tool for Step 3 or clerkship examinations.

For multiple-choice questions, the **one best** response to each question should be selected. For matching sets, a group of questions will be preceded by a list of lettered options. For each question in the matching set, select **one** lettered option that is **most** closely associated with the question. Each question in this book has a corresponding answer, a reference to a text that provides background to the answer, and a short discussion of various issues raised by the question and its answer.

To simulate the time constraints imposed by the qualifying examinations for which this book is intended as a practice guide, the student or physician should allot about one minute for each question. After answering all questions in a chapter, as much time as necessary should be spent in reviewing the explanations for each question at the end of the chapter. Attention should be given to all explanations, even if the examinee answered the question correctly. Those seeking more information on a subject should refer to the reference materials listed in the bibliography or to other standard texts in medicine.

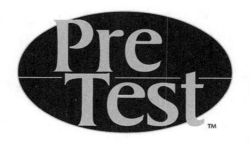

Pediatrics

PreTest™ Self-Assessment and Review

General Pediatrics

Questions

1. Two weeks after a viral syndrome, a 9-year-old boy presents to your clinic with a complaint of several days of weakness of his mouth. In addition to the drooping of the left side of his mouth, you note that he is unable to completely shut his left eye. His smile is asymmetric, but his examination is otherwise normal. Which of the following is the most likely diagnosis?

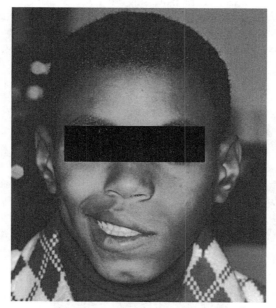

(Courtesy of Robin T. CoHon, MD, as printed with permission from Knoop KJ, Stack LB, Storrow AB. Atlas of Emergency Medicine. *2nd ed. New York, NY: McGraw-Hill; 2002.)*

   a. Guillain-Barré syndrome
   b. Botulism
   c. Cerebral vascular accident
   d. Brainstem tumor
   e. Bell palsy

2. An infant can regard his parent's face, follow to the midline, lift his head from the examining table, smile spontaneously, and respond to a bell. He does not yet regard his own hand, follow past the midline, nor lift his head to a 45° angle off the examining table. Which of the following is the most likely age of the infant?

a. 1 month
b. 3 months
c. 6 months
d. 9 months
e. 12 months

3. A child is brought to your clinic for a routine examination. She can put on a T-shirt but requires a bit of help dressing otherwise. She can copy a circle well but has difficulty in copying a square. Her speech is understandable and she knows four colors. She balances proudly on each foot for 2 seconds but is unable to hold the stance for 5 seconds. Which of the following is the most likely age of this child?

a. 1 year
b. 2 years
c. 3 years
d. 4 years
e. 5 years

4. A 4-year-old girl is noticed by her grandmother to have a limp and a somewhat swollen left knee. The parents report that the patient occasionally complains of pain in that knee. An ophthalmologic examination reveals findings as depicted in the photograph. Which of the following conditions is most likely to be associated with these findings?

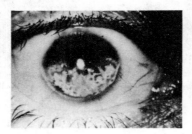

a. Juvenile rheumatoid arthritis
b. Slipped capital femoral epiphysis
c. Henoch-Schönlein purpura
d. Legg-Calvé-Perthes disease
e. Osgood-Schlatter disease

5. A previously healthy 4-year-old child pictured below presents to the emergency room (ER) with a 2-day history of a brightly erythematous rash and temperature of 40°C (104°F). The exquisitely tender, generalized rash is worse in the flexural and perioral areas. The child is admitted and over the next day develops crusting and fissuring around the eyes, mouth, and nose. The desquamation of skin shown in the photograph occurs with gentle traction. Which of the following is the most likely diagnosis?

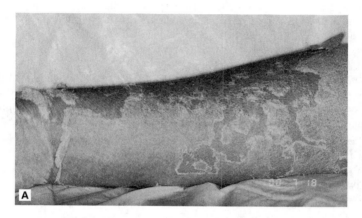

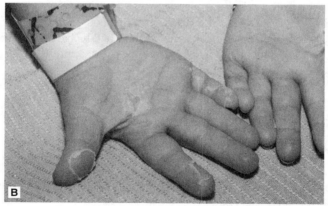

(Courtesy of Adelaide Hebert, MD.)

a. Epidermolysis bullosa
b. Staphylococcal scalded skin syndrome
c. Erythema multiforme
d. Drug eruption
e. Scarlet fever

6. A mother brings to your office an article from the Internet suggesting that infants in day care have a statistically higher incidence of upper respiratory infections ($p < 0.05$) as compared to children not in day care. You explain to her that this means which of the following?

a. Infants in day care are 5% more likely to have an upper respiratory tract infection than infants not in day care.
b. A critical threshold for medical significance has been reached.
c. Infants in day care will have an upper respiratory infection 5% of the time.
d. The odds are less than 1 in 20 that the differences in upper respiratory infection rates observed were only a chance variation.
e. The study suggests that day cares are not safe for children.

7. A patient comes to your office for a hospital follow-up. You had sent him to the hospital 3 weeks earlier for persistent fevers but no other symptoms; he was diagnosed with endocarditis and is currently being treated appropriately. Advice to this family should now include which of the following?

a. Restrict the child from all strenuous activities.
b. Give the child a no-salt-added diet.
c. Provide the child with antibiotic prophylaxis for dental procedures.
d. Test all family members in the home with repeated blood cultures.
e. Avoid allowing the child to get upset or agitated.

8. A mother calls you on the telephone and says that your 4-year-old son bit the hand of her 2-year-old son 48 hours previously. The area around the injury has become red, indurated, and swollen, and he has a temperature of 39.4°C (103°F). Which of the following is the most appropriate response?

a. Arrange for a plastic surgery consultation at the next available appointment.
b. Admit the child to the hospital immediately for surgical debridement and antibiotic treatment.
c. Prescribe penicillin over the telephone and have the mother apply warm soaks for 15 minutes four times a day.
d. Suggest purchase of bacitracin ointment to apply to the lesion three times a day.
e. See the patient in the ER to suture the laceration.

9. The adolescent shown presents with a 14-day history of multiple oval lesions over her back. The rash began with a single lesion over the lower abdomen (A); the other lesions developed over the next days (B). These lesions are slightly pruritic. Which of the following is the most likely diagnosis?

a. Contact dermatitis
b. Pityriasis rosea
c. Seborrheic dermatitis
d. Lichen planus
e. Psoriasis

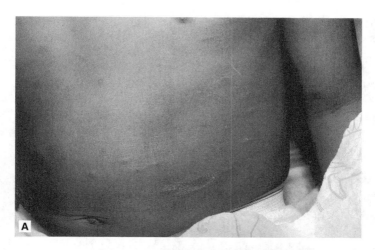

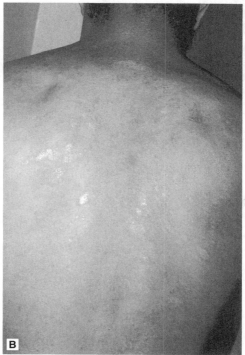

(Courtesy of Adelaide Hebert, MD.)

10. A chubby 6-month-old baby boy is brought to the clinic by his father. His father is concerned that his penis is too small (see photograph). The child is at the 95% for weight and the 50% for length; he has been developing normally and has had no medical problems. Which of the following is the most appropriate first step in management of this child?

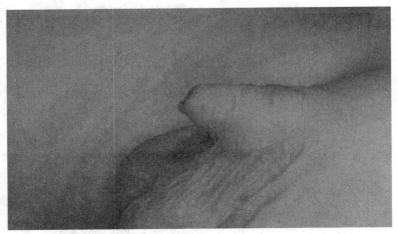

(Courtesy of Michaelene R. Ribbeck, NP, PhD.)

a. Surgical consultation
b. Evaluation of penile length after retracting the skin and fat lateral to the penile shaft
c. Ultrasound for uterus and ovaries
d. Weight loss
e. Serum testosterone levels

I I. A previously healthy 5-year-old boy has a 1-day history of low-grade fever, colicky abdominal pain, and a rash. He is well-appearing and alert. His vital signs, other than a temperature of 38°C (100.5°F) are completely normal. A diffuse, erythematous, maculopapular, and petechial rash is present on his buttocks and lower extremities, as shown in the photograph. He has no localized abdominal tenderness or rebound; bowel sounds are active. Laboratory data demonstrate

Urinalysis: 30 red blood cells (RBCs) per high-powered field, 2+ protein
Stool: Guaiac positive
Platelet count: 135,000/μL

These findings are most consistent with which of the following?

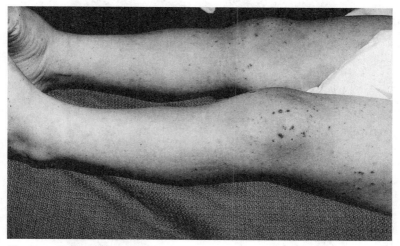

(Courtesy of Adelaide Hebert, MD.)

a. Anaphylactoid purpura
b. Meningococcemia
c. Child abuse
d. Leukemia
e. Hemophilia B

12. A 4-month-old baby boy arrives to the ER cold and stiff. The parents report that he had been healthy and that they put him to bed as usual for the night at the regular time. When they next saw him, in the morning, he was dead. Physical examination is uninformative. A film from a routine skeletal survey is shown below. Which of the following is the most likely diagnosis?

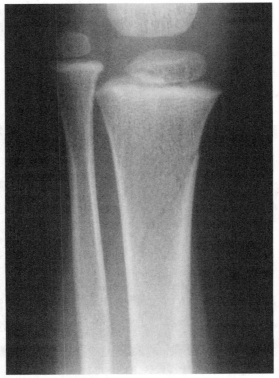

(Courtesy of Susan John, MD.)

a. Scurvy
b. Congenital syphilis
c. Sudden infant death syndrome (SIDS)
d. Osteogenesis imperfecta
e. Abuse

13. A 6-year-old boy is often teased at school because he has stooled in his underwear almost daily for the last 3 months. He was toilet trained at 2 years of age without difficulty, but over the last 2 years he had developed ongoing constipation. His family is frustrated because they cannot believe him when he says "I didn't know I had to go." He is otherwise normal; school is going well, and his home life is stable. His only finding on examination is significant for stool in the rectal vault. The plain radiograph of his abdomen is shown. Initial management of this problem should include which of the following?

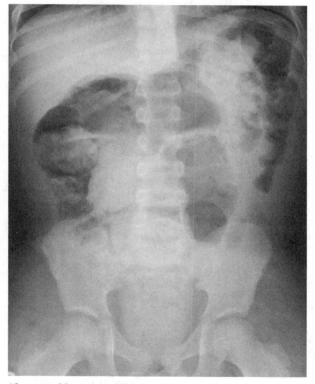

(Courtesy of Susan John, MD.)

a. Barium enema and rectal biopsy
b. Family counseling
c. Time-out when he stools in his underwear
d. Clear fecal impaction and short-term stool softener use
e. Daily enemas for 4 weeks

14. A 2-year-old child presents to the office with a paternal complaint of "bowlegs." The girl has always had bowlegs; her previous pediatrician told the family she would grow out of it. Now, however, it seems to be worsening. Her weight is greater than 95% for age, and she has significant bowing out of her legs and internal tibial torsion; otherwise, her examination is normal. A radiograph of her lower leg is shown. Which of the following is the most likely diagnosis?

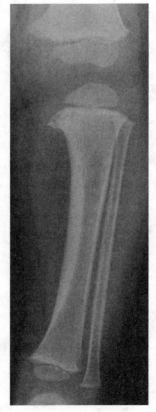

(Courtesy of Susan John, MD.)

a. Osgood-Schlatter disease
b. Physiologic genu varum
c. Slipped capital femoral epiphysis
d. Legg-Calvé-Perthes disease
e. Blount disease

15. A very concerned mother brings a 2-year-old child to your office because of two episodes of a brief, shrill cry followed by a prolonged expiration and apnea. You have been following this child in your practice since birth and know the child to be a product of a normal pregnancy and delivery, to be growing and developing normally, and to have no chronic medical problems. The first episode occurred immediately after the mother refused to give the child some juice; the child became cyanotic, unconscious, and had generalized clonic jerks. A few moments later the child awakened and had no residual effects. The most recent episode (identical in nature) occurred at the grocery store when the child's father refused to purchase a toy for her. Your physical examination reveals a delightful child without unexpected physical examination findings. Which of the following is the most likely diagnosis?

a. Seizure disorder
b. Drug ingestion
c. Hyperactivity with attention deficit
d. Pervasive development disorder
e. Breath-holding spell

16. A 10-year-old child arrives with the complaint of new-onset bed-wetting. He has had no fever, his urine culture is negative, and he has had no new stresses in his life. He is well above the 95th percentile for weight as is much of his family. Which of the following is most helpful in making a diagnosis?

a. Fasting plasma glucose of 135 mg/dL
b. Random plasma glucose of 170 mg/dL
c. Two-hour glucose during glucose tolerance test of 165 mg/dL
d. Acanthosis nigricans on the neck
e. Symptoms alone are enough to make the diagnosis

17. You are called to the ER to see one of your patients. The father of this 14-year-old mildly retarded child says that he found the child about 20 minutes ago in the neighbor's garden shed with an unknown substance in his mouth. The child first had a headache, but then became agitated and confused; while you are talking to the father in the ER the child begins to have a seizure and dysrhythmia on the cardiac monitor. The blood gas demonstrates a severe metabolic acidosis. Which of the following agents is most likely the culprit?

a. Organophosphate
b. Chlorophenothane (DDT)
c. Sodium cyanide
d. Warfarin
e. Paraquat

18. The mother of a 3-day-old infant brings her child to your office for an early follow-up visit. The mom notes that the child has been eating well, has had no temperature instability, and stools and urinates well. She notes that over the previous 3 days the child has had a progressive "rash" on the face as pictured here. Which of the following is the most likely diagnosis?

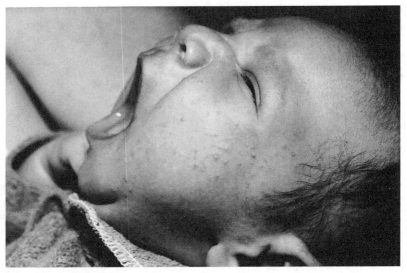

(Courtesy of Adelaide Hebert, MD.)

a. Herpes
b. Neonatal acne
c. Milia
d. Seborrheic dermatitis
e. Eczema

19. A 2-year-old child (A) presents with a 4-day history of a rash limited to the feet and ankles. The papular rash is both pruritic and erythematous. The 3-month-old sibling of this patient (B) has similar lesions also involving the head and neck. The most appropriate treatment for this condition includes which of the following?

a. Coal-tar soap
b. Permethrin
c. Hydrocortisone cream
d. Emollients
e. Topical antifungal cream

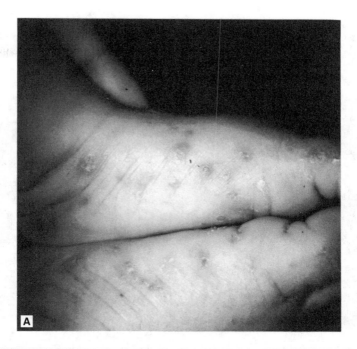

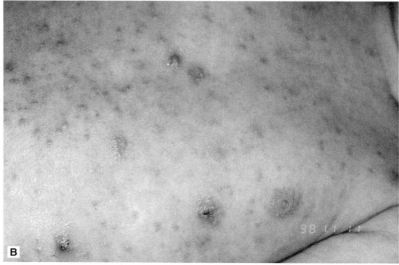

(Courtesy of Adelaide Hebert, MD.)

20. An 8-hour-old infant develops increased respiratory distress, hypothermia, and hypotension. A complete blood count (CBC) demonstrates a white blood cell (WBC) count of 2500/μL with 80% bands. The chest radiograph is shown below. Which of the following is the most likely diagnosis?

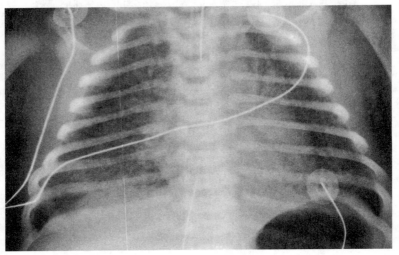

(Courtesy of Susan John, MD.)

a. Congenital syphilis
b. Diaphragmatic hernia
c. Group B streptococcal pneumonia
d. Transient tachypnea of the newborn
e. Chlamydial pneumonia

21. A 16-year-old arrives to your office soon after beginning basketball season. He states that he has had progressive pain in his knees. A physical examination reveals, in addition to tenderness, a swollen and prominent tibial tubercle. Radiographs of the area are unremarkable. Which of the following is the most likely diagnosis?

a. Osgood-Schlatter disease
b. Popliteal cyst
c. Slipped capital femoral epiphysis
d. Legg-Calvé-Perthes disease
e. Gonococcal arthritis

22. You are performing a well-child examination on the 1-year-old child shown in the picture. For this particular problem, which of the following is the most appropriate next step in management?

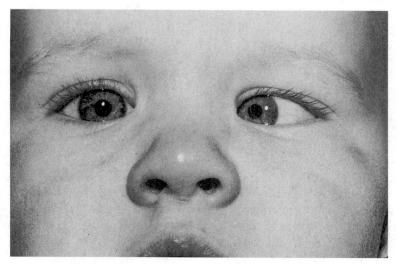

(Courtesy of Kathryn Musgrove, MD.)

a. Patch the eye with the greater refractive error
b. Patch the eye that deviates
c. Defer patching or ophthalmologic examination until the child is older and better able to cooperate
d. Reassure the mother that he will outgrow it
e. Refer immediately to ophthalmology

23. You are seeing a 2-year-old child, brought by his father for a well-child examination. In providing age-appropriate anticipatory guidance, you should tell him which of the following?

a. He should set his water heater to 71°C (160°F) to ensure the sterility of dishes and clothes, thereby decreasing the risk of infections.
b. Milk should be switched from whole to skim or low fat.
c. Continue rear facing car seats.
d. Purchase a bed alarm to assist with the child's nocturnal enuresis.
e. Teach the child to swim so that the parents have the ability to allow the child to be alone in pools.

24. A child can walk well holding on to furniture but is slightly wobbly when walking alone. She uses a neat pincer grasp to pick up a pellet, and she can release a cube into a cup after it has been demonstrated to her. She tries to build a tower of two cubes with variable success. She is most likely at which of the following age?

a. 2 months
b. 4 months
c. 6 months
d. 9 months
e. 1 year

25. You are called by a general practitioner to consult on a patient admitted to the hospital 4 days ago. The patient is a 7-month-old white boy with poor weight gain for the past 3 months, who has not gained weight in the hospital despite seemingly adequate nutrition. You take a detailed diet history from his foster mother, and the amounts of formula and baby food intake seem appropriate for age. Physical examination reveals an active, alert infant with a strong suck reflex who appears wasted. You note generalized lymphadenopathy with hepatomegaly. In addition, you find a severe case of oral candidiasis that apparently has been resistant to treatment. Which of the following is the most appropriate next step in the evaluation or treatment of this child?

a. Increase caloric intake because this is probably a case of underfeeding.
b. Order human immunodeficiency virus (HIV) polymerase chain reaction (PCR) testing because this is likely the presentation of congenitally acquired HIV.
c. Draw blood cultures because this could be sepsis.
d. Perform a sweat chloride test because this is probably cystic fibrosis.
e. Send stool for fecal fat because this is probably a malabsorption syndrome.

26. A 5-year-old boy presents with the severe rash shown in the photographs. The rash is pruritic, and it is especially intense in the flexural areas. The mother reports that the symptoms began in infancy (when it also involved the face) and that her 6-month-old child has similar symptoms. Which of the following is the most appropriate treatment of this condition?

a. Coal-tar soaps and shampoo
b. Topical antifungal cream
c. Ultraviolet light therapy
d. Moisturizers and topical steroids
e. Topical antibiotics

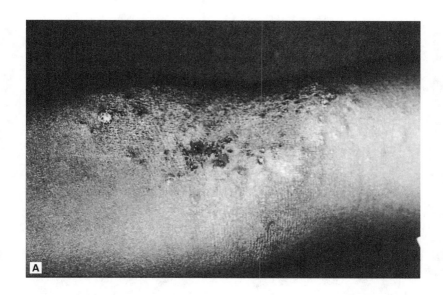

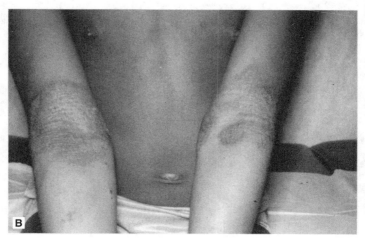

(Courtesy of Adelaide Hebert, MD.)

27. A 1-year-old presents for a well-child checkup, but the parents are concerned about giving the child his immunizations. Which of the following is a true contraindication to the administration of the fourth DTaP (diphtheria and tetanus toxoid and acellular pertussis) vaccine?

a. Child is currently on amoxicillin for an otitis media
b. Positive family history of adverse reactions to DTaP vaccine
c. A past history of infantile spasms
d. Child is currently febrile to 39°C (102.2°F)
e. Prolonged seizures 6 days after the last DTaP vaccine

28. A mother arrives to the clinic with her three children (ages 2 months, 18 months, and 36 months). The 18-month-old has an intensely pruritic scalp, especially in the occipital region, with 0.5-mm lesions noted at the base of hair shafts, as shown in the picture. Which of the following therapies should be avoided in this situation?

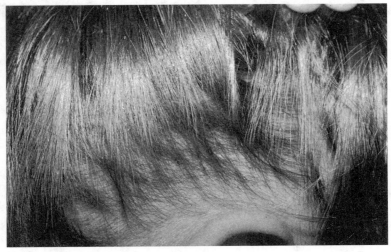

(Courtesy of Adelaide Hebert, MD.)

a. Treatment of all household contacts with 1% lindane (Kwell)
b. Use of 1:1 vinegar-water rinse for hair for nit removal
c. Washing of all clothing and bedding in very hot water
d. Replacement of all commonly used brushes
e. Advice to the mother that treatment will again be necessary in 7 to 10 days

29. A 2-year-old boy has been vomiting intermittently for 3 weeks and has been irritable, listless, and anorectic. His use of language has regressed to speaking single words. In your evaluation of this patient, which of the following is the most reasonable diagnosis to consider?

a. Expanding epidural hematoma
b. Herpes simplex virus (HSV) encephalitis
c. Tuberculous meningitis
d. Food allergy
e. Bacterial meningitis

30. You find a discrete, whitish polyp that extends through the tympanic membrane in a child with a history of recurrent otitis media. This most likely represents which of the following?

a. A cholesteatoma
b. Tympanosclerosis
c. Acute otitis media with perforation and drainage
d. Dislocation of the malleus from its insertion in the tympanic membrane
e. Excessive cerumen production

31. An 8-month-old infant arrives to the emergency department (ED) with a 2-day history of diarrhea and poor fluid intake. Your quick examination reveals a lethargic child; his heart rate is 180 beats per minute, his respiratory rate is 30 breaths per minute, and his blood pressure is low for age. He has poor skin turgor, 5-second capillary refill, and cool extremities. Which of the following fluids is most appropriate management for his condition?

a. Dextrose 5% in 1/4 normal saline (D5 1/4 NS)
b. Dextrose 5% in 1/2 normal saline (D5 1/2 NS)
c. Normal saline
d. Whole blood
e. Dextrose 10% in water (D10W)

32. During the examination of a 2-month-old infant, you note that the infant's umbilical cord is still firmly attached. This finding prompts you to suspect which of the following?

a. Occult omphalocele
b. Leukocyte adhesion deficiency
c. IgG subclass deficiency
d. Umbilical granuloma
e. Persistent urachus (urachal cyst)

33. You are seeing an established patient, a 4-year-old girl brought in by her mother for vaginal itching and irritation. She is toilet trained and has not complained of frequency or urgency, nor has she noted any blood in her urine. Her mother noted she has been afebrile and has not complained of abdominal pain. Mom denies the risk of inappropriate contact; the girl also denies anyone "touching her there." Your physical examination of the perineum is significant for the lack of foul odor or discharge. You do note some erythema of the vulvar area but no evidence of trauma. Which of the following is the most appropriate course of action?

a. Refer to pediatric gynecology for removal under anesthesia of a suspected foreign body in the vagina.
b. Counsel mother to stop giving the girl bubble baths, have the girl wear only cotton underwear, and improve hygiene.
c. Refer to social services for suspected physical or sexual abuse.
d. Swab for gonorrhea and plate on chocolate agar, and send urine for *Chlamydia*.
e. Treat with an antifungal cream for suspected yeast infection.

34. A 20-month-old child is brought to the ED because of fever and irritability and refusal to move his right lower extremity. Physical examination reveals a swollen and tender right knee that resists passive motion. Which of the following is the most likely to yield the diagnosis in this patient?

a. Examination of joint fluid
b. X-ray of the knee
c. Erythrocyte sedimentation rate (ESR)
d. CBC and differential
e. Blood culture

35. A 14-year-old high school student arrives to your clinic for well-child care. In reviewing his records you determine that his most recent immunization for tetanus was at 4 years of age. Which of the following should you recommend?

a. Tetanus toxoid
b. Adult tetanus and diphtheria toxoid (Td)
c. Diphtheria toxoid, whole cell pertussis, and tetanus toxoid (DPT) booster
d. Tetanus toxoid and tetanus immune globulin
e. Tetanus toxoid, reduced diphtheria toxoid, and acellular pertussis vaccine adsorbed (Tdap)

36. A 5-year-old boy is brought into the ER immediately after an unfortunate altercation with a neighbor's immunized Chihuahua that occurred while the child was attempting to dress the dog as a superhero. The fully immunized child has a small, irregular, superficial laceration on his right forearm that has stopped bleeding. His neuromuscular examination is completely normal, and his perfusion is intact. Management should include which of the following?

a. Irrigation and antimicrobial prophylaxis
b. Tetanus booster immunization and tetanus toxoid in the wound
c. Copious irrigation
d. Primary rabies vaccination for the child
e. Destruction of the dog and examination of brain tissue for rabies

37. Aunt Mary is helping her family move to a new apartment. During the confusion, 3-year-old Jimmy is noted to become lethargic. The contents of Aunt Mary's purse are strewn about on the floor. In the ER, the lethargic Jimmy is found to have miosis, bradycardia, and hypotension. He develops apnea, respiratory depression, and has to be intubated. His condition would most likely benefit from which of the following therapies?

a. Deferoxamine
b. Pediatric intensive care unit (PICU) support and trial of naloxone
c. N-acetylcysteine (Mucomyst)
d. Atropine
e. Dimercaptosuccinic acid (DMSA, succimer)

38. As a city public health officer, you have been charged with the task of screening high-risk children for lead poisoning. Which of the following is the best screen for this purpose?

a. Careful physical examination of each infant and child
b. Erythrocyte protoporphyrin levels (EP, FEP, or ZPP)
c. CBC and blood smear
d. Blood lead level
e. Environmental history

39. A 15-year-old is participating in high school football practice in August in Texas. He had complained of headache and nausea earlier in practice, but kept playing after a cup of water. He is now confused and combative. He is dizzy and sweating profusely. His temperature is 41°C (105.8°F). Therapy should consist of which of the following?

a. Provide oral rehydration solutions
b. Administer acetaminophen rectally
c. Order to rest on the bench until symptoms resolve
d. Initiate whole body cold water immersion
e. Tell him to go take a shower and rest until the next day's practice

40. As part of your anticipatory guidance to new parents of a healthy newborn, you suggest putting the child in which of the following positions for sleep?

a. Supine position
b. Prone position
c. Seated position
d. Trendelenburg position
e. A hammock

41. A mentally retarded 14-year-old boy has a long face, large ears, micropenis, and large testes. Chromosome analysis is likely to demonstrate which of the following?

a. Trisomy 21
b. Trisomy 18
c. Trisomy 13
d. Fragile X syndrome
e. Williams syndrome

42. A 5-month-old child with poor growth presents to the ER with generalized tonic-clonic seizure activity of about 30-minute duration that stops upon the administration of lorazepam. Which of the following historical bits of information gathered from the mother is most likely to lead to the correct diagnosis in this patient?

a. The child has had congestion without fever for the past 3 days
b. The child is developmentally normal, as are his siblings
c. The mother has been diluting the infant's formula to make it last longer
d. The mother reports there are two dogs and one cat at home.
e. The mother previously worked as an attorney in an energy-trading firm

Questions 43 to 48

Many rashes and skin lesions can be found first in the newborn period. For each of the descriptions listed below, select the most likely diagnosis. Each lettered option may be used once, more than once, or not at all.

a. Sebaceous nevus
b. Salmon patch
c. Neonatal acne
d. Pustular melanosis
e. Erythema toxicum
f. Seborrheic dermatitis
g. Milia

43. A 1-week-old child's mother complains that the child has a transient rash that has splotchy areas of erythema with a central clear pustule. Your microscopic examination of the liquid in the pustule reveals eosinophils.

44. An adolescent boy complains of a splotchy red rash on the nape of his neck, discovered when he had his head shaved for football season. The rash seems to become more prominent with exercise or emotion. His mother notes that he has had the rash since infancy, but that it became invisible as hair grew. He had a similar rash on his eyelids that resolved in the newborn period.

45. A nurse calls you to evaluate an African American newborn whom she thinks has a bacterial skin infection. The areas in question have many scattered pustules full of a milky fluid. Upon examining pustules, they easily wipe away, revealing a small hyperpigmented macule.

46. The obstetrical resident on call asks you to evaluate an area of a newborn's scalp that seems to have no hair and is scaly and yellowish.

47. A newborn's mother complains that her infant seems to have very small white dots all over his nose. The dots do not wipe off with bathing, but they are also not erythematous.

48. A newborn's father complains that his son has dandruff, with many waxy flakes of skin on the scalp. When he scrapes the lesions, hair often comes off with the flakes of skin. In addition, the baby has flaking of the eyebrows.

Questions 49 to 53

For each otherwise normal child presented, choose the sleep disturbance most consistent with the history. Each lettered option may be used once, more than once, or not at all.

a. Night terrors
b. Nightmares
c. Learned behavior
d. Obstructive sleep apnea
e. Somniloquy

49. A 3-year-old boy awakens every night around 2:00 AM screaming incoherently. His parents note that he is agitated, seems awake but unresponsive, and goes back to sleep within a few minutes. He has no memory of the episodes in the morning.

50. A 15-month-old toddler continues to wake up crying every night. Her parents give her a nighttime bottle, rock her, and sing to her to help her go back to sleep. Her parents are exhausted and ask you if she is having bad dreams.

51. Parents hear over their baby monitor that their 5-year-old girl regularly calls out during the night. When the parents check on her, she is sleeping comfortably and is in no apparent distress.

52. A 4-year-old boy occasionally wakes in the middle of the night crying. When his parents check on him, he seems visibly frightened and tells his parents that Chihuahuas were chasing him.

53. A 5-year-old child refuses to sleep in his bed, claiming there are monsters in his closet and that he has bad dreams. The parents allow him to sleep with them in their bed to avoid the otherwise inevitable screaming fit. The parents note that the child sleeps soundly, waking only at sunrise.

Questions 54 to 58

For each of the cases listed below, select the type of cold injury most likely to be causing the symptoms described. Each lettered option may be used once, more than once, or not at all.

a. Frostnip
b. Frostbite
c. Chilblain
d. Cold panniculitis
e. Hypothermia
f. Trench foot

54. A 6-year-old returns from playing all day in the snow with several erythematous, ulcerative lesions on his fingertips; he complains the lesions are painful and itchy.

55. A teen, just back from a skiing trip, has blistering and peeling of several areas on her face; she reports the lesions started as firm, cold, white areas that felt stinging at the time and are now more sensitive than the surrounding skin.

56. A 9-year-old girl presents during summer break with an area of erythematous, firm, and slightly swollen skin at the corner of her mouth and extending to her cheek. The area is not tender.

57. A 14-year-old on a mountain-climbing expedition in December becomes tired, clumsy, and begins to hallucinate. His heart rate is 45 beats per minute.

58. A skier recently rescued from a snowbank following an avalanche (caused by a barking Chihuahua) complains about his feet. Upon rescue they were whitish yellow and numb, but now they are blotchy and painful.

Questions 59 to 62

For each disorder below, select the dietary deficiency that is likely to be responsible. Each lettered option may be used once, more than once, or not at all.

a. Folate deficiency
b. Thiamine deficiency
c. Niacin deficiency
d. Vitamin D deficiency
e. Vitamin C deficiency
f. Vitamin B_{12} deficiency
g. Vitamin B_6 deficiency
h. Biotin deficiency
i. Riboflavin deficiency

59. Megaloblastic anemia, growth failure, paresthesias, sensory defects, developmental regression, weakness, and fatigue

60. Photophobia, blurred vision, burning and itching of eyes, poor growth, cheilosis

61. Irritability, convulsions, hypochromic anemia

62. Megaloblastic anemia, glossitis, pharyngeal ulcers, impaired immunity

Questions 63 to 66

Match each clinical presentation with the most likely syndrome. Each lettered option may be used once, more than once, or not at all.

a. Trisomy 13
b. Cri du chat syndrome
c. Angelman syndrome
d. VATER
e. Cornelia de Lange syndrome

63. A newborn infant is noted to have microcephaly with sloping forehead, cutis aplasia on the scalp, microphthalmia, and cleft lip and palate. His echocardiogram demonstrates a complex heart lesion including atrial septal defect (ASD), ventricular septal defect (VSD), and dextrocardia.

64. A 17-year-old boy has an unusual gait, large mouth with tongue protrusion, hypopigmentation with blond hair and pale blue eyes, and unprovoked bursts of laughter.

65. A 6-week-old boy was small for his birth weight and had intrauterine growth retardation. He is microcephalic, has a rounded face, hypertelorism, and epicanthal folds. His cry is high-pitched.

66. A 3-day-old infant who was found at birth to have anal atresia also has vertebral defects, a VSD, tracheoesophageal fistula, absent left kidney, and shortened arms.

Questions 67 to 70

For each case listed below, select the most likely diagnosis. Each lettered option may be used once, more than once, or not at all.

a. Legg-Calvé-Perthes disease
b. Slipped capital femoral epiphysis
c. Osteomyelitis
d. Septic arthritis of the hip
e. Transient synovitis

67. An afebrile, obese 14-year-old boy has developed pain at the right knee and a limp.

68. A 6-year-old boy has developed a limp and has limited mobility of the hip, but denies pain and fever.

69. A 2-year-old refuses to walk, has fever, has significant pain with external rotation of the right leg, and has an elevated WBC count.

70. A 3-year-old refuses to walk, is afebrile, had an upper respiratory tract infection a week ago, has right hip pain with movement, and has a normal WBC count.

Questions 71 to 75

For the most likely toxic substance involved in the cases below, select the appropriate treatment. Each lettered option may be used once, more than once, or not at all.

a. Atropine and pralidoxime (2-PAM)
b. N-acetylcysteine (Mucomyst)
c. Dimercaptosuccinic acid (DMSA, succimer)
d. Naloxone (Narcan)
e. Sodium bicarbonate

71. Over the past several weeks, a 2-year-old girl has exhibited developmental regression, abnormal sleep patterns, anorexia, irritability, and decreased activity. These symptoms have progressed to acute encephalopathy with vomiting, ataxia, and variable consciousness. The family recently moved, and they are in the process of restoring the interior of their home.

72. After a fight with her boyfriend, a 16-year-old girl took "some pills." At presentation she is alert and complains of emesis, diaphoresis, and malaise. Her initial liver function tests, obtained about 12-hour postingestion, are elevated. Repeat levels at 24-hours show markedly elevated aspartate aminotransferase (AST) and alanine aminotransferase (ALT), along with abnormal coagulation studies and an elevated bilirubin.

73. You are called to the delivery room. A newborn infant seems lethargic and has poor tone with only marginal respiratory effort, but his heart rate is above 100 beats per minute. The mother had an uncomplicated pregnancy, and delivery was uncomplicated and vaginal 10 minutes after spontaneous rupture of membranes. The mother received only pain medications while in labor.

74. A 4-year-old girl comes into the ER after eating a bottleful of small, chewable pills she found while at her grandfather's house. She has an increased respiratory rate, elevated temperature, vomiting, and is disoriented. She is intermittently complaining that "a bell is ringing" in her ears. She has a metabolic acidosis on an arterial blood gas.

75. After helping his father in the yard, a 14-year-old boy complains of weakness and feels like his muscles are twitching. He begins to drool, and then collapses in a generalized tonic-clonic seizure. Upon the arrival of EMS, his heart rate is found to be 40 beats per min and his pupils are pinpoint.

Questions 76 to 78

For the most likely toxic substance involved in the cases below, match the appropriate treatment. Each lettered option may be used once, more than once, or not at all.

a. Deferoxamine mesylate
b. Diphenhydramine (Benadryl)
c. Acetazolamide and sodium bicarbonate
d. Ethanol
e. Dimercaprol (BAL)

76. A 14-year-old male presents after taking a "happy pill" that his friend gave him. He is alert and oriented, but complains of a muscle spasm in his neck, making his head lean on his right shoulder. You also notice he is arching his back in an unusual manner.

77. A 2-year-old boy found a bottle of his mother's prenatal vitamins and consumed the majority of them. He now has hematemesis and abdominal pain. He is febrile, and laboratory tests reveal a leukocytosis and hyperglycemia.

78. A 17-year-old is brought into the ED by his friends at about 10:00 AM. They were at a party the night before and drank some "homemade" alcohol. He is disoriented and confused, and has an anion-gap acidosis. He begins to have seizures.

Questions 79 to 83

Excess vitamin intake has been shown to have deleterious effects. Match the vitamin with the toxic effect. Each lettered option may be used once, more than once, or not at all.

a. A 4-year-old with diarrhea, abdominal pain, and kidney stones which prove to be caused by calcium oxalate.
b. A 6-year-old who has developed ataxia and sensory neuropathy.
c. A 12-month-old presents with isolated edema of his hands and feet.
d. An irritable 8-year-old child with headache, vomiting, alopecia, dry/itchy skin with desquamation of the palms and soles, hepatosplenomegaly, and swelling of the bones.
e. A 2-year-old presents with nausea, vomiting, poor feeding, abdominal pain, and constipation. On electrocardiogram (ECG) he has decreased Q-T interval. He has calcifications in his kidneys noted on a CT scan done for his abdominal pain.
f. Upon lumbar puncture, a 12-year-old is found to have reduced cerebrospinal fluid (CSF) pressure.
g. After getting into his mother's bottle of vitamins, a 3-year-old has burning, tingling, and itching on his arms as well as a reddened face, arms, and chest.

79. Vitamin A

80. Nicotinic acid

81. Vitamin C

82. Vitamin D

83. Pyridoxine

Questions 84 to 88

The normal development of the fetus can be adversely affected by exposure to a number of environmental factors, including infectious agents, physical agents, chemical agents, and maternal metabolic and genetic agents. Match each maternal history of teratogen exposure with the most likely clinical presentation. Each lettered option may be used once, more than once, or not at all.

a. Small palpebral fissures, ptosis, midfacial hypoplasia, smooth philtrum
b. Hypoplasia of distal phalanges, small nails
c. Bilateral microtia or anotia
d. Spina bifida
e. Ebstein anomaly
f. Renal dysgenesis
g. Cataracts
h. Hemangiomatosis

84. A 15-year-old with severe acne on an oral preparation of retinoic acid.

85. A woman without prenatal care has a diet low in green vegetables and enriched grain products.

86. A woman with long-standing hypertension treated with angiotensin-converting enzyme (ACE) inhibitors.

87. A primiparous mother late in her first trimester has a fever and "3-day" measles.

88. A 23-year-old pregnant woman with manic-depressive disorder has had poor prenatal care and was maintained on lithium.

Questions 89 to 92

Match each common skin condition with the most appropriate therapy. Each lettered option may be used once, more than once, or not at all.

a. Mild cleansing cream, topical moisturizers, and topical steroids
b. Ivermectin
c. Oral antihistamines alone
d. Reassurance only
e. Permethrin 5% cream
f. Topical steroids or a selenium sulfide–containing product
g. Topical antifungal agents
h. Isoretinoid

89. An 18-year-old friend of the family returns from spring break from a coastal town in Central America. He has an intensely pruritic lesion on his foot. The lesion is raised, red, serpiginous, and has a few associated bullae.

90. A 2-week-old boy is brought by his mother to the clinic; he has scaly, yellow patches on his scalp with associated hair loss.

91. Two days after a backyard party where the children enjoyed limeade and the adults partook of margaritas, a father brings his 4-year-old child to your office for a well-child checkup. The child is healthy other than a slight sunburn and some hyperpigmentation around her face and on her chest. Her father mentions that he, too, has some splotchy hyperpigmentation on his chest.

92. A 4-month-old presents with a dry, scaly rash on his cheeks, arms, and upper chest. His 10-year-old sister had a similar rash when she was young, but the rash is now confined to her antecubital and popliteal fossa; her rash worsens in winter months.

Questions 93 to 95

Match each clinical condition with the most likely cause. Each lettered option may be used once, more than once, or not at all.

a. Glomerulonephritis
b. Severe anemia
c. Heart block
d. Ventricular septal defect (VSD)
e. Arteriovenous malformation
f. Coarctation of the aorta

93. A 6-month-old child has a loud systolic murmur at the left lower sternal border

94. A 14-year-old child has headache, hypertension, edema, and a change in urine output and color

95. A 3-day-old infant was born to a mother with active systemic lupus erythematosus (SLE)

Questions 96 to 102

The Committee on Nutrition of the American Academy of Pediatrics has concluded that children on a normal diet generally do not need vitamin supplements. There are, however, some clinical situations in which special needs do occur. Match each situation with the appropriate supplement. Each lettered option may be used once, more than once, or not at all.

a. All fat-soluble vitamins
b. Pyridoxine
c. Vitamin A
d. Vitamin D
e. Vitamin K
f. Folate

96. Isoniazid therapy in a pregnant teenager

97. Administration of phenytoin

98. Measles in developing countries

99. Liver disease

100. Breast-fed infant in Alaska

101. Sickle-cell disease

102. 1-day-old newborn

Questions 103 to 107

Match each clinical condition with the most appropriate diagnostic laboratory test. Each lettered option may be used once, more than once, or not at all.

a. ESR
b. Serum immunoglobulin levels
c. Nitroblue tetrazolium (NBT) test
d. CH50 assay
e. CBC demonstrating Howell-Jolly bodies
f. Platelet count
g. Intradermal skin test using *Candida albicans*

103. A 1-year-old boy has been admitted three times in the past with abscess formation requiring incision and drainage. He is now admitted for surgical drainage of a hepatic abscess identified on ultrasound.

104. A 5-month-old infant is admitted with severe varicella infection. The lesions cover the infant's entire body, and the infant is beginning to show symptoms of respiratory distress. Past medical history is significant for a history of atopic dermatitis. The family also notes frequent epistaxis; the last episode required nasal packing in the ED.

105. A 3-year-old has had repeated episodes of sinusitis and otitis media. He was recently admitted for osteomyelitis of his femur with *Staphylococcus aureus*. The family notes that while his first 4 or 5 months of life were normal, he has been persistently ill with multiple infections in the ensuing months. The mother notes that her brother had similar problems with infections and died at the age of 3 years from a "lung infection." Physical examination is significant for the absence of lymph nodes and tonsillar tissue.

106. A general practitioner refers to you for evaluation a 3-year-old boy with frequent infections. You note the child to have a loud systolic murmur, posteriorly rotated ears that are small and low-set, down-slanting and widely spaced eyes, a small jaw, and an upturned nose. At birth the child spent 2 weeks in the nursery for "low calcium" and seizures, and he still receives calcium supplementation, but the mother does not know why. You would like to order a rapid diagnostic test for this child.

107. A 2-year-old girl has had two episodes of *Neisseria meningitidis* septicemia and is now admitted for *Streptococcus pneumoniae* septicemia.

General Pediatrics

Answers

1. The answer is e. *(Kliegman et al, pp 2081-2082. McMillan et al, pp 1963-1964. Rudolph et al, p 2366.)* Bell palsy is an acute, unilateral facial nerve palsy that begins about 2 weeks after a viral infection. The exact pathophysiology is unknown, but it is thought to be immune or allergic. On the affected side, the upper and lower face are typically paretic, the mouth droops, and the patient cannot close the eye. Treatment consists of maintaining moisture to the affected eye (especially at night) to prevent keratitis. Complete, spontaneous resolution occurs in about 85% of cases, 10% of cases have mild residual disease, and about 5% of cases do not resolve. Occasionally infants will have a facial nerve palsy at birth; this is usually related to compression from forceps and spontaneously resolves over several weeks. As this is a compression neuropathy, it should not be called congenital Bell palsy.

2. The answer is a. *(Hay et al, p 81. Kliegman et al, pp 74-81. McMillan et al, pp 593-597. Rudolph et al, pp 14, 440.)* At one month infants typically regard face, follow items to the midline, begin to vocalize, respond to a bell, and lift their head from the examining table. An 8-week-old child normally should be able to smile and coo when smiled at or talked to. Not until about 3 months of age would an infant be expected to follow a moving toy from side to side and also in the vertical plane. Such skills as maintaining a seated position are developed at about 6 to 8 months of age.

3. The answer is d. *(Hay et al, p 81. Kliegman et al, pp 74-81. McMillan et al, pp 593-597. Rudolph et al, pp 14, 440.)* Four- and five-year-old children begin to be able to copy a square; children younger than this age have difficulty with this task. By 4 years of age the language should be fully understandable and children begin to be able to name four colors, define five words, and know three adjectives. A 4-year-old can stand on each leg for 2 seconds, and by 5 years of age that skill can be maintained for at least 5 seconds. A 4-year-old may require some help with some clothing, but by 5 years of age they are able to dress themselves independently.

4. The answer is a. (*Hay et al, pp 822-824. Kliegman et al, pp 1001-1011. McMillan et al, pp 2538-2543. Rudolph et al, pp 836-839.*) Pauciarticular rheumatoid arthritis asymmetrically involves large joints, especially the knee, and often has no other symptoms. A major morbidity of pauciarticular rheumatoid arthritis is chronic uveitis, resulting in blindness. About 20% of girls who have the monoarthritis or pauciarticular form of juvenile rheumatoid arthritis have iridocyclitis (anterior uveitis) as their only significant systemic manifestation. Because this eye disorder can require treatment with local or systemic steroids and develop without signs or symptoms, it is recommended that all children with this form of arthritis have frequent slit-lamp eye examinations. For none of the other conditions listed are ophthalmologic changes expected nor diagnostic.

5. The answer is b. (*Hay et al, pp 409-410. Kliegman et al, pp 2739-2740. McMillan et al, pp 499, 848. Rudolph et al, pp 1225-1226.*) Also known as Ritter disease, staphylococcal scalded skin disease is seen most commonly in children less than 5 years of age. The rash is preceded by fever, irritability, erythema, and extraordinary tenderness of the skin. Circumoral erythema; crusting of the eyes, mouth, and nose; and blisters on the skin can develop. Intraoral mucosal surfaces are not affected. Peeling of the epidermis in response to mild shearing forces (Nikolsky sign) leaves the patient susceptible to problems similar to those of a burn injury, including infection and fluid and electrolyte imbalance. Cultures of the bullae are negative, but the source site or blood often may be positive. Treatment includes antibiotics (to cover resistant *S aureus*) and localized skin care.

6. The answer is d. (*McMillan et al, pp 18-25.*) The probability given is an estimation of the odds that the observed differences could have occurred by chance alone. More precisely, assuming one therapy was no different than the other (relative risk = 1.0, termed the *null hypothesis*), the *p*-value is the probability of obtaining an association as strong as or stronger than the one observed. Typically, the *p*-value most often selected in the medical literature to test for "statistical significance" is 0.05; the smaller the *p*-value, the "more significant" the result. The interpretation of these results depends on an assessment of factors, such as the study design, the size of the sample, the type of controls used, the severity of the disease, the side effects, and the importance of the treatment. The tendency for negative results to remain unpublished should also be kept in mind.

7. The answer is c. (*Hay et al, p 1087. Kliegman et al, pp 1960-1961. McMillan et al, pp 1652-1655. Rudolph et al, pp 909-913.*) The guidelines for the use of prophylactic antibiotics are updated frequently by the American Heart Association. Among those currently recommended to receive antibiotic prophylactic treatment are patients for whom any heart infection would result in the highest incidence of adverse outcome: previous history of endocarditis, prosthetic valve or material for repair, heart transplant patients, and severe or partially repaired congenital heart defects. Activity is not usually limited unless there is extensive destruction of heart muscle or the conducting system leading to failure. Minimizing salt intake is generally a good idea, but not any more so in an individual who has endocarditis. Bed rest should be instituted only in the case of heart failure. Family members are not typically at risk.

8. The answer is b. (*Hay et al, pp 334-335. Kliegman et al, pp 2928–2931. McMillan et al, pp 709-711.*) Human bites can pose a significant problem. They can become infected with oropharyngeal bacteria, including *S aureus, Streptococcus viridans, Bacteroides* spp., and anaerobes. A patient with an infected human bite of the hand requires hospitalization for appropriate drainage procedures, Gram stain and culture of the exudate, vigorous cleaning, debridement, and appropriate antibiotics. The wound should be left open and allowed to heal by secondary intention (healing by granulation tissue rather than closure with sutures).

9. The answer is b. (*Hay et al, pp 416-417. Kliegman et al, pp 2704-2705. McMillan et al, pp 839-840. Rudolph et al, p 1181.*) Pityriasis rosea is a benign condition that usually presents with a herald patch, a single round or oval lesion appearing anywhere on the body. Usually about 5 to 10 days after the appearance of the herald patch, a more diffuse rash involving the upper extremities and trunk appears. These lesions are oval or round, slightly raised, and pink to brown in color. The lesion is covered in a fine scale with some central clearing possible. The rash can appear in the Christmas tree pattern on the back, identified by the aligning of the long axis of the lesions with the cutaneous cleavage lines. The rash lasts 2 to 12 weeks and can be pruritic. This rash is commonly mistaken for tinea corporis, and the consideration of secondary syphilis is important. Treatment is usually unnecessary but can consist of topical emollients and oral antihistamines, as needed. More uncommonly, topical steroids can be helpful if the itching is severe.

Lichen planus is rare in children. It is intensely pruritic, and additional lesions can be induced with scratching. The lesion is commonly found on the flexor surfaces of the wrists, forearms, inner thighs, and occasionally on the oral mucosa.

Seborrheic dermatitis can begin anytime during life; it frequently presents as cradle cap in the newborn period. This rash is commonly greasy, scaly, and erythematous and, in smaller children, involves the face, neck, axilla, and diaper area. In older children, the rash can be localized to the scalp and intertriginous areas. Pruritus can be marked.

Contact dermatitis is characterized by redness, weeping, and oozing of the affected skin. The pattern of distribution can be helpful in identification of the offending agent. The rash can be pruritic; removal of the causative agent and use of topical emollients or steroids is curative.

Psoriasis consists of red papules that coalesce to form plaques with sharp edges. A thick, silvery scale develops on the surface and leaves a drop of blood upon its removal (Auspitz sign). Additional lesions develop upon scratching older lesions. Commonly affected sites include scalp, knees, elbows, umbilicus, and genitalia.

10. The answer is b. (*Kliegman et al, p 2257. McMillan et al, pp 1829-1830. Rudolph et al, pp 1739-1740.*) Many boys, especially those who are chubby, have an inconspicuous penis; when skin and fat lateral to the penis shaft are retracted, a normally sized and shaped penis is revealed. If, after performing this maneuver, the penis is found to be more than 2.5 standard deviations below the mean in size for age, and especially if other abnormal physical examination findings are noted, then further evaluation would be initiated.

11. The answer is a. (*Hay et al, pp 690-691, 871. Kliegman et al, pp 1043-1045, 2178-2179. McMillan et al, pp 1860-1861, 2559-2562. Rudolph et al, pp 842-844.*) The clinical presentation described supports the diagnosis of anaphylactoid purpura (also known as Henoch-Schönlein purpura or HSP), a generalized, acute vasculitis of unknown cause involving small blood vessels. In this condition, the skin lesion, which is classic in character (palpable purpura) and distribution, is often accompanied by arthritis, usually of the large joints, and by gastrointestinal symptoms. Colicky abdominal pain, vomiting, and melena are common. Renal involvement occurs in a significant number of patients and is potentially the most serious manifestation of the disease. Although most children with this complication recover, a few will develop chronic nephritis. Laboratory studies are not diagnostic. Serum complement and IgA levels can be normal or elevated. Coagulation studies and platelets are normal. Meningococcal infection and leukemia should be in the differential diagnosis, as both can cause purpura, but in a well-appearing child with normal vital signs and normal blood count they are unlikely. Child abuse and hemophilia will typically result in bruises, not petechiae.

12. The answer is e. (*Hay et al, pp 219-224. Kliegman et al, pp 171-178. McMillan et al, pp 147-156, 2503-2504. Rudolph et al, pp 463-469.*) The x-ray showing a fracture (or an x-ray showing multiple fractures in various stages of healing) indicates trauma. This information should be reported to the medical examiner and appropriate social agencies, including the police, so that an investigation can be started and other children in the home or under the care of the same babysitter can be protected. Although an autopsy (and death-scene investigation) should be done in every such case, there is a tendency for medical examiners to diagnose SIDS without an autopsy, particularly if the parents object to one, unless further information is provided by the ER staff, as in this case. For none of the other conditions (except osteogenesis) would bone injuries at various levels of healing be expected. Osteogenesis would be expected to present with symptoms of a broken bone and not to present with death.

13. The answer is d. (*Hay et al, pp 206-207. Kliegman et al, pp 114-115. McMillan et al, pp 672-674, 1920-1923. Rudolph et al, pp 1368-1370.*) Encopresis is defined as the passage of feces in inappropriate locations after bowel control would be expected (usually older than 4 years). Encopresis is seen both with chronic constipation and overflow incontinence (retentive encopresis), and without constipation (nonretentive encopresis). Retentive encopresis is more common, and is the source of this child's problem. There is leakage of liquid stool around a large fecal impaction, resulting in fecal soiling. The radiograph demonstrates a dilated, stool-filled colon consistent with retentive encopresis. Treatment involves clearing the fecal mass, maintaining soft stools for a short period of time with mineral oil or stool softeners (3-6 months), and behavioral modification. Most children will grow out of this condition. Time-out would be ineffective, because these children usually have dysfunctional anal sphincters and little control over the problem; they do not know they are soiling their clothes until it is too late. Daily enemas could potentially be harmful. A rectal biopsy would help diagnose Hirschsprung disease, but the story presented is not consistent with that diagnosis.

14. The answer is e. *(Kliegman et al, pp 2788-2790. McMillan et al, pp 2480-2481. Rudolph et al, pp 2431-2432.)* Genu varum (bowlegs) is a common finding in infants and toddlers younger than 2 years of age. Improvement occurs spontaneously with time, and most children have straight legs by the time they are 2 years old. A few children with bowlegs, however, continue to progress and worsen, and in some cases the bowing is unilateral. This is termed Blount disease and is characterized by an abnormality in the medial aspect of the proximal tibial epiphysis. Radiographically there is a prominent step abnormality with beaking at the proximal tibial epiphysis. Aggressive treatment is essential, as the disease can be rapidly progressive and lead to permanent growth disturbances. Bracing can be effective up to the age of 3; later correction may require surgery. Blount disease can occur in several forms: infantile (ages 1-3 years), juvenile (ages 4-10 years), and adolescent (age 11 years and older). Clinically, the findings are the same; in the adolescent group, radiograph findings are less prominent. Legg-Calvé-Perthes disease is avascular necrosis of the femoral head, caused by an interruption of the blood supply by a currently unknown cause. Onset is usually between 2 and 12 years of age and classically presents with a painless limp, although mild pain of the thigh is common. Repeated microfracture of the tibial tubercle at the insertion of the patellar tendon is called Osgood-Schlatter disease. This is an overuse injury, and presents with swelling and knee pain localized to the tubercle. Improvement occurs with rest. Slipped capital femoral epiphysis (SCFE) typically occurs in overweight adolescents, and presents with a limp. Radiographically, the capital femoral epiphysis is separated from the neck of the femur and remains in the acetabulum as the rest of the femur moves anteriorly.

15. The answer is e. *(Hay et al, pp 90-92. Kliegman et al, pp 2476-2477. Rudolph et al, p 2274.)* The child in this question most likely has breath-holding spells. Two forms exist. Cyanotic spells consist of the symptoms outlined and are predictable upon upsetting or scolding the child. They are rare before 6 months of age, peak at about 2 years of age, and resolve by about 5 years of age. Avoidance of reinforcing this behavior is the treatment of choice. Pallid breath-holding spells are less common and are usually caused by a painful experience (such as a fall). With these events, the child will stop breathing, lose consciousness, become pale and hypotonic, and may have a brief tonic episode. Although the family may be concerned that these "tonic episodes" are seizures, the temporal relationship with an inciting event make this diagnosis highly unlikely. These pallid events, too, resolve spontaneously. Again, avoidance of reinforcing behavior is indicated. Assuring the family that this is a benign condition is important.

16. The answer is a. *(Hay et al, p 979. Kliegman et al, pp 2411-2412. McMillan et al, p 1793. Rudolph et al, pp 2103-2104.)* The criteria for diagnosis of diabetes mellitus, as established by the Expert Committee on the Diagnosis and Classification of Diabetes Mellitus (sponsored by the American Diabetes Association) include a fasting glucose level ≥ 126 mg/dL, a 2-hour plasma glucose during an oral glucose tolerance test ≥ 200 mg/dL, or symptoms of diabetes mellitus plus a random plasma glucose ≥ 200 mg/dL. Acanthosis nigricans in children usually suggests insulin resistance, but is not, in and of itself, diagnostic, nor are symptoms alone diagnostic. Previous standards suggested a fasting glucose between 110 and 125 mg/dL or a 2-hour glucose during an oral glucose tolerance test between 140 and 200 mg/dL indicated impaired glucose tolerance. Impaired (not yet diabetic) glucose levels include fasting values between 100 and 125 mg/dL and impaired 2-hour values between 140 and 200 mg/dL. The bed-wetting in the question can be explained by increased liquid consumption due to the hyperosmolar state caused by hyperglycemia.

17. The answer is c. *(Hay et al, pp 350-351. Kliegman et al, pp 354-355. McMillan et al, p 621. Rudolph et al, pp 752-753, 766.)* The description in the question is that of cyanide poisoning, a rodenticide still found in some rural areas. A more common exposure to cyanide occurs in fire victims; rapid treatment with a cyanide antidote kit along with high levels of oxygen potentially are life saving. Another agent likely to be found in a garden shed is organophosphate; signs and symptoms of poisoning to this agent includes constricted pupils, bradycardia, and muscle fasciculations associated with the sudden onset of neurologic symptoms, progressive respiratory distress, diaphoresis, diarrhea, and overabundant salivation.

18. The answer is b. *(Hay et al, p 403. Kliegman et al, p 2763. McMillan et al, pp 462, 830. Rudolph et al, pp 1169, 1210.)* The pictured infant has a classic case of neonatal acne, which peaks at 2 to 4 weeks of age. The condition results from maternal hormone transmission. It resolves in a few weeks to months, and occasionally is severe enough to require treatment with agents such as tretinoin or benzoyl peroxide.

Neonatal herpes infection can occur in 3-day-old infants, but the clinical scenario is of a healthy child; children with neonatal herpes are usually ill. Milia are benign, tiny white bumps on the nose. Seborrheic dermatitis is a weepy rash that can be found on the face or on the scalp (cradle cap); it is not usually found at 3 days of age but rather later in infancy. Eczema commonly occurs on the face of children in the early years of life (later occurring in the more "adult" pattern of extremities), but would be unusual in a 3-day-old infant.

19. The answer is b. (*Hay et al, pp 413, 1272. Kliegman et al, pp 2756-2758. McMillan et al, pp 847, 863, 1382-1383. Rudolph et al, pp 1153-1154, 1233-1234.*) Scabies is caused by the mite *Sarcoptes scabiei var. hominis.* Most older children and adults present with intensely pruritic and threadlike burrows in the interdigital areas, groin, elbows, and ankles; the palms, soles, face, and head are spared. Infants, however, usually present with bullae and pustules, and the areas spared in adults are often involved in infants. The clinical manifestations closely resemble those of atopic dermatitis. Gamma benzene hexachloride (lindane) can cause neurotoxicity through percutaneous absorption, especially in small infants and those with abnormal skin (impetigo, etc), and is, therefore, not recommended in children as first-line therapy for scabies. An excellent alternative—5% permethrin cream (Elimite)—is safer and is more often recommended.

20. The answer is c. (*Hay et al, pp 49-53, 1156-1158. Kliegman et al, pp 1145-1150. McMillan et al, pp 482-483, 501-506. Rudolph et al, pp 999-1001.*) The rapid onset of the symptoms, the low WBC count with left shift, and the depicted chest x-ray findings are typical of a patient with group B streptococcus (GBS) pneumonia. Appropriate management would include rapid recognition of symptoms, cardiorespiratory support, and rapid institution of appropriate antibiotics. Despite these measures, mortality from this infection is not uncommon. The other infectious causes listed do not present so early, and the noninfectious causes listed do not cause elevations in the band count. GBS disease in the infant is decreasing in incidence with better prevention strategies in the perinatal period, including early screening in pregnancy and treatment with antibiotics just prior to delivery to eliminate GBS colonization and, thus, markedly decrease the risk to the infant.

Congenital syphilis can cause pneumonia, but it is diagnosed at birth along with other features including hepatosplenomegaly, jaundice, rashes, hemolytic anemia, and others. Diaphragmatic hernia presents with early respiratory distress, but the diagnosis is confirmed clinically with bowel sounds heard in the chest and a radiograph that has loops of bowel located above the normal placement of the diaphragm. Transient tachypnea of the newborn (TTN) causes an increase in respiratory rate and occasionally a low oxygen requirement; the history is often positive for a cesarean delivery, and the radiograph shows retained fluid in the fissures. TTN does not cause temperature instability nor is the CBC abnormal. Chlamydial pneumonia is not a condition that occurs in an 8-hour-old infant; it is generally a mild pneumonia that can develop in an exposed infant at several weeks of life.

21. The answer is a. *(Hay et al, p 819. Kliegman et al, pp 2798-2799. McMillan et al, p 2109. Rudolph et al, p 2479.)* This history is typical of Osgood-Schlatter disease. Microfractures in the area of the insertion of the patellar tendon into the tibial tubercle are common in athletic adolescents. Swelling, tenderness, and an increase in size of the tibial tuberosity are found. Radiographs can be necessary to rule out other conditions. Treatment consists of rest.

Legg-Calvé-Perthes disease is avascular necrosis of the femoral head. This condition usually produces mild or intermittent pain in the anterior thigh but can also present as a painless limp. Gonococcal arthritis, although common in this age range, is uncommon in this anatomic site. More significant systemic signs and symptoms, including chills, fever, migratory polyarthralgia, and rash, are commonly seen. Slipped capital femoral epiphysis is usually seen in a younger, more obese child (mean age about 10 years) or in a thinner, older child who has just undergone a rapid growth spurt. Pain upon movement of the hip is typical. Popliteal (Baker) cysts are found on the posterior aspect of the knee. Observation is usually all that is necessary, as they typically resolve over several years. Surgical excision is indicated if the cyst progressively enlarges or if there are unacceptable symptoms associated with the cyst.

22. The answer is e. *(Hay et al, p 445. Kliegman et al, pp 2578-2595. McMillan et al, pp 662, 672-673. Rudolph et al, pp 815-817.)* To prevent monocular blindness and to ensure the development of normal binocular vision, early recognition and treatment of strabismus are essential. Infants can be screened for strabismus by observing the location of a light reflection in the pupils when the patient fixes on a light source. Normally, it should be in the center or just nasal of the center in each pupil. Persistence of a transient or fixed deviation of an eye beyond 4 months of age requires referral to an ophthalmologist. Another method of testing for strabismus is the "cover" or "cover-uncover" test, using the principle that children with strabismus will use the "good" eye for fixation. By covering the good eye, the other eye will deviate. The aim of treatment is to prevent loss of central vision from foveal suppression of a confusing image in the deviating eye. This is accomplished by surgery, eyeglasses, or patching of the normal eye. The prognosis for normal vision if diagnosis is delayed beyond 6 years of age is guarded. Routine vision and strabismus screening is essential at age 3 to 4 years.

23. The answer is b. (*Hay et al, pp 204-206, 236-237, 303-304. Kliegman et al, pp 222-223, 370-372, 2249-2250. McMillan et al, pp 117-118, 140, 143, 670-672. Rudolph et al, pp 32-33, 37-38, 1742-1743, 1891.*) Water temperature should be set to about 49°C (120°F); this will minimize the risk of accidental scald burns. In the older child, limiting fat to less than 35%, saturated fats and polyunsaturated fats each less than 10% of total calories, and cholesterol intake to less than 100 mg/1000 kcal/d usually results in switching from whole to skim or low-fat milk. As many as 15% of 5-year-old children have enuresis "normally"; it is unrealistic for a 2-year-old child to be expected to have no enuresis. Rear facing infant seats are recommended for a child less than 20 lb and 1 year of age with the switch to a forward-facing seat to occur between 20 to 40 lb and older than 1 year. Infants and young children should never be left alone in water, even if they "know" how to swim; a child may drown in as little as 1 to 2 in of water and swimming lessons are not preventative.

24. The answer is e. (*Hay et al, p 75. Kliegman et al, pp 31-37. McMillan et al, pp 756-761. Rudolph et al, p 14.*) At 6 to 6½ months of age, infants will be able to sit alone, leaning forward to support themselves with arms extended, in the so-called tripod position. They can reach for an object by changing the orientation of the torso. They can purposefully roll from a prone to a supine as well as from a supine to a prone position. By 12 months, they usually can complete all of the motor tasks outlined in the question. Thus, motor development occurs in a cephalocaudal and central-to-peripheral direction; truncal control precedes arm control, which precedes finger dexterity.

25. The answer is b. (*Hay et al, pp 244-245. Kliegman et al, pp 184-187. McMillan et al, pp 900-906. Rudolph et al, pp 1046-1048.*) This child is presenting with failure to thrive (FTT), and the differential diagnosis of this problem is extensive. While any of the answers provided may have a place in an FTT evaluation, the best single recommendation in this case would be to evaluate for HIV. In this case, the natural mother was in jail for unknown reasons (possibly for prostitution, drugs, or other high-risk activities), this child has an increased risk for congenital HIV. In addition, the presenting symptoms (lymphadenopathy, hepatomegaly, and oral candidiasis) are most consistent with HIV. An HIV ELISA may still reflect maternal antibody at this age; thus, an antigen test like the HIV PCR is preferred.

26. The answer is d. (*Hay et al, pp 413-414, 1062-1067. Kliegman et al, pp 970-975. McMillan et al, pp 2423-2427. Rudolph et al, pp 1177-1179.*) Eczema is a chronic dermatitis that occurs in a population with a strong personal or family history of atopy. The skin presents initially as an erythematous, papulo-vesicular, weeping eruption, which progresses over time to a scaly, lichenified dermatitis. From about 3 months to about 2 years of age, the rash is prominent on the cheeks, wrists, scalp, postauricular areas, and arms and legs. In a young child 2 to 12 years of age, mainly the extensor surfaces of arms, legs, and neck are involved. Pruritus is a predominant feature, and scratching leads to excoriation, secondary infection, and lichenification of the skin. The rash has a chronic and relapsing course, and treatment is determined by the major clinical features. Cutaneous irritants (bathing in hot water, scrubbing vigorously with soap, wearing wool or synthetic clothing) should be avoided, and maximal skin hydration with emollients is essential. Topical moisturizers, steroids, and topical calcineurin inhibitors (tacrolimus and pimecrolimus) are the mainstays of therapy for atopic dermatitis. The use of antihistamines can provide additional relief from pruritus.

27. The answer is e. (*Hay et al, pp 258-259. Kliegman et al, pp 1156-1157. McMillan et al, pp 124-129. Rudolph et al, p 44.*) There are few true contraindications to vaccines, but many misconceptions about contraindications. The one contraindication for all vaccines is a prior history of a severe allergic reaction to a component of the vaccine. For the DTaP, another contraindication is the occurrence of encephalopathy (such as coma, altered level of consciousness, or prolonged seizures) within 7 days of administration of the previous dose. Minor illnesses; current antibiotic therapy; history of local reaction (such as erythema or swelling) after previous immunizations; family history of seizures, SIDS, or adverse events due to DTaP; and stable, nonprogressive neurologic conditions (eg, cerebral palsy, controlled seizure disorder, or developmental delay) are not contraindications.

28. The answer is a. (*Hay et al, p 413. Kliegman et al, pp 2758-2759. McMillan et al, pp 1384-1385. Rudolph et al, pp 1155-1156.*) The photo and history are consistent with head lice (Pediculosis capitis). All the treatments outlined for this patient are appropriate for the treatment of lice except for use of 1% lindane in the 2-month-old family member, because of the potential of neurotoxicity from transdermal absorption. The treatment of choice for these small children is permethrin 1% cream rinse (Nix).

29. The answer is c. *(Hay et al, pp 1197-1200. Kliegman et al, pp 1248-1249. McMillan et al, p 1149. Rudolph et al, p 953.)* Of the options, tuberculous (TB) meningitis is most likely to linger for 3 weeks; the other infectious causes lead to rapid deterioration, as would the epidural hematoma. A food allergy does not typically cause the central nervous system (CNS) manifestations described. Unfortunately, the seriousness of the illness in a child as presented in the vignette often will be unrecognized with a diagnosis of an incipient nondisease being made and symptomatic treatment provide. While many patients with nonspecific complaints have trivial diseases that resolve spontaneously, the patient presented here has a 3-week history with potentially grave implications. Diagnoses that cause a slowly progressive course should be considered foremost.

30. The answer is a. *(Hay et al, p 471. Kliegman et al, p 2644. Rudolph et al, p 1255.)* A cholesteatoma may be congenital or acquired. It is a small sac lined with epithelium-containing debris. Acquired cholesteatoma can present in children with recurrent otitis media, or in the face of a chronically draining ear. The mass can grow aggressively, leading to CNS complications like facial nerve damage, hearing loss, and intracranial extension. Referral to an otolaryngologist is required; a CT scan of the temporal bones can define the extent of disease.

Tympanosclerosis would present with scarring on the surface of the tympanic membrane. Acute otitis media with perforation and drainage would present with a hole in the tympanic membrane and with (often) purulent drainage. Dislocation of the malleus from its insertion in the tympanic membrane can occur, but would not produce a mass extending through the tympanic membrane. Excessive cerumen production would result in waxy buildup that is removable with washing.

31. The answer is c. *(Hay et al, pp 1277-1279. Kliegman et al, pp 313-316. McMillan et al, pp 63-65. Rudolph et al, pp 1643-1647.)* The patient has severe dehydration, probably in the 10% to 15% range and requires rapid expansion of the vascular space to prevent death. Appropriate intravenous (IV) fluids include Ringer's lactate and normal saline. Albumin, plasma, and blood offer no significant advantages over the cheaper and more available Ringer's lactate or normal saline. If this patient is in shock, it is vital to restore circulatory volume quickly, thereby improving tissue perfusion and shifting anaerobic toward aerobic metabolism. The restoration of vascular volume would also improve functioning of the intestines so that diarrhea will abate and would improve circulation to the kidney so that renal function would be restored. A volume of 20 mL/kg is about one-quarter the blood volume of the patient; therefore, it should be given at a rate that will not produce pulmonary edema. An emergency phase (where further boluses of fluids to establish appropriate perfusion) lasting 1 to 2 hours or less has worked well in practice. The dextrose fluids listed are various forms of maintenance fluids and would not result in the rapid expansion of the vascular volume required.

32. The answer is b. (*Hay et al, pp 930-931. Kliegman et al, pp 775-777. McMillan et al, pp 2454-2455. Rudolph et al, p 90.*) The umbilical cord typically separates from a newborn 10 to 14 days after birth, although some will remain for 3 weeks. An intact cord after 1 month of age is considered "delayed separation." Leukocyte adhesion deficiency type 1 (LAD-1) has been described with delayed cord separation. These children are at risk for overwhelming bacterial infection. Diagnosis is made by measuring surface CD11b using flow cytometry. Most patients with LAD-1 have normal antibody production. An omphalocele is an abdominal wall defect with intestine or liver protruding into the base of the umbilical cord, covered by peritoneum but not by skin. It should be readily recognizable at birth. Umbilical granulomas form after the cord has separated, and are easily treated with application of silver nitrate. A persistent urachus will produce ongoing clear or yellow fluid from the umbilicus.

33. The answer is b. (*Hay et al, pp 142-143. Kliegman et al, p 2275.*) A nonspecific vulvovaginitis is common in this age group, often caused by chemical irritants such as bubble baths or by poor hygiene. Mothers should be counseled to use only cotton underwear for young children, stop bubble baths (or at least splash fresh, clean water in the vaginal area at the end of a bath), and reemphasize wiping front to back after urination or bowel movements. Vaginal foreign bodies in young girls are usually either toilet paper or stool, and are accompanied by a foul odor and discharge that is sometimes bloody. Removal of vaginal foreign bodies is frequently done under general anesthesia in the operating room. While child sexual abuse is always a possibility, there is no verbal or physical evidence that this is a problem in this child. Gonorrhea and *Chlamydia* would go along with abuse and are usually accompanied by a mild discharge in the prepubertal child.

34. The answer is a. *(Hay et al, p 799. Kliegman et al, pp 2845-2847. McMillan et al, pp 2499-2450. Rudolph et al, pp 907-908.)* All of the answers may ultimately be done, but examination of the joint fluid is the key to diagnosis. The joint tap will reveal cloudy fluid containing a predominance of polymorphonuclear leukocytes. Organisms are readily seen on Gram stain examination; cultures of joint fluid and blood are usually positive. X-ray reveals a widened joint space. Finding pus in the joint indicates the need for immediate surgical drainage and prompt institution of IV antibiotic therapy to avoid serious damage to the joint and permanent loss of function. The most common organism found to cause septic arthritis is *S aureus*. Since immunization against *Haemophilus influenzae* type B has become an established practice, invasive disease such as septic arthritis caused by this organism is rarely seen. In sexually active adolescents, *Neisseria gonorrhoeae* is a common cause of septic arthritis.

35. The answer is e. *(Hay et al, p 249. Kliegman et al, p 1063. McMillan et al, pp 120, 129-130. Rudolph et al, pp 1007-1008.)* Until recently, the correct answer would have been a booster immunization with adult Td (which generally is given every 10 years to maintain immunity against both diphtheria and tetanus). However, recognition of an increased incidence of pertussis in adolescents and young adults (and this group's serving as a reservoir for disease in infants) has lead to a vaccine that incorporates immunity also against pertussis. Current recommendations are for the new Tdap to replace the Td to help eliminate pertussis.

36. The answer is c. *(Hay et al, pp 333-334. Kliegman et al, pp 2928-2931. McMillan et al, pp 709-710.)* Mammalian bites should be promptly and thoroughly scrubbed with soap and water and debrided. The decision to suture depends on the location, age, and nature of the wound. Antibiotic prophylaxis is extremely controversial. Most experts suggest a short course of antibiotics should be started for cat, human, or monkey bites. Only 4% of dog bites become infected (and therefore do not necessarily need antibiotic prophylaxis), compared with 35% of cat bites and 50% of monkey bites (which require antibiotics in most cases). Cat bites are usually deep punctures. Human bites almost invariably become infected. The etiologies of these infections are polymicrobial. *Pasteurella multocida* is a common organism in infected cat and dog bites. Infected human bites tend to have positive cultures for *S viridans*, *S aureus*, and *Bacteroides* spp. Treatment with oral amoxicillin-clavulanate or erythromycin is recommended. Antibiotic prophylaxis is recommended for any bite sustained by an infant, a diabetic, or an immunocompromised patient because of the higher risk of infection in these persons. Since the child is fully immunized, tetanus boosters are not required. Similarly, as the dog was provoked and was fully immunized, rabies should not be a concern.

37. The answer is b. (*Hay et al, pp 216-217. Kliegman et al, p 350. Rudolph et al, p 364.*) Poisoning with clonidine is becoming more commonplace since it is used not only in adults for hypertension but in some children for attention-deficit/hyperactivity disorder and tic disorders. Symptoms described in the vignette often occur within 1 hour of the ingestion. Treatment includes aggressive PICU support and naloxone (which has variable effect). Young children often ingest poisons and drugs during times of household disruption. Visitors' handbags are a great temptation for the inquisitive toddler. Defer-oxamine is used to treat iron overdose and N-acetylcysteine treats aceta-minophen ingestions. In addition, Aunt Mary should be encouraged not to carry organophosphates (antidote is atropine) and arsenic (antidote includes dimercaptosuccinic acid) in her purse along with her other medications.

38. The answer is d. (*Hay et al, pp 232-233. Kliegman et al, pp 2913-2918. McMillan et al, pp 767-772. Rudolph et al, pp 23-24.*) Impaired cognitive function can occur at blood lead levels previously thought to be safe; the toxic concen-tration of lead in whole blood was revised downward in 1991 from 25 μg/dL to 10 μg/dL. The blood erythrocyte protoporphyrin concentration is not elevated in such low-level poisoning rendering this test useless as a valid screening test. The definitive screen, then, is the blood lead level, preferably via venous sampling which avoids the risk of environmental contamination with lead that is more likely with finger sticks. Most lead poisoning is clin-ically inapparent. A careful history will help to identify sources of lead in the environment. However, neither the history nor the anemia that accompa-nies severe lead poisoning is an appropriate means of screening for lead poisoning. In most areas, lead screening recommendations are made by the state or local health department, based on local risk factors (eg, number of older houses potentially containing lead-based paint).

39. The answer is d. (*Hay et al, p 331. Kliegman et al, p 2864. McMillan et al, pp 882-883. Rudolph et al, pp 388-390.*) Hyperthermia with dry, hot skin and mental status changes characterizes classic heat stroke, typically seen in the elderly with a gradual onset. Young athletes exerting themselves in a hot environment may develop acute heat stroke with signs and symptoms of hyperthermia and mental status changes; the difference, however, is that the athletes will continue to sweat profusely. Heat stroke is a medical emergency. These otherwise healthy athletes should be rapidly rehydrated with IV fluids, undergo aggressive cooling (cold water immersion, cool mist fans, removal of clothing), and perhaps oxygen, laboratory evaluation, and ICU admission. Heat stroke can have a high mortality; prevention is certainly the best option, but prompt recognition is essential. Oral rehydration therapy might have been preventive if instituted before symptoms of heat stroke were manifest, but once the syndrome has started IV fluids are indicated.

40. The answer is a. (*Hay et al, pp 539-541. Kliegman et al, pp 1736-1742. McMillan et al, pp 722-729. Rudolph et al, p 1936.*) Much research in infants suggests the prone (facedown) sleeping position to be a risk factor for SIDS. A higher risk of SIDS in the prone position has been noted when the infant sleeps on a soft, porous mattress or in an overheated room, is swaddled, or has recently been ill. The American Academy of Pediatrics recommends that healthy infants be positioned on their back when being put down for sleep. (The prone position is still recommended for infants with certain medical conditions.) The rate of SIDS has declined in areas where the change from prone to supine (faceup) sleeping positions has been effected.

41. The answer is d. (*Hay et al, pp 98-99, 1041. Kliegman et al, p 515. McMillan et al, pp 2636-2637. Rudolph et al, p 720.*) The physical features associated with the fragile X syndrome become more obvious after puberty. They include a long face, large ears, prominent jaw, macroorchidism, hypotonia, repetitive speech, gaze avoidance, and hand flapping. Even in the absence of physical findings, boys of all ages with developmental delay, autism, and abnormal temperament of unknown cause probably should be tested for the fragile X syndrome. The genetics of the fragile X syndrome are unique. Most males who carry the fragile X mutation are mentally impaired and show the clinical phenotype; however, 20% of males who inherit the genetic mutation are normal in intelligence and physical appearance. They are also cytogenetically normal in that the fragile site on their X chromosome is not seen by the karyotyping method. These normal transmitting males (NTMs) transmit the fragile X mental retardation (*FMR-1*) gene to all of their daughters and often have severely affected grandchildren. It is thought that a premutation carried by these NTMs must go through oogenesis in their daughters to become a full mutation. Daughters of NTMs are usually normal but are obligate carriers of the *FMR-1* gene. Daughters who inherit the gene from the mother are mentally retarded about one-third of the time. Because both males and females can be affected, the fragile X syndrome is best described as a dominant X-linked disorder with reduced penetrance in females. Direct DNA analysis is available for diagnosis of phenotypically affected persons as well as suspected carriers of fragile X; it has supplanted cytogenetic testing for the fragile site on the X chromosome. The DNA test can also be used for prenatal testing.

Trisomy 21 (Down syndrome) has a wide variety of features including hypotonia, epicanthal folds, simian crease, cardiac lesions (VSD or atrioventricular [AV] canal), mental retardation, and a propensity for leukemia. Trisomy 18 (Edwards syndrome) features include small for age gestation, micrognathia, low-set ears, a variety of cardiac defects, small palpebral fissures, microcephaly, cleft lip/palate, and rocker bottom feet. Trisomy 13 (Patau syndrome) features include microcephaly, cutis aplasia of the scalp, a variety of cardiac defects, holoprosencephaly, cleft lip/palate, and coloboma. Williams syndrome features include short stature, blue irides, a variety of cardiac abnormalities involving the pulmonary vessels, hypercalcemia in infancy, and a friendly attitude.

42. The answer is c. (*Hay et al, p 1279. Kliegman et al, pp 275-279. McMillan et al, p 60. Rudolph et al, pp 1650-1651.*) The differential diagnosis of seizure activity is extensive, and a detailed history is essential. While knowing the occupation of the mother and the developmental status of the children are important, the most helpful historical detail for acute management of this patient is the dilution of the formula, especially in light of the history of poor growth. Over time, inappropriate dilution can cause hyponatremia and water intoxication, leading to seizure activity. Slow correction of the sodium is curative. The technique used to correct the patient's hyponatremia depends on the etiology. In this case the child likely has chronic hyponatremia from poor intake. If the child continues to seize, 3% sodium chloride may be used to rapidly increase serum sodium and, theoretically, decrease cerebral edema. Otherwise, starting the child on a regular formula and eliminating excess water will correct the deficiency over time.

43 to 48. The answers are 43-e, 44-b, 45-d, 46-a, 47-g, 48-f. (*Hay et al, pp 5, 402-405, 415. Kliegman et al, pp 2661-2664, 2678, 2696-2697. McMillan et al, pp 829-831, 833-834, 853-854. Rudolph et al, pp 86-87, 1169, 1175-1176.*) Erythema toxicum is a benign, self-limited condition of unknown etiology. It is found in about 50% of term newborns. Lesions are yellow-white and 1 to 2 mm in size, with a surrounding edge of erythema. This rash waxes and wanes over the first days to weeks of life. Examination of the fluid from these lesions demonstrates eosinophils. No therapy is indicated.

Salmon patches (aka nevus simplex or flameus) are flat vascular lesions that occur in the listed regions and appear more prominent during crying. The lesions on the face fade over the first weeks of life. Lesions found over the nuchal and occipital areas often persist. No therapy is indicated.

Pustular melanosis is another benign, self-limited disease of unknown etiology of the newborn period. It is more common in blacks than in whites. These lesions are usually found at birth and consist of 1- to 2-mm pustules that result in a hyperpigmented lesion upon rupture of the pustule. The pustular stage of these lesions occurs during the first few days of life, with the hyperpigmented stage lasting for weeks to months. No therapy is indicated.

Sebaceous nevi (nevus of Jadassohn) are small, sharply edged lesions that occur most commonly on the head and neck of infants. These lesions are yellow-orange in color and are slightly elevated. They usually are hairless. Malignant degeneration is possible, most commonly after adolescence.

Milia are fine, yellowish white, 1- to 2-mm lesions scattered over the face and gingivae of the neonate. They are cysts that contain keratinized material. Commonly, these lesions resolve spontaneously without therapy. When on the palate, they are called Epstein pearls.

Seborrheic dermatitis can begin anytime during life and frequently presents as cradle cap in the newborn period. This rash is commonly greasy, scaly, and erythematous and in smaller children involves the face, neck, axilla, and diaper area. In older children, the rash can be localized to the scalp and intertriginous areas. Pruritus can be marked.

49 to 53. The answers are 49-a, 50-c, 51-e, 52-b, 53-c. (Hay et al, pp 88-90, 536-537, 739-740. Kliegman et al, pp 92-100. McMillan et al, pp 662-668. Rudolph et al, pp 417-420.) Sleep disturbances are fairly common in childhood. Many children resist going to bed, and parents frequently give in just to get the child to sleep by allowing the child to sleep in the parents' bed or allowing them to stay up late. Unfortunately, children learn remarkably well how to get what they want, and the parents' concessions only make the problem worse. Learned behavior is the root of many sleep disturbances in young children.

Other types of sleep disturbance in children fall into the category of sleep disruptions, such as nightmares and night terrors. A nightmare is a scary or disturbing dream that usually awakens the child and causes agitation about the content of the dream. Nightmares occur during rapid eye movement (REM) sleep. Many children and adults have an occasional nightmare; recurrent or frequent nightmares, however, may be indicative of an ongoing stress in the child's life. Night terrors (pavor nocturnus) are non-REM phenomena seen less commonly than nightmares, occurring in 1% to 6% of all children. The child will be described as apparently awake but unresponsive; they can have evidence of autonomic arousal such as tachycardia, sweating, and tachypnea, and appear frightened and agitated. Attempts at calming the child are usually not effective, and the child will eventually go back to sleep. Although usually a problem in early childhood, night terrors can sometimes continue through adolescence.

Somnambulism, or sleepwalking, occurs in 15% of children and is described as recurrent episodes of rising from bed and walking around. The child is typically hard to arouse and will have amnesia after the event. This usually happens in the first third of the sleep cycle, during stage 4 non-REM sleep. Somniloquy, or sleeptalking, can occur at any sleep stage and is seen in all ages.

54 to 58. The answers are 54-c, 55-a, 56-d, 57-e, 58-b. *(Kliegman et al, pp 458-460.)* Frostnip is manifest by small, firm, white, cold patches of skin in exposed areas; treatment is rewarming the areas before they become numb. Trench foot occurs with prolonged exposure to cold and/or moisture. The foot will become cold, numb, pale, edematous, and clammy. A prolonged autonomic disturbance after this condition can persist for years. Frostbite is the condition in which tissue is frozen and destroyed. There is initial stinging, followed by aching, culminating in numb areas. Once rewarmed, the area becomes red, blotchy, and painful. Gangrene may develop. Hypothermia can develop in any cold weather exposure. As the core temperature drops, the individual becomes lethargic, tired, uncoordinated, apathetic, mentally confused, irritable, and bradycardic. Chilblains are small, ulcerated lesions on exposed areas such as the ears and fingers. Lesions may last 1 to 2 weeks. Cold panniculitis is destruction of fat cells caused by exposure to cold weather or a cold object; in this case, the child had "Popsicle panniculitis," which is usually a benign condition that self-resolves.

59 to 62. The answers are 59-f, 60-i, 61-g, 62-a. *(Hay et al, pp 299, 838-839. Kliegman et al, pp 243, 247, 249-250. McMillan et al, pp 113-114. Rudolph et al, pp 1322-1323.)* Vitamin B_{12} or cobalamin deficiency is unusual, but can be seen in those ingesting a strict vegetarian diet or in a breast-fed baby whose mother has undiagnosed pernicious anemia or other cobalamin-malabsorption syndromes, or in a child with pernicious anemia. Neurologic symptoms in a child include weakness, failure to thrive, irritability, fatigue, sensory defect, delayed or loss of milestones, seizures, and neuropsychiatric changes; hematologic changes include megaloblastic anemia.

Isolated riboflavin deficiency is rare but can occur with deficiencies of other B-complex vitamins. It occurs because of poor intake, reduced absorption in patients with biliary atresia or hepatitis, or poor absorption in those receiving probenecid, phenothiazine, or oral contraceptives. Signs and symptoms of riboflavin deficiency include cheilosis, glossitis, a variety of ocular problems (keratitis, conjunctivitis and corneal vascularization) and seborrheic dermatitis.

Vitamin B_6 or pyridoxine deficiency occurs in patients with low levels of this vitamin in their diet, because of a vitamin B_6–dependent syndrome whereby enzyme structure problems result in poor absorption, or a result vitamin inhibition due to drug ingestion including isoniazid, penicillamine, corticosteroids, and anticonvulsants. Seizures, peripheral neuritis, dermatitis, and microcytic anemia are commonly seen evidence of deficiency.

Folate deficiency can occur from a number of etiologies including poor intake or absorption; in high-demand diseases such as sickle cell; and in inborn errors of metabolism. It also can be seen in conjunction with a variety of medication uses included high dose nonsteroidal anti-inflammatory drugs (NSAIDs), methotrexate, and dilantin. It produces megaloblastic anemia, glossitis, pharyngeal ulcers, and impaired immunity.

Deficiencies of the other vitamins listed include: thiamine and beriberi; niacin and pellagra; vitamin D and rickets; vitamin C and scurvy; biotin deficiency and dermatitis/seborrhea.

63 to 66. The answers are 63-a, 64-c, 65-b, 66-d. (*Hay et al, pp 97, 961, 1031-1034. Kliegman et al, pp 135, 509, 511, 513, 1543-1544, 2451. McMillan et al, pp 2634, 2637, 2639, 2644, 2663, 2251. Rudolph et al, pp 735, 737-740, 752.*) Trisomy 13 occurs in about 1:5000 to 12,000 live births. In most cases all or a majority of the extra 13 chromosome is present. The survival of these infants is poor with less than 5% survival after 6 months of age. Failure to thrive, seizures, and severe mental retardation are seen. Advanced maternal age is commonly noted. Translocation can be a cause, thus imparting ~10% risk of recurrence and the need for parental testing.

Angelman syndrome is also called "happy puppet syndrome" because of the unusual gait and the unprovoked outbursts of laughter. In most case it is caused by an interstitial deletion of chromosome 15q1-q13; the deleted material always comes from the maternal side (the same deleted segment from the paternal side results in Prader-Willi).

The distinctive, catlike cry associated with cri du chat syndrome is likely caused by abnormal laryngeal development; it tends to resolve with time. Profound mental retardation, self-injury behavior, hypersensitivity to sound, and repetitive behaviors are commonly seen. Deletion of the short arm of chromosome 5 is the etiology. About 85% of cases are paternal in origin.

VATER (or VACTERL) is an association of commonly seen findings of unknown etiology. The patents affected have vertebral defect, anal atresia, cardiac defects, tracheoesophageal fistula, renal/radial defect (or both), and limb abnormalities. Intelligence is normal.

Features of Cornelia de Lange include bushy eyebrows, hirsutism, limb defects, VSD, and mental retardation.

67 to 70. The answers are 67-b, 68-a, 69-d, 70-e. *(Hay et al, pp 792-793, 797-801. Kliegman et al, pp 2805-2811, 2841-2947. McMillan et al, pp 2474-2476, 2497-2500. Rudolph et al, pp 907-908, 2436-2439.)* Slipped capital femoral epiphysis is a disease of unknown etiology and occurs typically in adolescents; the disorder is most common among obese boys with delayed skeletal maturation or in thin, tall adolescents having recently enjoyed a growth spurt. Onset of this disorder is frequently gradual; pain referred to the knee in 20% of cases can mask the hip pathology.

Legg-Calvé-Perthes disease is avascular necrosis or idiopathic osteonecrosis of the femoral head; the cause of this disorder is unknown. Boys between the ages of 2 and 12 years are most frequently affected (incidence in boys is greater by four- to fivefold), with a mean of 6 to 7 years old. Presenting symptoms include a limp and pain in the anterior thigh, groin, or knee, although classic symptoms include a painless limp.

Septic arthritis requires urgent intervention to preserve joint mobility. Joint aspiration is diagnostic and can be helpful in treatment. Opening the joint space may be required in a septic hip to assist in draining purulent material. These children need treatment for 4 to 6 weeks.

Transient synovitis is a disorder of unknown etiology, affecting children usually from 2 to 6 years of age. These children usually present with a painful limp. This is a diagnosis of exclusion; septic hip and osteomyelitis must be ruled out. While the WBC count and ESR may be normal, or they also may be slightly elevated. Early aspiration of the joint space may assist in diagnosis. Transient synovitis is a self-limited disorder.

Osteomyelitis usually presents with focal bone tenderness and fever. Early evaluation is best done through nuclear medicine studies, as plain film bony changes usually take a week or so before becoming evident.

71 to 75. The answers are 71-c, 72-b, 73-d, 74-e, 75-a. (*Hay et al, pp 339-340, 350-354, 357. Kliegman et al, pp 341-345, 354-355, 2913-2918. McMillan et al, pp 210, 752-764, 767-772. Rudolph et al, pp 360, 368-371, 373-376.*) The most important aspect of the management of lead poisoning is the identification and withdrawal of the source of the lead. Patients with symptomatic lead poisoning or extremely high lead levels in the blood (> 70 µg/dL) should be treated with both dimercaprol and calcium EDTA. With milder poisoning, intravenous or intramuscular calcium EDTA or, more likely, oral dimercaptosuccinic acid can be used.

N-acetylcysteine (NAC) is an effective treatment for acetaminophen poisoning and acts by removing hepatotoxic metabolites. It should be given within 16 hours of ingestion; after 36 hours it is probably ineffective.

Morphine and other narcotics used in the labor and delivery process produce their major toxic effect by suppression of ventilation. Ventilatory support can be necessary initially, but naloxone is a specific antidote and can be very rapidly effective. The effect of naloxone can wear off more quickly than the effects of the drug for which it was given, so careful observation and repeated doses may be necessary.

Salicylate poisoning produces metabolic acidosis and respiratory alkalosis (although this latter feature is often missed in young children), hyperglycemia or hypoglycemia, paradoxical aciduria, dehydration, and lethargy. Excretion of salicylates in the urine can be markedly enhanced by the administration of acetazolamide and IV sodium bicarbonate. Hemodialysis can also be used.

Organophosphate insecticides are absorbed from all sites and act by inhibiting cholinesterases, thereby leading to the accumulation of high levels of acetylcholine. This affects the parasympathetic nervous system, muscle, and the CNS. Treatment of a patient contaminated with organophosphate insecticide will include thorough washing of the pesticide from the skin, inducing emesis or performing gastric lavage, supporting ventilation, and administering atropine followed by pralidoxime (2-PAM).

76 to 78. The answers are 76-b, 77-a, 78-d. (*Hay et al, pp 351-352, 354-355, 360. Kliegman et al, pp 350-351, 353, 2492-2493. McMillan et al, pp 751-752, 2371-2373. Rudolph et al, pp 347, 367-368, 371-372.*) Phenothiazine can cause an idiosyncratic reaction causing extrapyramidal symptoms such as oculogyric crisis, tremors, torticollis, opisthotonus, and dysphagia. These dystonic symptoms respond surprisingly quickly to the intravenous or intramuscular administration of diphenhydramine (Benadryl).

Iron in the form of salts, such as ferrous sulfate or gluconate, used to treat iron deficiency anemia can be highly toxic to infants; as few as 3 tablets can cause severe symptoms and as few as 10 tablets can be lethal to young children. Symptoms occur in two phases: gastrointestinal symptoms such as bloody vomiting or diarrhea and abdominal pain, followed by a latent period of up to 12 hours or more and terminating with cardiovascular collapse. Deferoxamine given intravenously or intramuscularly forms a complex with the iron and is excreted in the urine, to which it imparts the color of *vin rosé* (red wine).

Methanol, also known as methyl alcohol or wood alcohol, is present in a number of household products and is a frequent contaminant of bootleg alcohol. Toxicity causes a profound metabolic acidosis. Treatment includes emptying the stomach by inducing emesis or by gastric lavage, the IV infusion of ethanol to saturate the enzyme systems that convert methanol to toxins, and, in severe poisoning, the use of hemodialysis to remove the methanol.

Acetazolamide and sodium bicarbonate might be used for aspirin ingestion, and dimercaprol (BAL) would be used for heavy metal ingestions.

79 to 83. The answers are 79-d, 80-g, 81-a, 82-e, 83-b. *(Hay et al, p 293. Kliegman et al, pp 242-245, 247-249, 251-253, 262-263. McMillan et al, pp 113-114. Rudolph et al, pp 1322-1323.)* In general, little scientific data support the use of large doses of vitamins beyond the levels found in a regular, balanced diet. Vitamin excess can be dangerous. Vitamin A in large doses slows normal growth and causes hyperostosis (excess bone growth), hepatomegaly, increased CSF pressure, and drying of skin. Nicotinic acid, a vasodilator, causes skin flushing and pruritus; long-term use can cause tachycardia, liver damage, hyperglycemia, and hyperuricemia. Excessive doses of vitamin C, in addition to causing kidney stones, diarrhea, and cramps, also causes an increase the normal requirement for the vitamin when large doses are discontinued. Prolonged excessive intake of vitamin D can cause nausea, diarrhea, weight loss, polyuria, and soft-tissue calcification of heart, kidney, blood vessels, bronchi, and stomach. Excessive intake of pyridoxine (B_6) can result in sensory neuropathy with altered sensation of touch, pain, and fever.

84 to 88. The answers are 84-c, 85-d, 86-f, 87-g, 88-e. *(Hay et al, pp 1045-1046. Kliegman et al, pp 692-693, 1340, 2012-2013. McMillan et al, pp 173, 175, 2633. Rudolph et al, pp 774-779.)* The use of lithium early in pregnancy has been associated with Ebstein anomaly. The class of antihypertensive medications that include ACE inhibitors has been associated with renal dysgenesis, oligohydramnios, and skull ossification defect. Isotretinoin, a very effective medication for nodular cystic acne, if taken when a woman is pregnant commonly results in teratogenic effects including fetal death, hydrocephalus, CNS defects, microtia/anotia, small or missing thymus, conotruncal heart defect, and micrognathia.

Ensuring adequate folate supplementation before and during pregnancy is associated with a reduction in the incidence of neural tube defects.

The congenital rubella syndrome, now rare in the United States, can result in infants born with deafness, cataracts, mental retardation, and heart defects.

89 to 92. The answers are 89-b, 90-f, 91-d, 92-a. (*Hay et al, pp 415, 1062-1067, 1232. Kliegman et al, pp 970-975, 1498-1499, 2696-2699. McMillan et al, pp 466, 852-854, 860, 864-865, 1362-1363. Rudolph et al, pp 1104, 1174-1175, 1177-1180, 1193-1194.*) Cutaneous larva migrans (also known as creeping eruption) is caused primarily by dog or cat hookworms. After exposure (such as walking barefoot on a beach and stepping where an infected dog has recently been) the larvae penetrate the skin at the epidermal-dermal junction and migrate at about 1 to 2 cm/d. The result is an intensely pruritic lesion as described in the vignette. Left untreated the larvae die, but treatment with antihelminthic medications hastens resolution of symptoms.

Seborrheic dermatitis is a common condition in newborn infants, arising in the first weeks after delivery. The description is as in the vignette. Chronic seborrheic dermatitis, particularly if it is associated with failure to thrive, can result from histiocytosis X. Treatment for common seborrheic dermatitis consists of antiseborrheic shampoos and in some cases topical corticosteroids.

Photosensitive or photoallergic reactions are seen when the offending agent is found on the skin and the patient is exposed to sunlight. In the vignette, lime juice (a common offender) is found in the lime-aid and in the margaritas. The distribution on the face and chest of the child would be expected, as might spilling on the chest of her father.

Atopic dermatitis, an immediate hypersensitivity reaction to common environmental irritants, has a prevalence of 2% to 3% in children. Inflammatory patches and weeping, crusted plaques on the neck, face, groin, and extensor surfaces characterize the infantile form. In older children, dermatitis of the flexural areas is common. Soaps and hot water are common irritants. Therapy is based on avoidance of irritants, adequate hydration of the skin, and use of topical steroids, as well as treatment of infected lesions.

93 to 95. The answers are 93-d, 94-a, 95-c. (*Hay et al, pp 556-558, 689-690, 825-827. Kliegman et al, pp 1015-1019, 1888-1891, 2173-2175. McMillan* *et al, pp 1575-1578, 1856-1858, 2543-2546. Rudolph et al, pp 1677-1681, 1788-1791.*) VSD is the most common congenital cardiac malformation. Although small lesions result in insignificant left-to-right shunts, the murmur associated with them can be significantly louder as a result of turbulent blood flow. Larger lesions result in significant left-to-right shunting of blood and can result in dyspnea, poor growth, and heart failure, usually during early infancy.

The classic presentation of acute poststreptococcal glomerulonephritis consists of the sudden onset of change in urine color (bloody), edema, hypertension, and renal insufficiency. This disease follows an infection of the throat or the skin with a nephrogenic strain of group A streptococci. The oliguria can progress to heart failure if fluid overload occurs.

Neonatal lupus can be responsible for a variety of problems in the newborn. Mothers with antibodies to Ro/SSA and some with antibodies to La/SSB can deliver infants with rashes, thrombocytopenia, and congenital heart block, among the more common problems. Whereas the other symptoms usually resolve during the first months of life, the congenital heart block can be irreversible and can result in heart failure, need for early pacemakers, and an increased incidence of early death.

96 to 102.   The answers are 96-b, 97-f, 98-c, 99-a, 100-d, 101-f, 102-e.
(*Hay et al, pp 8, 294-298. Kliegman et al, pp 242-245, 249, 253-265, 450, 1595, 1599, 1815. McMillan et al, pp 113-114, 1429, 1992-1993, 2014-2015. Rudolph et al, pp 31, 105, 956-957, 1055, 1513, 1529.*) Isoniazid therapy can cause peripheral neuritis as a result of competitive inhibition of pyridoxine metabolism when the dose is high and the patient is poorly nourished or is an alcoholic. It is seldom seen in childhood. To be safe, vitamin B_6 supplements should be given to adolescents. Children maintained on anticonvulsants such as phenytoin can develop low folate levels that, rarely, can be associated with megaloblastic anemia. Folic acid supplementation may be indicated.

The World Health Organization (WHO) recommends that, in communities where vitamin A deficiency is prevalent, vitamin A can be given to all children with measles. Compliance with this recommendation has resulted in a definite reduction in measles-related morbidity and mortality. In the United States, vitamin A supplements should be considered for use in measles patients with immunodeficiency, impaired intestinal absorption, and malnutrition. Recent immigrants from areas with a high mortality from measles and who show ophthalmologic evidence of vitamin A deficiency (blindness, Bitot spots, or xerophthalmia) should also be included in that group.

Fat malabsorption occurs (1) in the absence of pancreatic enzymes, as in cystic fibrosis; (2) as a result of failure of micellar solubilization by bile salts, as in chronic liver disease; and (3) with a problematic mucosal uptake, as in celiac sprue. For people with these conditions, attention must be paid to the provision of fat-soluble vitamins A, D, E, and K.

Both human and cow's milk are low in vitamin D content. Cow's milk and infant formulas are fortified with this vitamin. Breast-fed infants require supplementation with vitamin D when adequate exposure to sunlight cannot be ensured, such as in urban areas where pollutants obscure ultraviolet light, in northern areas with long periods of darkness, and in patients with darkly pigmented skin.

Patients with hemolytic anemia, such as sickle-cell disease, have an ongoing compensatory erythropoiesis. To supply the increased need of rapidly dividing RBC precursors for folate, supplementation is necessary.

In newborns, a lack of free vitamin K in the mother and the absence of bacterial intestinal flora that synthesizes vitamin K result in a transient deficiency in vitamin K–dependent factors (II, VII, IX, X). Milk is a poor source of vitamin K. Vitamin K administered shortly after birth prevents hemorrhagic disease of the newborn.

103 to 107. The answers are 103-c, 104-f, 105-b, 106-g, 107-e. (Hay et al, pp 917-925. Kliegman et al, pp 867-873. McMillan et al, pp 2441-2444, 2467-2468. Rudolph et al, pp 793-802.) The bulk of immunodeficiencies can be ruled out with little cost. The nitroblue tetrazolium (NBT) or other respiratory burst assay will help identify phagocytic-cell defects such as chronic granulomatous disease (causing the frequent liver abscess in the child in the question). Wiskott-Aldrich syndrome is unlikely if the platelet count is normal; Wiskott-Aldrich syndrome must be considered in a patient with severe eczema, thrombocytopenia, and unusual infections. B-cell defects are likely to result in low immunoglobulin A, G, and M levels and result in multiple infections such as that described in the 3-year-old with otitis media and sinusitis. An intradermal skin test using Candida albicans will result in no response in the patient with T-cell deficiencies, such as in the question of the dysmorphic child who possibly has DiGeorge syndrome. Asplenia results in Howell-Jolly bodies and also an increased risk for encapsulated organisms such as pneumococcus or meningococcus; a CBC with a peripheral smear can rule out this disease. Should any of these tests prove to be positive, more extensive, invasive, and expensive testing can be undertaken.

The Newborn Infant

Questions

108. The term infant pictured below weighs 2200 g (4 lb, 14 oz). He is found to have a ventricular septal defect on cardiac evaluation. This infant appears to have features consistent with which of the following?

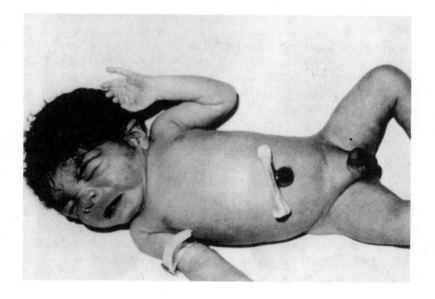

a. Perinatal phenytoin exposure
b. Trisomy 21
c. Alport syndrome
d. Fetal alcohol syndrome
e. Infant of diabetic mother

109. A newborn is noted to be quite jaundiced at 3 days of life. Laboratory data demonstrate his total bilirubin to be 17.8 mg/dL (direct bilirubin is 0.3 mg/dL). Which of the following factors is associated with an increased risk of neurologic damage in a jaundiced newborn?

a. Metabolic alkalosis
b. Increased attachment of bilirubin to binding sites caused by drugs such as sulfisoxazole
c. Hyperalbuminemia
d. Neonatal sepsis
e. Maternal ingestion of phenobarbital during pregnancy

110. A 2-hour-old full-term newborn infant is noted by the nursing staff to be having episodes of cyanosis and apnea. Per nursery protocol they place an oxygen saturation monitor on him. When they attempted to feed him, his oxygen levels drop into the 60s. When he is stimulated and cries, his oxygen levels increase into the 90s. Which of the following is the most important next step to quickly establish the diagnosis?

a. Echocardiogram
b. Ventilation perfusion scan
c. Passage of catheter into nose
d. Hemoglobin electrophoresis
e. Bronchoscopic evaluation of palate and larynx

111. A mother calls you frantic because she has just been diagnosed with chicken pox. She delivered 7 days ago a term infant that appears to be eating, stooling, and urinating well. The child has been afebrile and seems to be doing well. Which of the following is the most appropriate step in management?

a. Isolate the infant from the mother.
b. Hospitalize the infant in the isolation ward.
c. Administer acyclovir to the infant.
d. Administer varicella-zoster immunoglobulin to the infant.
e. Advise the mother to continue regular well-baby care for the infant.

112. A mother wishes to breast-feed her newborn infant, but is worried about medical conditions that would prohibit her from doing so. You counsel her that of her listed conditions, which of the following is a contraindication to breast-feeding?

a. Upper respiratory tract infection
b. Cracked and bleeding nipples
c. Mastitis
d. Inverted nipples
e. HIV infection

113. A mother delivers a neonate with meconium staining and Apgar scores of 3 at 1 and 5 minutes of life. She had no prenatal care and the delivery was by emergency cesarean section for what the obstetricians report as "severe fetal bradycardia." Which of the following sequelae could be expected to develop in this intubated neonate with respiratory distress?

a. Sustained rise in pulmonary arterial pressure
b. Hyperactive bowel sounds
c. Microcephaly with micrognathia
d. Cataracts
e. Thrombocytosis

114. A 2-year-old boy is being followed for congenital cytomegalovirus (CMV) infection. He is deaf and developmentally delayed. The child's mother informs you that she has just become pregnant and is concerned that the new baby will be infected and may develop serious consequences. Which of the following is true?

a. The mother has antibodies to CMV that are passed to the fetus.
b. The mother's infection cannot become reactivated.
c. The likelihood that the new baby will become clinically ill is approximately 80%.
d. Termination of pregnancy is advised.
e. The new infant should be isolated from the older child.

115. A full-term infant is born after a normal pregnancy; delivery, however, is complicated by marginal placental separation. At 12 hours of age, the child, although appearing to be in good health, passes a bloody meconium stool. For determining the cause of the bleeding, which of the following diagnostic procedures should be performed first?

a. A barium enema
b. An Apt test
c. Gastric lavage with normal saline
d. An upper gastrointestinal series
e. A platelet count, prothrombin time, and partial thromboplastin time

116. As you are about to step out of a newly delivered mother's room, she mentions that she wants to breast-feed her healthy infant, but that her obstetrician was concerned about one of the medicines she was taking. Which of the woman's medicines, listed below, is clearly contraindicated in breast-feeding?

a. Ibuprofen as needed for pain or fever
b. Labetalol for her chronic hypertension
c. Amphetamines for her attention deficit disorder
d. Carbamazepine for her seizure disorder
e. Acyclovir for her HSV outbreak

117. A recovering premature infant who weighs 950 g (2 lb, 1 oz) is fed breast milk to provide 120 cal/kg/d. Over the ensuing weeks, the baby is most apt to develop which of the following?

a. Hypernatremia
b. Hypocalcemia
c. Blood in the stool
d. Hyperphosphatemia
e. Vitamin D toxicity

118. A primiparous woman whose blood type is O positive gives birth at term to an infant who has A-positive blood and a hematocrit of 55%. A total serum bilirubin level obtained at 36 hours of age is 12 mg/dL. Which of the following additional laboratory findings would be characteristic of ABO hemolytic disease in this infant?

a. A normal reticulocyte count
b. A positive direct Coombs test
c. Crescent-shaped red blood cells in the blood smear
d. Elevated hemoglobin
e. Petechiae

119. The nurse from the level 2 neonatal intensive care nursery calls you to evaluate a baby. The infant, born at 32 weeks' gestation, is now 1 week old and had been doing well on increasing nasogastric feedings. This afternoon, however, the nurse noted that the infant has vomited the last two feedings and seems less active. Your examination reveals a tense and distended abdomen with decreased bowel sounds. As you are evaluating the child, he has a grossly bloody stool. The plain film of his abdomen is shown. The next step in your management of this infant should include which of the following?

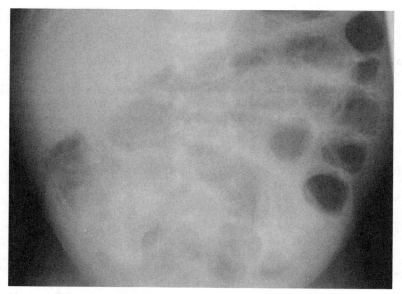

(Courtesy of Susan John, MD.)

a. Surgical consultation for an emergent exploratory laparotomy.
b. Continued feeding of the infant, as gastroenteritis is usually self-limited.
c. Stool culture to identify the etiology of the bloody diarrhea and an infectious diseases consultation.
d. Stopping feeds, beginning intravenous fluids, ordering serial abdominal films, and initiating systemic antibiotics.
e. Removal of nasogastric tube, placement of a transpyloric tube and, after confirmation via radiograph of tube positioning, switching feeds from nasogastric to nasoduodenal.

120. An infant weighing 1400 g (3 lb) is born at 32 weeks' gestation. Initial evaluation was benign, and the infant was transferred to the level 2 nursery for prematurity. The nurse there calls at 1 hour of life and reports the infant is tachypneic. Vital signs include a heart rate of 140 beats per minute, a respiratory rate of 80 breaths per minute, a temperature of 35°C (95°F), and a peripheral oxygen saturation of 98%. The lungs are clear with bilateral breath sounds and there is no murmur; the infant is in no distress. The child's chest radiograph is shown. Which of the following is the most appropriate next step in evaluating the infant?

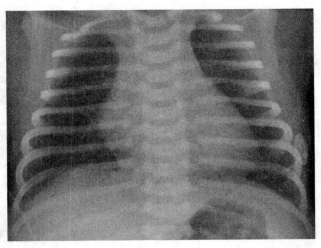

(Courtesy of Susan John, MD.)

a. Obtain a complete blood count and differential.
b. Perform a lumbar puncture.
c. Administer intravenously 5cc of $D_{50}W$.
d. Place the infant under a warmer.
e. Administer supplemental oxygen.

121. Two new mothers are discussing their infants outside the neonatal intensive care unit. Both were born at 36 weeks' gestation. One infant weighs 2600 g (5 lb, 12 oz) while the other infant weighs 1600 g (3 lb, 8 oz). The mother of the second infant should be told that her child is more likely to have which of the following conditions?

a. Congenital malformations
b. Low hematocrit
c. Hyperglycemia
d. Surfactant deficiency
e. Rapid catch-up growth

122. A 3-day-old infant, born at 32 weeks' gestation and weighing 1700 g (3 lb, 12 oz), has three episodes of apnea, each lasting 20 to 25 seconds and occurring after a feeding. During these episodes, the heart rate drops from 140 to 100 beats per minute, and the child remains motionless; between episodes, however, the child displays normal activity. Blood sugar is 50 mg/dL and serum calcium is normal. Which of the following is most likely true regarding the child's apneic periods?

a. They are due to an immature respiratory center.
b. They are a part of periodic breathing.
c. They are secondary to hypoglycemia.
d. They are manifestations of seizures.
e. They are evidence of underlying pulmonary disease.

123. You have an 11-day-old term infant in your office for a well-child visit. The mother notes that she received a letter that day from the state's Department of Health reporting that her child's newborn screen had come back abnormal, indicating possible galactosemia. Which of the following is the most appropriate management at this point?

a. Discontinue oral feeds and begin total parenteral nutrition.
b. Supplement her breast-feeding with a multivitamin.
c. Refer to endocrinology for evaluation.
d. Discontinue breast-feeding and initiate soy formula feedings.
e. Ultrasound of pancreas.

124. The father of a 1-week-old infant comes to the office in a panic. He has just noticed on his child a right anterior shoulder mass that seems tender. The father is an osteosarcoma survivor and fears the child has the same malignancy. In reviewing the baby's discharge papers, you note the child was a term, appropriate-for-gestational-age vaginal delivery with a birth weight of 3200 g (7 lb, 1 oz). Apgar scores were 9 at 1 and 5 minutes. Your examination is significant for a large firm mass on the right clavicle; the rest of the examination is normal. Management of this problem should include which of the following?

a. Magnetic resonance imaging of the right shoulder
b. Reassurance and supportive care
c. A biopsy of the mass for culture and cytology
d. Referral to an orthopedic surgeon
e. Skin biopsy to test for osteogenesis imperfecta

125. A 1-day-old infant who was born by a difficult forceps delivery is alert and active. She does not move her left arm spontaneously or during a Moro reflex. Rather, she prefers to maintain it internally rotated by her side with the forearm extended and pronated. The rest of her physical examination is normal. This clinical scenario most likely indicates which of the following?

a. Fracture of the left clavicle
b. Fracture of the left humerus
c. Left-sided Erb-Duchenne paralysis
d. Left-sided Klumpke paralysis
e. Spinal injury with left hemiparesis

126. You are examining a newborn infant in the well-baby nursery. The infant was the product of a benign pregnancy and vaginal delivery; he appears to be in no distress. Interestingly, your measurement of fronto-occipital head circumference is about 2 cm larger than the initial measurement done several hours before. Your examination otherwise is significant for tachycardia and a "squishy" feel to the entire scalp. You can elicit a fluid wave over the scalp. Management of this condition should include which of the following?

a. Transfer to the newborn ICU
b. Observation and parental reassurance
c. CT scan of the skull with bone windows
d. Surgical drainage
e. Elevation of the head of the crib

127. A 19-year-old primiparous woman develops toxemia in her last trimester of pregnancy and during the course of her labor is treated with magnesium sulfate. At 38 weeks' gestation, she delivers a 2100-g (4-lb, 10-oz) infant with Apgar scores of 1 at 1 minute and 5 at 5 minutes. Laboratory studies at 18 hours of age reveal a hematocrit of 79%, platelet count of 100,000/µL, glucose 41 mg/dL, magnesium 2.5 mEq/L, and calcium 8.7 mg/dL. Soon after, the infant has a generalized convulsion. Which of the following is the most likely cause of the infant's seizure?

a. Polycythemia
b. Hypoglycemia
c. Hypocalcemia
d. Hypermagnesemia
e. Thrombocytopenia

128. An infant who appears to be of normal size is noted to be lethargic and somewhat limp after birth. The mother is 28 years old, and this is her fourth delivery. The pregnancy was uncomplicated, with normal fetal monitoring prior to delivery. Labor was rapid, with local anesthesia and intravenous meperidine (Demerol) administered for maternal pain control. Which of the following therapeutic maneuvers is likely to improve this infant's condition most rapidly?

a. Intravenous infusion of 10% dextrose in water
b. Administration of naloxone (Narcan)
c. Administration of vitamin K
d. Measurement of electrolytes and magnesium levels
e. Neurologic consultation

129. At 43 weeks' gestation, a long, thin infant is delivered. The infant is apneic, limp, pale, and covered with "pea soup" amniotic fluid. Which of the following is the best first step in the resuscitation of this infant at delivery?

a. Intubation and suction of the trachea; provision of oxygen
b. Artificial ventilation with bag and mask
c. Chest compressions
d. Administration of 100% oxygen by mask
e. Catheterization of the umbilical vein

130. The newborn pictured below was born at home and has puffy, tense eyelids; red conjunctivae; a copious amount of purulent ocular discharge; and chemosis 2 days after birth. Which of the following is the most likely diagnosis?

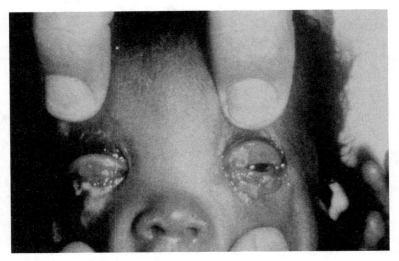

(Courtesy of Kathryn Musgrove, MD.)

a. Dacryocystitis
b. Chemical conjunctivitis
c. Pneumococcal ophthalmia
d. Gonococcal ophthalmia
e. Chlamydial conjunctivitis

131. After an uneventful labor and delivery, an infant is born at 32 weeks' gestation weighing 1500 g (3 lb, 5 oz). Respiratory difficulty develops immediately after birth and increases in intensity thereafter. At 6 hours of age, the child's respiratory rate is 60 breaths per minute. Examination reveals grunting, intercostal retraction, nasal flaring, and marked cyanosis in room air. Auscultation reveals poor air movement. Physiologic abnormalities compatible with these data include which of the following?

a. Decreased lung compliance, reduced lung volume, left-to-right shunt of blood
b. Decreased lung compliance, reduced lung volume, right-to-left shunt of blood
c. Decreased lung compliance, increased lung volume, left-to-right shunt of blood
d. Normal lung compliance, reduced lung volume, left-to-right shunt of blood
e. Normal lung compliance, increased lung volume, right-to-left shunt of blood

132. A term infant is born to a known HIV-positive mother. She has been taking antiretroviral medications for the weeks prior to the delivery of her infant. Routine management of the healthy infant should include which of the following?

a. Admission to the neonatal intensive care unit for close cardiovascular monitoring
b. HIV ELISA on the infant to determine if congenital infection has occurred
c. A course of zidovudine for the infant
d. Chest radiographs to evaluate for congenital *Pneumocystis carinii*
e. Administration of IVIG to the baby to decrease the risk of perinatal HIV infection

133. Initial examination of a full-term infant weighing less than 2500 g (5 lb, 8 oz) shows edema over the dorsum of her hands and feet. Which of the following findings would support a diagnosis of Turner syndrome?

a. A liver palpable to 2 cm below the costal margin
b. Tremulous movements and ankle clonus
c. Redundant skin folds at the nape of the neck
d. A transient, longitudinal division of the body into a red half and a pale half
e. Softness of the parietal bones at the vertex

134. You have been recently named as the medical director of the normal newborn nursery in your community hospital and have been asked to write standardized admission orders for all pediatricians to follow. Which of the following vaccines will you include on these orders?

a. Hepatitis A vaccine
b. Hepatitis B vaccine
c. Combination diphtheria, tetanus, and acellular pertussis vaccine
d. Inactivated polio virus
e. Haemophilus influenza B vaccine

135. A 1-week-old black infant presents to you for the first time with a large, fairly well-defined, purple lesion over the buttocks bilaterally, as shown in the photograph. The lesion is not palpable, and it is not warm nor tender. The mother denies trauma and reports that the lesion has been present since birth. This otherwise well-appearing infant is growing and developing normally and appears normal upon physical examination. Which of the following is the most appropriate course of action in this infant?

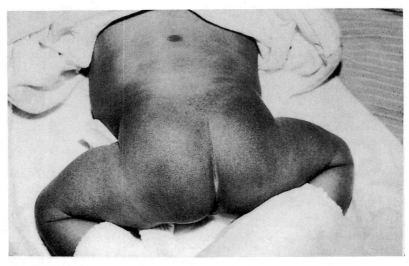

(Courtesy of Adelaide Hebert, MD.)

a. Report the family to child protective services
b. Reassurance of the normalcy of the condition
c. Soft tissues films of the buttocks to identify calcifications
d. Administration of vitamin K
e. Measurement of bleeding time as well as factor VII and XI levels

136. A newborn infant develops respiratory distress immediately after birth. His abdomen is scaphoid. No breath sounds are heard on the left side of his chest, but they are audible on the right. Immediate intubation is successful with little or no improvement in clinical status. Emergency chest x-ray is shown (A) along with an x-ray 2 hours later (B). Which of the following is the most likely explanation for this infant's condition?

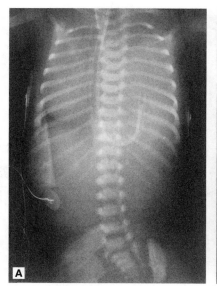 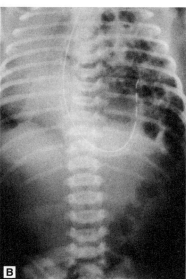

(Courtesy of Susan John, MD.)

a. Pneumonia
b. Cystic adenomatoid malformation
c. Diaphragmatic hernia
d. Choanal atresia
e. Pneumothorax

137. Shortly after birth, an infant develops abdominal distention and begins to drool. When she is given her first feeding, it runs out the side of her mouth, and she coughs and chokes. Physical examination reveals tachypnea, intercostal retractions, and bilateral pulmonary rales. The esophageal anomaly that most commonly causes these signs and symptoms is illustrated by which of the following?

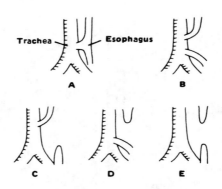

a. Figure A
b. Figure B
c. Figure C
d. Figure D
e. Figure E

138. You are advised by the obstetrician that the mother of a baby she has delivered is a carrier of hepatitis B surface antigen (HBsAg-positive). Which of the following is the most appropriate action in managing this infant?

a. Screen the infant for HBsAg.
b. Isolate the infant with enteric precautions.
c. Screen the mother for hepatitis B "e" antigen (HBeAg).
d. Administer hepatitis B immune globulin and hepatitis B vaccine to the infant.
e. Do nothing because transplacentally acquired antibody will prevent infection in the infant.

139. You are called to a delivery of a term infant, about to be born via cesarean section to a mother with multiple medical problems, including a 1-month history of a seizure disorder, for which she takes phenytoin; rheumatic heart disease, for which she must take penicillin daily for life; hypertension, for which she takes propranolol; acid reflux, for which she takes aluminum hydroxide; and a deep venous thrombosis in her left calf diagnosed 2 days ago, for which she was started on a heparin infusion. The obstetrician is concerned about the possible effects of the mother's multiple medications on the newborn infant. Which of the following medications is most likely to cause harm in this newborn infant at delivery?

a. Propranolol
b. Penicillin
c. Aluminum hydroxide
d. Phenytoin
e. Heparin

140. Your older sister, her husband, their 2-day-old infant, and their pet Chihuahua arrive at your door. The parents of the child are concerned because the pediatrician noted the child was "yellow" and ordered some studies. They produce a wad of papers for you to review. Both the mother and baby have O-positive blood. The baby's direct serum bilirubin is 0.2 mg/dL, with a total serum bilirubin of 11.8 mg/dL. Urine bilirubin is positive. The infant's white blood cell count is 13,000/μL with a differential of 50% polymorphonuclear cells, 45% lymphocytes, and 5% monocytes. The hemoglobin is 17 g/dL, and the platelet count is 278,000/μL. Reticulocyte count is 1.5%. The peripheral smear does not show fragments or abnormal cell shapes. Which of the following is the most likely explanation for this infant's skin color?

a. Rh or ABO hemolytic disease
b. Physiologic jaundice
c. Sepsis
d. Congenital spherocytic anemia
e. Biliary atresia

141. At the time of delivery, a woman is noted to have a large volume of amniotic fluid. At 6 hours of age, her baby begins regurgitating small amounts of mucus and bile-stained fluid. Physical examination of the infant is normal, and an abdominal x-ray is obtained (see below). Which of the following is the most likely diagnosis of this infant's disorder?

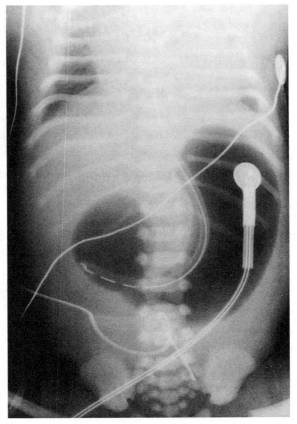

(Courtesy of Susan John, MD.)

a. Gastric duplication
b. Pyloric stenosis
c. Esophageal atresia
d. Duodenal atresia
e. Midgut volvulus

142. The mother and father of a newborn come in for the 2-week checkup. The mother complains of "colic" and asks if she can switch to goat's milk instead of breast milk. Which of the following should be your main concern about using goat's milk instead of breast milk or cow's milk?

a. It has insufficient calories.
b. It has insufficient folate.
c. It has insufficient whey.
d. It has insufficient casein.
e. It has insufficient fat.

143. You see the newborn baby shown below for the first time in the nursery. You consult plastic and reconstructive surgeon as well as the hospital's speech therapist. Understandably, the parents have many questions. Which of the following statements is appropriate anticipatory guidance for this family?

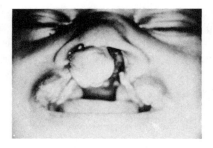

a. Parenteral alimentation is recommended to prevent aspiration.
b. Surgical closure of the palatal defect should be done before 3 months of age.
c. Good anatomic closure will preclude the development of speech defects.
d. Recurrent otitis media and hearing loss are likely complications.
e. The chance that a sibling also would be affected is 1 in 1000.

144. The mother of a 2-week-old infant reports that since birth, her infant sleeps most of the day; she has to awaken her every 4 hours to feed, and she will take only an ounce of formula at a time. She also is concerned that the infant has persistently hard, pellet-like stools. On your examination you find an infant with normal weight and length, but with an enlarged head. The heart rate is 75 beats per minute and the temperature is 35°C (95°F). The child is still jaundiced. You note large anterior and posterior fontanelles, a distended abdomen, and an umbilical hernia. This clinical presentation is likely a result of which of the following?

a. Congenital hypothyroidism
b. Congenital megacolon (Hirschsprung disease)
c. Sepsis
d. Infantile botulism
e. Normal development

145. A routine prenatal ultrasound reveals a male fetus with meningomyelocele. The 24-year-old primigravid mother is told the infant will require surgery shortly after birth. You counsel her about the etiology of this defect and the risk of further pregnancies being similarly affected, and state which of the following?

a. The hereditary pattern for this condition is autosomal recessive.
b. The prenatal diagnosis can be made by the detection of very low levels of alpha-fetoprotein in the amniotic fluid.
c. Subsequent pregnancies are not at increased risk compared to the general population.
d. Supplementation of maternal diet with folate leads to a decrease in incidence of this condition.
e. Neither environmental nor social factors have been shown to influence the incidence.

146. A term, 4200-g (9-lb, 4-oz) female infant is delivered via cesarean section because of cephalopelvic disproportion. The amniotic fluid was clear, and the infant cried almost immediately after birth. Within the first 15 minutes of life, however, the infant's respiratory rate increased to 80 breaths per minute, and she began to have intermittent grunting respirations. The infant was transferred to the level 2 nursery and was noted to have an oxygen saturation of 94%. The chest radiograph is shown. Which of the following is the most likely diagnosis?

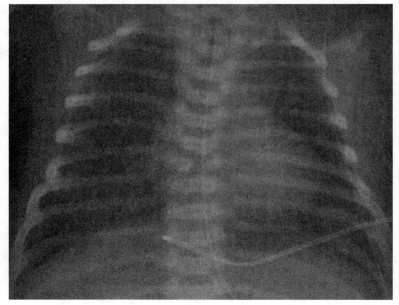

(Courtesy of Susan John, MD.)

a. Diaphragmatic hernia
b. Meconium aspiration
c. Pneumonia
d. Idiopathic respiratory distress syndrome
e. Transient tachypnea of the newborn

147. The infant in the following picture presents with hepatosplenomegaly, anemia, persistent rhinitis, and a maculopapular rash. Which of the following is the most likely diagnosis for this child?

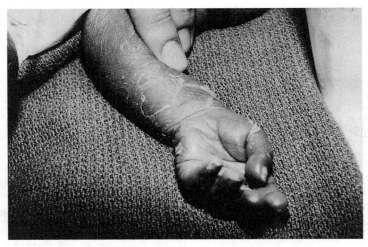

(Courtesy of Adelaide Hebert, MD.)

a. Toxoplasmosis
b. Glycogen storage disease
c. Congenital hypothyroidism
d. Congenital syphilis
e. Cytomegalovirus disease

148. A well-appearing, 3200-g (7-lb, 1-oz) black infant is noted to have fifth finger (postaxial) polydactyly. The extra digit has no skeletal duplications and is attached to the rest of the hand by a threadlike soft tissue pedicle (see photograph). Appropriate treatment for this condition includes which of the following?

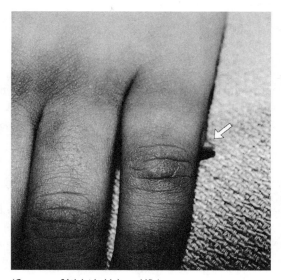

(Courtesy of Adelaide Hebert, MD.)

a. Chromosomal analysis
b. Excision of extra digit
c. Skeletal survey for other skeletal abnormalities
d. Echocardiogram
e. Renal ultrasound

149. An infant born at 35 weeks' gestation to a mother with no prenatal care is noted to be jittery and irritable, and is having difficulty feeding. You note coarse tremors on examination. The nurses report a high-pitched cry and note several episodes of diarrhea and emesis. You suspect which of the following?

a. Fetal alcohol syndrome
b. Prenatal exposure to marijuana
c. Heroin withdrawal syndrome
d. Cocaine exposure *in utero*
e. Tobacco use by the mother

150. A previously healthy full-term infant has several episodes of duskiness and apnea during the second day of life. Diagnostic considerations should include which of the following?

a. Hemolytic anemia
b. Congenital heart disease
c. Idiopathic apnea
d. Harlequin syndrome
e. Hyperglycemia

151. The signs and symptoms of meningitis in an infant can be different than those in an adult. Which of the following signs and symptoms of meningitis is more helpful in an adult patient than in a 4-month-old?

a. Lethargy
b. Jaundice
c. Vomiting
d. Brudzinski sign
e. Hypothermia

152. A woman gives birth to twins at 38 weeks' gestation. The first twin weighs 2800 g (6 lb, 3 oz) and has a hematocrit of 70%; the second twin weighs 2100 g (4 lb, 10 oz) and has a hematocrit of 40%. Which of the following statements is correct?

a. The second twin is at risk for developing respiratory distress, cyanosis, and congestive heart failure.
b. The first twin is more likely to have hyperbilirubinemia and convulsions.
c. The second twin is at risk for renal vein thrombosis.
d. The second twin probably has hydramnios of the amniotic sac.
e. The second twin is likely to be pale, tachycardic, and hypotensive.

153. Parents bring a 5-day-old infant to your office. The mother is O negative and was Coombs positive at delivery. The term child weighed 3055 g (6 lb, 1 oz) at birth and had measured baseline hemoglobin of 16 g/dL and a total serum bilirubin of 3 mg/dL. He passed a black tarlike stool within the first 24 hours of life. He was discharged at 30 hours of life with a stable axillary temperature of 36.5°C (97.7°F). Today the infant's weight is 3000 g, his axillary temperature is 35°C (95°F), and he is jaundiced to the chest. Parents report frequent yellow, seedy stool. You redraw labs and find his hemoglobin is now 14 g/dL, and his total serum bilirubin is 13 mg/dL. The change in which of the following parameters is of most concern?

a. Hemoglobin
b. Temperature
c. Body weight
d. Bilirubin
e. Stool

154. You are called to a delivery of a woman with no prenatal care; she is in active labor but has no history of amniotic rupture. The biophysical profile done in the emergency center revealed severe oligohydramnios. When you get this infant to the nursery, you should carefully evaluate him for which of the following?

a. Anencephaly
b. Trisomy 18
c. Renal agenesis
d. Duodenal atresia
e. Tracheoesophageal fistula

155. A newborn infant becomes markedly jaundiced on the second day of life, and a faint petechial eruption, first noted at birth, is now a generalized purpuric rash. Hematologic studies for hemolytic diseases are negative. Acute management should include which of the following?

a. Liver ultrasound
b. Isolation of the infant from pregnant hospital personnel
c. Urine drug screen on the infant
d. Discharge with an early follow-up visit in 2 days to recheck bilirubin
e. Thyroid hormone assay

Questions 156 to 159

For each clinical scenario below, select the most likely diagnosis. Each lettered option may be used once, more than once, or not at all.

a. Congenital toxoplasmosis
b. Congenital syphilis
c. Congenital rubella
d. Congenital cytomegalovirus
e. Congenital herpes simplex virus

156. A newborn has bilateral cataracts and microphthalmia, intrauterine growth retardation, hemorrhagic skin lesions scattered throughout the body, and a harsh systolic murmur heard at the left sternal border and radiating to the lung fields.

157. A week-old infant presents with fever and focal seizure.

158. A newborn has hydrocephalus, chorioretinitis, intracranial calcifications, and anemia.

159. A newborn has microcephaly, intracranial calcifications, hepato-splenomegaly, and marked hyperbilirubinemia and thrombocytopenia.

Questions 160 to 163

For each clinical scenario below, select the most likely diagnosis. Each lettered option may be used once, more than once, or not at all.

a. Bronchopulmonary dysplasia
b. Respiratory distress syndrome (hyaline membrane disease)
c. Pulmonary interstitial emphysema
d. Bronchiolitis
e. Primary pulmonary hypoplasia
f. Pneumothorax
g. Asthma
h. Meconium aspiration
i. Phrenic nerve paralysis
j. Bacterial pneumonia

160. A large-for-gestation-age term infant is delivered via scheduled cesarean section develops, at 15 minutes of age, tachypnea, grunting, flaring, and retractions. The child does not move his left arm well, but you find no clavicular fracture. A chest radiograph shows the left diaphragm to be markedly higher than the right.

161. A postterm infant is born at home after a prolonged and difficult labor. The maternal grandmother brings the infant to the hospital at 1 hour of life because of fast breathing. Grandmother notes that the child seemed well for a while, but then developed increased work of breathing. Physical examination reveals an infant in moderate respiratory distress with diminished breath sounds on the left. Chest radiograph reveals the heart to be pushed to the right side and loss of lung markings in the left lung field.

162. An infant of uncertain but seemingly term dates is born via emergent cesarean section for nonreassuring heart tones; the obstetrician has noted little or no amniotic fluid. The infant is small, has abnormally shaped limbs, and an unusual facies. The child has immediate respiratory distress. A chest radiograph reveals a poorly developed chest with little lung tissue.

163. A preterm infant is now 7 weeks old. She was intubated for 2 weeks and was weaned off oxygen at 3 weeks of age. You are about to leave your office for Thanksgiving holiday when the emergency room calls to tell you she has new hypoxia, respiratory distress, wheezes, and runny nose. A chest radiograph reveals patchy infiltrates and hyperexpansion in both lung fields. The newborn's 2-year-old sibling has an upper respiratory infection.

Questions 164 to 167

Blood samples of a 3-day-old full-term infant are sent for screening to identify diseases that would have serious, permanent consequences without prompt and appropriate treatment. Select the most appropriate treatment for each disease below. Each lettered option may be used once, more than once, or not at all.

a. Special infant formula
b. Hormone therapy
c. Vitamin therapy
d. Antibiotic prophylaxis
e. Sunlight

164. Galactosemia

165. Phenylketonuria

166. Biotinidase deficiency

167. Hypothyroidism

Questions 168 to 171

For each of the following descriptions of a patient with a congenital anomaly, select the major abnormality with which it is most likely to be associated. Each lettered option may be used once, more than once, or not at all.

a. Deafness
b. Seizures
c. Wilms tumor
d. Congestive heart failure
e. Optic glioma

168. A child's left arm and leg seem bigger than those on the right. In addition, the child has aniridia. None of the family members have aniridia or hemihypertrophy, nor do they know of anyone else in the family with these conditions.

169. An infant has fusion of the eyebrows, heterochromic irises, a broad nasal root with lateral displacement of the medial canthi, and a white forelock.

170. An infant presents with a large, flat vascular malformation over the left face and scalp. The mother notes that her other child was born with a capillary hemangioma on his arm and asks if this is the same thing. You explain that this vascular malformation is different, and that you will want to monitor him for another condition.

171. A new mother points out several hypopigmented oval macules over the child's trunk and extremities. She notes that these have been present since birth. She is concerned because she had a brother with the same spots whom she thinks had "growths" in his brain.

Questions 172 to 174

For each description of head injury that follows, select the major abnormality with which it is most likely to be associated. Each lettered option may be used once, more than once, or not at all.

a. Intraventricular hemorrhage
b. Caput succedaneum
c. Subdural hemorrhage
d. Subarachnoid hemorrhage
e. Subgaleal hemorrhage

172. A 1-day-old infant has a fronto-occipital head circumference that is 2 cm larger than the initial measurement done several hours before, the scalp has a "squishy" feel to it, and the infant has developed tachycardia.

173. A 6-month-old comatose infant has multiple broken bones in various stages of healing, a bulging anterior fontanelle, and retinal hemorrhages.

174. Previous premature infant born at 27 weeks' gestation and now 6 months of age presents with macrocephaly and hydrocephalus on ultrasonogram.

The Newborn Infant

Answers

108. The answer is d. (*Hay et al, pp 17-18, 99-100, 474, 1031, 1045-1046. Kliegman et al, pp 507-509, 692, 780-785, 2172-2173. McMillan et al, pp 338, 423-427, 1875-1878, 2632, 2635. Rudolph et al, pp 124-126, 527, 732-734, 775, 776, 1699-1700.*) Fetal alcohol syndrome is a preventable cause of birth defects. Prenatal exposure to ethanol is the cause. Findings include small-for-gestation birth, microcephaly, small palpebral fissures, short nose, smooth philtrum, thin upper lip, ptosis, microphthalmia, cleft lip and palate, and central nervous system abnormalities including mental retardation (average IQ = 67).

Common findings with trisomy 21 include protruding tongue, Brushfield spots, redundant neck skin, mental retardation, brachycephaly, upslanting palpebral fissures, epicanthal folds, flat face, small ears, cardiac abnormalities (especially ventricular septal defect or endocardial Cushing defect), palmar creases, and clinodactyly of the fifth digit.

Dilantin exposure causes midface hypoplasia, low nasal bridge, ocular hypertelorism, and accentuated Cupid's bow of the upper lip. Other features include cleft lip and palate, growth retardation, mental deficiency, distal phalangeal hyperplasia, cardiovascular anomalies, and skeletal defects.

Alport syndrome is the most common of the hereditary nephritis conditions, frequently leading to end-stage renal disease. In 85% of patients with Alport syndrome, an X-linked dominant form of inheritance is found; about 15% are autosomal recessive. All cause hematuria and progressive nephritis. Other findings include deafness and ocular defects.

Infants of diabetic mothers have an increased chance of congenital heart disease, caudal regression syndrome, and a small left colon. Besides, they are large-for-gestation age and have a number of biochemical abnormalities such as hypoglycemia or hypocalcemia.

109. The answer is d. (*Hay et al, pp 11-17. Kliegman et al, pp 756-766. McMillan et al, pp 235-245. Rudolph et al, pp 164-169.*) Significant unconjugated serum bilirubin levels in full-term newborn infants can lead to diffusion of bilirubin into brain tissue and to neurologic damage. Sulfisoxazole and other drugs compete with bilirubin for binding sites on albumin;

therefore, the presence of these drugs can cause dislocation, not increased affinity, of bilirubin to tissues. Metabolic acidosis also reduces binding of bilirubin, and neonatal sepsis interrupts the blood–brain barrier, thus allowing diffusion of bilirubin into the brain. Administration of phenobarbital has been used to induce glucuronyl transferase in newborn infants and can reduce, rather than exacerbate, neonatal jaundice. Other factors that reduce the amount of unconjugated bilirubin bound to albumin (and therefore cause an increase in free unconjugated bilirubin) include hypoalbuminemia and certain compounds (eg, nonesterified fatty acids, which are elevated during cold stress) that compete with bilirubin for albumin-binding sites.

110. The answer is c. *(Hay et al, p 479. Kliegman et al, p 1743. McMillan et al, p 197. Rudolph et al, p 1260.)* It is important to make the diagnosis of choanal atresia quickly because it responds to treatment but can be lethal if unrecognized and untreated. Most neonates are obligate nose breathers and cannot breathe adequately through their mouths. Infants with choanal atresia have increased breathing difficulty during feeding and sleeping and improved respirations when crying. A variety of temporizing measures to maintain an open airway have been used, including oropharyngeal airways, positioning, tongue fixation, and endotracheal intubation, but surgical correction with placement of nasal tubes is most effective. The diagnosis can be made by failure to pass a catheter through the nose to the pharynx or by checking for fog developing on a cold metal instrument placed under each nares. Bronchoscopy would help diagnose lower airway anomalies. A ventilation-perfusion scan would be the appropriate examination if you were concerned about mismatch (eg, that associated with pulmonary embolism). A newborn with a hemoglobinopathy such as sickle cell or thalassemia would not present as this infant did, so an electrophoresis would not be helpful. An echocardiogram would be useful if you suspected congenital cyanotic heart disease. The lack of a murmur in a newborn does not rule out pathology; this would be a reasonable next step if the catheter passed through both nares without difficulty.

111. The answer is e. *(Hay et al, pp 1117-1119. Kliegman et al, pp 1367-1368. McMillan et al, pp 520-522. Rudolph et al, pp 1043, 1224.)* Per CDC recommendations, varicella-zoster immunoglobulin (VZIG) should be administered to the infant immediately after delivery if the mother had the onset of varicella within 5 days prior to delivery, and immediately upon diagnosis if her chicken pox started within 2 days after delivery. If untreated, about half of these infants will develop serious varicella as early as 1 day of age.

If a normal full-term newborn is exposed to chicken pox 2 or more days postnatally, VZIG and isolation are not necessary because these babies appear to be at no greater risk for complications than older children. Acyclovir may be used in infants at risk for severe varicella, such as those infants exposed perinatally.

112. The answer is e. *(Hay et al, pp 299-301. Kliegman et al, pp 215-216, 218. McMillan et al, p 116. Rudolph et al, p 104.)* There are few contraindications to breast-feeding. Active pulmonary tuberculosis and HIV are two examples of infectious contraindications in developed countries, as well as malaria, typhoid fever, and septicemia. In underdeveloped countries, the risk of infectious diarrhea due to use of contaminated water to mix formula or the unavailability of formula can preclude this recommendation. All medications taken by the mother will be secreted in breast milk, but usually not in amounts significant enough to affect the infant. Mothers taking antineoplastic agents should not breast-feed. Mothers with mastitis can continue to breast-feed; frequent feedings may help the condition by preventing engorgement. Mothers with mild viral illness may also continue to breast-feed. Cracked or bleeding nipples may make breast-feeding uncomfortable, but are not contraindications. Inverted nipples usually can be remedied, and only rarely prohibit breast-feeding.

113. The answer is a. *(Hay et al, pp 551-552. Kliegman et al, p 1727. McMillan et al, pp 315-319. Rudolph et al, pp 98-99, 188.)* The low Apgar scores, meconium staining, and ensuing respiratory distress suggest that asphyxia has occurred. During a period of asphyxia, the resulting hypoxemia, acidosis, and poor perfusion can damage a neonate's brain, heart, kidney, liver, and lungs. The resulting clinical abnormalities include cerebral edema, irritability, seizures, cardiomegaly, heart failure, renal failure, poor liver function, disseminated intravascular coagulopathy, and respiratory distress syndrome. There can be excessively high pulmonary arterial pressure at the same time systemic blood pressure begins to fall, resulting in a persistent right-to-left shunt across a patent ductus arteriosus or foramen ovale.

114. The answer is a. *(Hay et al, pp 1120-1123. Kliegman et al, pp 1377-1379. McMillan et al, pp 511-516. Rudolph et al, pp 1031-1035.)* Cytomegalovirus infection is the most common cause of congenital infection, occurring in 0.2% to 2.4% of all live births. Cytomegalic inclusion disease is a constellation of findings including hepatomegaly, splenomegaly, jaundice, petechiae, purpura, and microcephaly. In the United States, 20% to 90% of women of childbearing age have serologic evidence of a past infection with CMV. Symptomatic congenital disease usually occurs when a mother has a primary CMV infection in the first trimester of pregnancy. Many of these babies die, and those who survive are severely affected. In the event of reactivation of CMV infection during pregnancy, maternal IgG, passed transplacentally, protects the infant from serious infection. Although most infants infected during this secondary maternal infection are asymptomatic, about 10% of them eventually manifest hearing and neurologic problems. Some recommend keeping a child with congenital CMV infection away from susceptible pregnant (or about to become pregnant) women because CMV excretion can persist for months to years; at the very least, good hand-washing practices should be instituted. If infected shortly after birth, the younger sibling will probably be asymptomatic since he or she has maternal IgG in the circulation. CMV is primarily an occult infection. Of toddlers in day-care centers, 20% to 80% acquire CMV and shed it in saliva and urine for years. Diagnosis is made with isolation of the virus from urine, saliva, or other secretions, although several rapid tests also are available.

115. The answer is b. *(Hay et al, p 631. Kliegman et al, p 774. McMillan et al, pp 1928-1929. Rudolph et al, p 1372.)* Hematemesis and melena are not uncommon in the neonatal period, especially if gross placental bleeding has occurred at the time of delivery. The diagnostic procedure that should be done first is the Apt test, which differentiates fetal from adult hemoglobin in a bloody specimen. The test is based upon the finding that fetal hemoglobin is alkali resistant, while adult hemoglobin will convert to hematin upon exposure to alkali. If the blood in an affected infant's gastric contents or stool is maternal in origin, further workup of the infant is obviated.

116. The answer is c. *(Hay et al, p 301. Kliegman et al, p 682. McMillan et al, p 198.)* Most medications are secreted to some extent in breast milk, and some lipid-soluble medications may be concentrated in breast milk. Although the list of contraindicated medications is short, caution should always be exercised when giving a medication to a breast-feeding woman. Medications that are clearly contraindicated include lithium, cyclosporin, antineoplastic agents, illicit drugs including cocaine and heroin, amphetamines, lithium, ergotamines, and bromocriptine (which suppresses lactation). Although some suggest that oral contraceptives may have a negative impact on milk production, the association has not been proven conclusively. In general, antibiotics are safe, with only a few exceptions (such as tetracycline). While sedatives and narcotic pain medications are probably safe, the infant must be observed carefully for sedation. All of the medications listed in the question are considered safe, except for amphetamines.

117. The answer is b. *(Hay et al, pp 33-34. Kliegman et al, pp 706-707. McMillan et al, pp 180-181.)* It usually is impossible with any combination of parenteral and enteral nutrition to match what the infant would have accumulated *in utero*. The average, healthy, low-birth-weight infant of this size requires a daily intake of calcium of about 200 mg/kg. Breast milk has much less calcium (and phosphorus) than do commercial formulas. The breast milk can be directly supplemented with calcium, or it can be supplemented with commercial fortifiers. Alternatively, it can be mixed with formulas designed for the premature infant. Breast milk promotes gut maturation and prevents intestinal atrophy induced by lack of enteral feeding; however, it is likely to have insufficient calcium and phosphorus for catch-up growth.

118. The answer is b. *(Hay et al, p 13. Kliegman et al, p 772. McMillan et al, pp 242-243. Rudolph et al, pp 177, 1531-1532.)* If a mother is O positive and her baby is A positive, the baby has a chance of developing hemolytic disease. Hemolytic disease and jaundice caused by a major blood-group incompatibility are usually less severe than with Rh incompatibility. Although the hematocrit of affected infants usually is normal, elevation of the reticulocyte count and the presence of nucleated red blood cells and microspherocytes in the blood smear provide evidence of hemolysis. In comparison with hemolytic disease caused by Rh incompatibility, where it is usually strongly positive, major blood-group incompatibility is often associated with a direct Coombs test that is frequently weakly positive. Petechiae are usually associated with decreased number of platelets. Crescent-shaped (sickled) red blood cells are found with sickle-cell disease.

119. The answer is d. *(Hay et al, pp 38-39. Kliegman et al, pp 755-756. McMillan et al, pp 389-397. Rudolph et al, pp 140-143.)* The infant presented in the question has necrotizing enterocolitis (NEC), a potentially life-threatening disease of the neonate; the radiograph demonstrates distended loops of bowel with air in the bowel wall. NEC is more common in premature infants, but has been described in term infants as well. Although several organisms have been isolated from NEC patients, no clear cause for this condition has been identified. Patients present with feeding intolerance and a distended abdomen; about a quarter have grossly bloody stool. Pneumatosis intestinalis is found on plain radiograph of the abdomen and is diagnostic for NEC in this age group. Management depends initially on the presence or absence of perforation; if no evidence of free peritoneal air is found, the infant should be put on bowel rest with nasogastric decompression, and systemic antibiotics are initiated. Electrolytes and vital signs should be monitored closely, and serial abdominal films should be performed to evaluate for perforation. If free air is identified on plain radiographs or if the infant clinically worsens with medical management, surgical consultation is required. An exploratory laparotomy is usually performed, and any necrotic intestinal tissue is removed. Occasionally, removal of necrotic gut will result in an infant without adequate intestinal surface area to absorb nutrition, a condition known as *short bowel syndrome*.

120. The answer is d. *(Hay et al, p 32. Kliegman et al, p 724. McMillan et al, p 259. Rudolph et al, pp 84-85, 123.)* The radiograph is normal. However, the vignette describes a cold infant. A room temperature of 24°C (approximately 75°F) provides a cold environment for newborn infants. Aside from the fact that these infants emerge from a warm, 37.6°C (99.5°F) intrauterine environment, at birth, infants (and especially preterm infants) are wet, have a relatively large surface area for their weight, and have little subcutaneous fat. Within minutes of delivery, the infants are likely to become pale or blue and their body temperatures will drop. In order to bring body temperature back to normal, they must increase their metabolic rate; ventilation, in turn, must increase proportionally to ensure an adequate oxygen supply. Because a preterm infant is likely to have respiratory problems and be unable to oxygenate adequately, lactate can accumulate and lead to a metabolic acidosis. Infants rarely shiver in response to a need to increase heat production. If the tachypnea persists after warming the infant, sepsis, pneumonia, and primary surfactant deficiency are all possible; thus, several of the alternative answers then may be appropriate.

121. The answer is a. *(Kliegman et al, p 703. McMillan et al, pp 274-181. Rudolph et al, pp 122, 2022-2023.)* Small-for-dates infants are subject to a different set of complications than preterm infants whose size is appropriate for gestational age. The small-for-dates infants have a higher incidence of major congenital anomalies and are at increased risk for future growth retardation, especially if length and head circumference as well as weight are small for gestational age. Also more common are neonatal asphyxia and the meconium aspiration syndrome, which can lead to pneumothorax, pneumomediastinum, or pulmonary hemorrhage. These, rather than hyaline membrane disease, are the major pulmonary problems in small-for-gestational-age infants. Because neonatal symptomatic hypoglycemia is more commonly found in small-for-dates infants, careful blood glucose monitoring and early feeding are appropriate precautions. Normal or elevated hematocrit is also more common in these infants.

122. The answer is a. (*Hay et al, pp 34-35. Kliegman et al, pp 729-730. McMillan et al, pp 318-320. Rudolph et al, p 1934.*) Apneic episodes are characterized by an absence of respirations for more than 20 seconds and may be accompanied by bradycardia and cyanosis. A large number of conditions can cause apnea. Periods of apnea are generally thought to be secondary to an incompletely developed respiratory center, particularly when they are seen, as is common, associated with prematurity. Although seizures, hypoglycemia, and pulmonary disease accompanied by hypoxia can lead to apnea, these causes are less likely in the infant described, given that no unusual movements occur during the apneic spells, the blood sugar level is more than 40 mg/dL, and the child appears well between episodes. Other, less common, explanations for central apnea include congenital central hypoventilation syndrome (formerly known as Ondine's curse), Arnold-Chiari malformations, and congenital infections. Periodic breathing, a common pattern of respiration in low-birth-weight babies, is characterized by recurrent breathing pauses of 3 to 10 seconds.

123. The answer is d. (*Hay et al, pp 992-993. Kliegman et al, pp 609-610. McMillan et al, pp 2187-2188. Rudolph et al, p 1486.*) All 50 states in the United States, as well as most developed countries, screen in the neonatal period infants for a variety of conditions, among them galactosemia. The condition is autosomal recessive (about 1:40,000 live births); if not identified on newborn screening, affected infants can present with jaundice, hepatomegaly, vomiting, hypoglycemia, convulsions, lethargy, irritability, feeding problems, poor weight gain, aminoaciduria, cataracts, liver cirrhosis/failure, and mental retardation. Early treatment is essential and consists of galactose avoidance (soy or casein hydrolysate infant formula). With appropriate treatment, many of the features listed can be avoided. However, affected children often have ovarian failure, reduced bone mineral density, and developmental delay.

124. The answer is b. (*Hay et al, p 797. Kliegman et al, p 727. McMillan et al, p 425. Rudolph et al, pp 185-186.*) The clavicle is the most commonly fractured bone in the delivery process. While some fractures are identified at birth, others may not be identified until callus formation is noted at about a week of age. Clavicular fracture may happen in any delivery, although there is higher risk with large-for-gestational-age infants. Initial presentation of a fractured clavicle may include a pseudoparalysis, in which the infant refuses to move the ipsilateral arm, mimicking an Erb-Duchenne paralysis.

125. The answer is c. (*Hay et al, p 23. Kliegman et al, pp 720-721, 2826. McMillan et al, p 2492. Rudolph et al, p 2447.*) In a difficult delivery in which traction is applied to the head and neck, several injuries, including all those listed in the question, may occur. Erb-Duchenne paralysis affects the fifth and sixth cervical nerves; the affected arm cannot be abducted or externally rotated at the shoulder, and the forearm cannot be supinated. Injury to the seventh and eighth cervical and first thoracic nerves (Klumpke paralysis) results in palsy of the hand and also can produce Horner syndrome. Fractures in the upper limb are not associated with a characteristic posture, and passive movement usually elicits pain. Spinal injury causes complete paralysis below the level of injury. When paralysis of an upper extremity from injury to the brachial plexus is found in a neonate, injury to the phrenic nerve should also be suspected because the nerve roots are close together and can be injured concurrently. The paralyzed diaphragm can be noted to remain elevated on a chest x-ray taken during deep inspiration when it will contrast with the opposite normal diaphragm in its lower normal position; on expiration, this asymmetry cannot be seen. On inspiration, not only is breathing impaired since the paralyzed diaphragm does not contract, but also the negative pressure generated by the intact diaphragm pulls the mediastinum toward the normal side, impairing ventilation further. The diagnosis can easily be made by fluoroscopy, where these characteristic movements on inspiration and expiration can be seen. Rarely, both diaphragms can be paralyzed, producing much more severe ventilatory impairment. Fortunately, these injuries frequently improve spontaneously.

126. The answer is a. (*Hay et al, p 5. Kliegman et al, p 714. McMillan et al, p 197. Rudolph et al, pp 186-187.*) The child has a subgaleal or subaponeurotic hemorrhage which can be life threatening; infants may lose a third or more of their blood volume into this potential space, leading to hypovolemic shock. A subgaleal hemorrhage will feel like a cephalohematoma that crosses the midline, but rapidly expands and can have cardiovascular complications. Careful monitoring is essential. Observation alone in this case would be appropriate, but should be accomplished in an ICU setting.

127. The answer is a. *(Hay et al, p 60. Kliegman et al, p 773. McMillan et al, p 445. Rudolph et al, pp 192-193.)* An infant of 2100 g (4 lb, 10 oz) at 38 weeks would be considered small for gestational age (SGA), a not uncommon consequence of maternal toxemia. Pregnancy-induced hypertension can produce a decrease in uteroplacental blood flow and areas of placental infarction. This can result in fetal nutritional deprivation and intermittent fetal hypoxemia, with a decrease in glycogen storage and a relative erythrocytosis, respectively. Hence, neonatal hypoglycemia and polycythemia are common clinical findings in these infants. A blood glucose level of 30 to 40 mg/dL in a full-term infant, however, is probably normal during the first postnatal day, and an infant is very unlikely to have a convulsion as a result of a level of 41 mg. Serum calcium levels usually decline during the first 2 to 3 postnatal days, but will only be considered abnormally low in a term infant when they fall below 7.5 to 8 mg/dL. Neonatal hypermagnesemia is common in an infant whose mother has received $MgSO_4$ therapy, but is usually asymptomatic or produces decreased muscle tone or floppiness. A persistent venous hematocrit of greater than 65% in a neonate is regarded as polycythemia and will be accompanied by an increase in blood viscosity.

Manifestations of the "hyperviscosity syndrome" include tremulousness or jitteriness that can progress to seizure activity because of sludging of blood in the cerebral microcirculation or frank thrombus formation, renal vein thrombosis, necrotizing enterocolitis, and tachypnea. Simple phlebotomy, while decreasing blood volume, will also decrease systemic arterial pressure and thus increase viscosity (based on Poiseuille law of flow). Therapy by partial exchange transfusion with saline or lactated Ringer solution is preferred, and may be more likely to be useful if performed prophylactically before significant symptoms have developed, but literature evaluating outcomes in these infants is lacking.

128. The answer is b. *(Hay et al, pp 29-30. Kliegman et al, pp 723-725. McMillan et al, pp 209-210. Rudolph et al, p 102.)* In the description provided, the most likely cause of the neonatal depression is maternal analgesic narcotic drug administration. While controlling the pain of the delivery in the mother, use of narcotics can result in depression of the newborn via crossing of the placenta. The appropriate first step in the management of this infant (after managing the ABCs of airway, breathing, and circulation) is the administration of naloxone, 0.1 mg/kg, IM, IV, or endotracheal. The other possibilities are unlikely, given the clinical information provided.

129. The answer is a. *(Hay et al, p 30. Kliegman et al, pp 725-726. McMillan et al, p 211. Rudolph et al, p 196.)* Infants who are postmature (more than 42 weeks' gestation) and show evidence of chronic placental insufficiency (low birth weight for gestational age and wasted appearance) have a higher than average chance of being asphyxiated, and passage of meconium into the amniotic fluid thus places these infants at risk for meconium aspiration. Ideally the obstetrician suctions the mouth, nose, and hypopharynx immediately after delivery of the infant's head but before delivery of the reminder of the body. If the infant's heart rate is more than 100 beats per minute and respirations are unlabored, routine neonatal management is appropriate. However, if the heart rate is less than 100 beats per minute in a floppy, depressed infant then endotracheal intubation is accomplished along with suctioning and providing oxygen.

130. The answer is d. *(Hay et al, p 432. Kliegman et al, pp 2588-2589. McMillan et al, pp 811-812. Rudolph et al, p 2370.)* The time of onset of symptoms is somewhat helpful in the diagnosis of ophthalmia neonatorum. Chemical conjunctivitis is a self-limited condition that presents within 6 to 12 hours of birth and lasts for the first day or so of life; it is a consequence of ocular silver nitrate (no longer available in the United States) or erythromycin prophylaxis. Gonococcal conjunctivitis has its onset within 2 to 5 days after birth and is the most serious of the bacterial infections. Prompt and aggressive topical treatment and systemic antibiotics are indicated to prevent serious complications such as corneal ulceration, perforation, and resulting blindness. Parents should be treated to avoid the risk to the child of reinfection.

Chlamydial conjunctivitis occurs 5 to 14 days after birth; to avoid the risk of chlamydial pneumonia, treatment in an infant with conjunctivitis is with systemic antibiotics (parents, too, require treatment). However, asymptomatic infants born to chlamydia-positive mothers are not routinely treated with oral antibiotics at birth as prophylaxis, but rather watched closely for signs of infection, due to an increased incidence of hypertrophic pyloric stenosis among neonates having received erythromycin.

131. The answer is b. *(Hay et al, pp 35-36. Kliegman et al, pp 731-741. McMillan et al, pp 305-310. Rudolph et al, pp 127-134.)* For the child described in the question, prematurity and the clinical picture presented make the diagnosis of hyaline membrane disease (infant respiratory distress syndrome) likely. HMD is caused by surfactant deficiency, and the incidence is increased with decreasing gestational age and birth weight. In this disease, lung compliance is reduced; lung volume is also reduced, and a significant right-to-left shunt of blood can occur. Some of the shunt can result from a patent ductus arteriosus or foramen ovale, and some can be due to shunting within the lung. Minute ventilation is higher than normal, and affected infants must work harder in order to sustain adequate respiration.

132. The answer is c. *(Hay et al, pp 1140-1151. Kliegman et al, pp 1435-1436. McMillan et al, pp 942-952. Rudolph et al, pp 1046, 1052.)* The transmission of HIV from mother to infant has decreased in recent years, due in large part to perinatal administration of antiretroviral medications to the mother and a course of zidovudine to the exposed infant. Studies suggest that a better than 50% decrease in transmission can be seen with appropriate medications as outlined.

An ELISA is an antibody test and will be positive in the infant born to an HIV-infected mother due to maternal antibodies that are passed through the placenta; it is not a useful test in the newborn infant to determine neonatal infection because of this expected transfer of maternal (and not infant) immunoglobulin. IVIG has not been shown to have a role in decreasing perinatal transmission. Healthy asymptomatic term infants born to HIV-infected mothers do not need special monitoring, nor do they need routine radiographs.

133. The answer is c. *(Hay et al, p 1032. Kliegman et al, pp 2386-2389. McMillan et al, pp 2635-2636. Rudolph et al, pp 2087-2089.)* Turner syndrome is a genetic disorder; the 45,XO karyotype is the most common. At birth, affected infants have low weights, short stature, edema over the dorsum of the hands and feet, and loose skin folds at the nape of the neck. Some other findings with this syndrome include sexual infantilism, streak gonads, typical faces, shield chest, low hairline, coarctation of the aorta, hypertension, bicuspid aortic valve, high palate, and horseshoe kidney. Coarse, tremulous movements accompanied by ankle clonus; vascular instability as evidenced, for example, by a harlequin color change (a transient, longitudinal division of a body into red and pale halves); softness of parietal bones at the vertex (craniotabes); and a liver that is palpable down to 2 cm below the costal margin are all findings often demonstrated by normal infants and are of no diagnostic significance in the clinical situation presented.

134. The answer is b. *(Hay et al, pp 271-273. Kliegman et al, pp 1682-1685. McMillan et al, pp 533-534. Rudolph et al, p 1498.)* The only vaccine routinely given in the newborn nursery is the hepatitis B vaccine. The other vaccines listed typically are administered beginning at 2 months of age. The other injection typically included on standardized order sheets and given to all hospitalized newborns is vitamin K, which is provided prophylactically to prevent a danger drop in vitamin K-dependent coagulation factors. Failure to provide vitamin K (especially those fed human breast milk) can result in vitamin K levels low enough to produce classic hemorrhagic manifestations (melena, hematuria, bleeding from circumcision site, intracranial hemorrhage, hypovolemic shock) on the second to seventh day of life.

135. The answer is b. *(Hay et al, p 404. Kliegman et al, p 2662. McMillan et al, p 828. Rudolph et al, p 1192.)* The pictured lesion is a Mongolian spot, a bluish-gray lesion located over the buttocks, lower back, and occasionally, the extensor surfaces of the extremities. These are common in blacks, Asians, and Latin Americans. They tend to disappear by 1 to 2 years of age, although those on the extremities may not fully resolve. Child abuse is unlikely to present with bruises alone; children frequently present with more extensive injuries. Subcutaneous fat necrosis, which may ultimately result in subcutaneous calcifications in the affected area, is usually found as a sharply demarcated, hard lesion on the cheeks, buttocks, and limbs but it usually is red. Hemophilia and vitamin K deficiency rarely present with subcutaneous lesions as described and are more likely to present as a bleeding episode.

136. The answer is c. *(Hay et al, p 609. Kliegman et al, pp 746-749. McMillan et al, pp 211-212. Rudolph et al, pp 189-191.)* Diaphragmatic hernia occurs with the transmittal of abdominal contents across a congenital or traumatic defect in the diaphragm. In the newborn, this condition results in profound respiratory distress with significant mortality. Prenatal diagnosis is common and, when found, necessitates that the birth take place at a tertiary-level center. In the neonate, respiratory failure in the first hours of life, a scaphoid abdomen, and presence of bowel sounds in the chest are common findings. Intensive respiratory support, including high-frequency oscillatory ventilation and extracorporeal membrane oxygenation (ECMO), has increased survival. Mortality can be as high as 50% despite aggressive treatment. While surgery may correct the diaphragmatic defect, the lung on the affected side remains hypoplastic and continues to contribute to morbidity.

Pneumonia and pneumothorax may cause respiratory distress with decreased breath sounds, but the radiograph in diaphragmatic hernia shows the nasogastric tube curving into the left thorax, clearly an abnormal placement. A congenital cystic adenomatoid malformation will frequently look like a diaphragmatic hernia on radiographs, but the nasogastric tube would be in the correct location. Choanal atresia is an upper airway abnormality and does not cause these radiographic changes; it would have been difficult to place the nasogastric tube in the first place with this condition, in which there is a bony or membranous septum between the nose and pharynx.

137. The answer is d. (*Hay et al, p 46. Kliegman et al, pp 1543-1544. McMillan et al, pp 369-371. Rudolph et al, pp 1385-1387.*) Abdominal distention, choking, drooling, and coughing associated with feedings are symptoms of esophageal anomalies. The anomaly illustrated by **D** is the most common; that of **A** can be diagnosed after repeated episodes of pneumonia. The anomalies in **E** and **C** are associated with all the same symptoms except abdominal distention, which cannot develop because air cannot enter the gastrointestinal tract. **B** and **C** are the least common; in these, the upper esophageal segment is connected directly to the trachea, and massive entry of fluid into the lungs occurs.

VATER association, a complex of cardiovascular malformations, skeletal malformations, and renal abnormalities, has tracheoesophageal fistula as a common finding.

138. The answer is d. (*Hay et al, pp 271-273. Kliegman et al, pp 1682-1685. McMillan et al, pp 533-534. Rudolph et al, pp 49-50.*) The infant of a mother, who is a carrier of hepatitis B surface antigen, has a significant risk of acquiring infection. This usually occurs at the time of delivery, but infection can also be acquired during pregnancy and postnatally. A small percentage of infected neonates develop acute icteric hepatitis, but the majority remains asymptomatic. Of these infected asymptomatic infants, 80% or more will develop chronic infection, the long-term consequences of which are chronic liver disease and, possibly, hepatocellular carcinoma. Combined passive-active immunoprophylaxis in the form of hepatitis B immune globulin and hepatitis B vaccine affords protection not only from immediate perinatal infection but also from infection that may be acquired as a result of continued exposure in the household of a chronic carrier.

Immunization in this infant is indicated regardless of the presence of hepatitis B "e" antigen (HBeAg) in the mother. Although the presence of HBeAg, especially in the absence of antibody to HBeAg, is associated with high rates of transmission to neonates, any woman positive for hepatitis B surface antigen (HBsAg) is potentially infectious. It is not necessary to isolate infants born to carriers of HBsAg, and screening of neonates for HBsAg is not indicated. Testing for HBsAg and anti-HBsAg at least 1 month after the third dose of hepatitis B vaccine will determine the efficacy of these measures.

139. The answer is a. (*Hay et al, p 25. Kliegman et al, p 693. McMillan et al, pp 171-173.*) The effect of a drug on the fetus is determined by the nature of the drug and by the timing and degree of exposure. Heparin does not cross the placental barrier and does not appear to directly affect the fetus once pregnancy is well established. Phenytoin may cause birth defects when given during the first trimester. Penicillin and aluminum hydroxide have not been found to affect the fetus. Propranolol, which may cause growth retardation when given throughout pregnancy, diminishes the ability of an asphyxiated infant to increase heart rate and cardiac output. It has also been associated with hypoglycemia and apnea.

140. The answer is b. (*Hay et al, pp 12-15. Kliegman et al, pp 758-759. McMillan et al, pp 240-241. Rudolph et al, pp 164-169.*) The development of jaundice in a healthy full-term baby may be considered the result of a normal physiologic process in certain circumstances. It may be normal if the time of onset and duration of the jaundice and the pattern of serially determined serum concentrations of bilirubin are in conformity with currently accepted safe criteria. Physiologic jaundice becomes apparent on the second or third day of life, peaks to levels no higher than about 12 mg/dL on the fourth or fifth day, and disappears by the end of the week. The rate of rise is less than 5 mg/dL per 24 hours and levels of conjugated bilirubin do not exceed about 1 mg/dL. Concern about neonatal jaundice relates to the risk of the neurotoxic effects of unconjugated bilirubin.

The precise level and duration of exposure necessary to produce toxic effects are not known, but bilirubin encephalopathy, or kernicterus, is rare in term infants whose bilirubin level is kept below 18 to 20 mg/dL. Certain risk factors affecting premature or sick newborns increase their susceptibility to kernicterus at much lower levels of bilirubin. The diagnosis of physiologic jaundice is made by excluding other causes of hyperbilirubinemia by means of history, physical examination, and laboratory determinations.

Jaundice appearing in the first 24 hours is usually a feature of hemolytic states and is accompanied by an indirect hyperbilirubinemia, reticulocytosis, and evidence of red-cell destruction on smear. In the absence of blood group or Rh incompatibility, congenital hemolytic states (eg, spherocytic anemia) or G6PD deficiency should be considered. With infection, hemolytic and hepatotoxic factors are reflected in the increased levels of both direct and indirect bilirubin. Studies should include maternal and infant Rh types and blood groups and Coombs tests to detect blood-group or Rh incompatibility and sensitization.

Measurements of total and direct bilirubin concentrations help to determine the level of production of bilirubin and the presence of conjugated hyperbilirubinemia. Hematocrit and reticulocyte count provide information about the degree of hemolysis and anemia, and a complete blood count screens for the possibility of sepsis and the need for cultures.

Examination of the blood smear is useful in differentiating common hemolytic disorders. Except for determinations of total and direct bilirubin, tests of liver function are not particularly helpful in establishing the cause of early-onset jaundice. Transient elevations of transaminases (AST and ALT) related to the trauma of delivery and to hypoxia have been noted.

Biliary atresia and neonatal hepatitis can be accompanied by elevated levels of transaminase, but characteristically present as chronic cholestatic jaundice with mixed hyperbilirubinemia after the first week of life.

141. The answer is d. *(Hay et al, p 47. Kliegman et al, pp 1559-1560. McMillan et al, p 373. Rudolph et al, pp 1403-1404.)* The finding of polyhydramnios suggests high intestinal obstruction, signs of which include abdominal distention and early and repeated regurgitation. Distention usually is not present, as vomiting keeps the intestine decompressed. The bile-stained vomitus of the infant places the obstruction distal to the ampulla of Vater, eliminating esophageal atresia and pyloric stenosis from consideration. The "double bubble" sign on the x-ray is characteristic of duodenal atresia, which is compatible with the history. Midgut volvulus, which may obstruct the bowel in the area of the duodenojejunal junction, most often produces signs after an affected infant is 3 or 4 days old with acute onset of bilious vomitus. Gastric duplication does not usually produce intestinal obstruction; a cystic mass may be palpated on abdominal examination. Patients with duodenal atresia should be examined closely for evidence of other conditions such as Down syndrome or heart disease.

142. The answer is b. *(Kliegman et al, pp 939-940, 1611-1612. McMillan et al, pp 1448-1449. Rudolph et al, p 1332.)* Goat's milk, by itself, is not an ideal source of infant nutrition as it contains inadequate folate and iron, potentially contributing to anemia. Caloric content is actually more dense than cow's milk–based formulas (about 30 kcal/oz, compared to 20 kcal/oz for formula and breast milk). Casein and whey are the protein sources in goat's milk, as they are for many formulas. Some manufacturers in different countries produce a goat milk–based formula that contains supplemental vitamins and iron. Unpasteurized goat's milk should never be used as an infant formula because of the risk of brucellosis.

143. The answer is d. (*Hay et al, pp 450-451. Kliegman et al, pp 1532-1533. McMillan et al, pp 469-472, 2661-2662. Rudolph et al, pp 748-753.*) The infant pictured has bilateral cleft lip and palate. This defect occurs in about 4% of the siblings of affected infants; its incidence in the general population is 1 in 1000. Evaluation for other structural and chromosomal abnormalities is indicated. Although affected infants are likely to have feeding problems initially, these problems usually can be overcome by feeding in a propped-up position and using special nipples. Complications include recurrent otitis media and hearing loss as well as speech defects, which may be present despite good anatomic closure. Repair of a cleft lip usually is performed within the first 2 to 3 months of life; the palate is repaired later, usually between the ages of 6 months and 5 years.

144. The answer is a. (*Hay et al, pp 947-950. Kliegman et al, pp 2319-2325. McMillan et al, pp 421-422, 2126-2128. Rudolph et al, pp 2065-2070.*) The clinical findings of congenital hypothyroidism are subtle, and may not be present at all at birth; this is thought to be a result of passage of some T_4 transplacentally. Infants with examination findings will usually have an umbilical hernia and a distended abdomen. The head may be large, and the fontanelles will be large as well. The child may be hypothermic and have feeding difficulties; constipation and jaundice may be persistent. Skin may be cold and mottled, and edema may be found in the genitals and extremities. The heart rate may be slow, and anemia may develop. As these findings may be subtle or nonexistent, neonatal screening programs are extremely important for early diagnosis of these infants.

Sepsis can cause hypothermia and poor feeding, but the 2-week time makes this choice unlikely. Hirschsprung disease may cause chronic constipation and abdominal distension, but not the other findings. Botulism can cause a flaccid paralysis and poor feeding, but the large fontanelles and umbilical hernia are not caused by this infection.

145. The answer is d. (*Hay et al, pp 1024, 1044. Kliegman et al, pp 697, 2444-2447. McMillan et al, pp 175, 265-266. Rudolph et al, pp 2186-2187.*) Diseases that are due to defects in a single gene are designated as autosomal or X-linked, depending on whether the affected gene is located on an autosome or an X chromosome. Genetically determined diseases that are multifactorial in origin (ie, neural tube defects) do not conform to the Mendelian pattern of inheritance but exhibit a variable outcome that reflects the interaction between a particular genotype and an environment. The relatives of persons with diseases of multifactorial origin have an increased risk of having similar abnormalities.

The recurrence risk for most single primary defects of multifactorial inheritance (eg, neural tube defects) is increased with each child affected. This increased risk forms the basis for assuming that genetic factors play a role in the occurrence of these abnormalities. Other factors, such as race, sex, and ethnic and racial background, influence the frequency with which an abnormality of multifactorial inheritance occurs in relatives. The prenatal diagnosis of neural tube defects (anencephaly and meningomyelocele) can be made by the detection of elevated levels of alpha-fetoprotein in the amniotic fluid. To reduce the risk of neural tube defects, it is now recommended that all women capable of becoming pregnant take 400 mcg of folic acid daily.

146. The answer is e. (*Hay et al, p 20. Kliegman et al, p 741. McMillan et al, p 311. Rudolph et al, pp 179-181.*) Transient tachypnea of the newborn is usually seen after a normal vaginal or, especially, after a cesarean delivery. The condition is a result of retained fetal lung fluid. These patients have tachypnea, retractions, grunting, and sometimes cyanosis. The chest examination is usually normal; the chest radiograph demonstrates prominent pulmonary vascular markings with fluid in the fissures and hyperexpansion (flat diaphragms). Therapy is supportive, with maintenance of normal oxygen saturation. Resolution usually occurs in the first 3 days of life.

Diaphragmatic hernia would demonstrate intestinal contents located in the chest on plain radiograph. Meconium aspiration would present in a patient who is born with meconium at the delivery and the radiograph would have patchy infiltrates. Pneumonia in a patient of this age is more likely to have diffuse infiltrates on radiograph and clinical findings of temperature instability. Idiopathic respiratory distress syndrome occurs in premature infants whose radiographs demonstrate a "ground glass appearance."

147. The answer is d. (*Hay et al, pp 1205-1208. Kliegman et al, pp 1263-1269. McMillan et al, pp 1135-1142. Rudolph et al, pp 1004-1005.*) The clinical presentation of congenital syphilis is varied. Many newborns appear normal at birth and continue to be asymptomatic for the first few weeks or months of life. Most untreated infants will develop skin lesions, the usual one being an infiltrative, maculopapular peeling rash that is most prominent on the face, palms, and soles. Involvement of the nasal mucous membranes causes rhinitis with a resultant serous, and occasionally purulent, blood-tinged discharge (snuffles). This, as well as scrapings from the skin lesions, contains abundant viable treponemes. Hepatosplenomegaly and lymphadenopathy are common, and early jaundice is a manifestation of syphilitic hepatitis. Liver function tests are elevated; hemolytic anemia and thrombocytopenia are common. Infants may have a saddle nose, a result of destruction of bone from syphilitic rhinitis. Among the later manifestations, or stigmata, of congenital syphilis is interstitial keratitis, which is an acute inflammation of the cornea that begins in early childhood (most commonly between 6 and 14 years of age). Interstitial keratitis represents the response of the tissue to earlier sensitization. Findings include marked photophobia, lacrimation, corneal haziness, and eventual scarring. Hutchinson teeth (peg or barrel-shaped upper central incisors), abnormal enamel, and mulberry molars (first lower molars with an abnormal number of cusps) are dental manifestations of syphilis.

148. The answer is b. (*Kliegman et al, pp 2829-2930. McMillan et al, p 2123. Rudolph et al, p 2493.*) Fifth-finger polydactyly is 10 times more common in black than in white children and is typically familial. This finding in otherwise healthy black children should raise no special concern. In a white child, careful examination of the cardiac system is warranted. Similarly, preaxial (or thumb-side) polydactyly is unusual and should be further investigated. Some syndromes that are associated with polydactyly are trisomy 13, Rubinstein-Taybi syndrome, Meckel-Gruber syndrome, and Ellis-van Creveld syndrome. Simple postaxial polydactyly without bone involvement may be surgically removed shortly after birth. Simply tying these appendages off with string will usually leave a nub.

149. The answer is c. (*Kliegman et al, p 693. Rudolph et al, p 2196.*) Infants born to narcotic addicts are more likely than other children to exhibit a variety of problems, including perinatal complications, prematurity, and low birth weight. The onset of withdrawal commonly occurs during an infant's first 2 days of life and is characterized by hyperirritability and coarse tremors, along with vomiting, diarrhea, fever, high-pitched cry, and hyperventilation; seizures and respiratory depression are less common. The production of surfactant can be accelerated in the infant of a heroin-addicted mother.

In utero exposure to alcohol leads to a fetal alcohol syndrome consisting of growth retardation, microcephaly, flat philtrum, thin upper lip, cardiac defects, and hypoplastic fifth fingernails. Maternal cocaine use puts the infant at risk for vascular accidents and premature delivery, but not a withdrawal syndrome. Similarly, marijuana is not associated with neonatal withdrawal. Maternal tobacco use can result in small-for-gestation age infants, but not a neonatal withdrawal syndrome as described in the question.

150. The answer is b. (*Kliegman et al, p 711. McMillan et al, p 346. Rudolph et al, pp 1934-1936.*) Idiopathic apnea is common in premature infants but is not expected in the full-term newborn. When apnea occurs in the term infant, there is almost always an identifiable cause. Sepsis, gastroesophageal reflux, congenital heart disease, seizures, hypoglycemia, and airway obstruction can cause apnea in term newborns. Harlequin syndrome is a transient change in the skin color of the otherwise asymptomatic newborn (usually preterm) in which the dependent side of the entire body turns red while the upper side remains pale.

151. The answer is d. (*Hay et al, pp 49-53, 763, 1088-1090. Kliegman et al, pp 2515-2516. McMillan et al, pp 493-496. Rudolph et al, pp 106-107.*) Neonatal sepsis, a clinical syndrome of systemic illness accompanied by bacteremia, often results in spread of infection to the meninges and other distant sites. The diagnosis of serious infection, including meningitis, in a neonate is difficult because the signs and symptoms are subtle and nonspecific. They include lethargy; feeding problems including abdominal distention, vomiting, and diarrhea; temperature instability; respiratory distress or apnea; and jaundice. Nuchal rigidity and Kernig and Brudzinski signs are frequently not present in the neonate with meningitis.

152. The answer is b. (*Hay et al, pp 25-26. Kliegman et al, pp 699-701. Rudolph et al, pp 63, 68, 118-119.*) Twin-to-twin transfusions occur in about 15% of monochorionic twins and commonly cause intrauterine death. This disorder should be suspected when the hematocrits of twins differ by more than 15 mg/dL. The donor twin is likely to have oligohydramnios, anemia, and hypovolemia with evidence of shock if the hematocrit is significantly reduced; the recipient twin is likely to have hydramnios and plethora and to be larger than the donor twin. A 20% difference in body weight may result. As the central venous hematocrit rises above 65%, infants can develop hyperviscosity, respiratory distress, hyperbilirubinemia, hypocalcemia, renal vein thrombosis, congestive heart failure, and convulsions.

153. The answer is b. (*Hay et al, pp 32-34. Kliegman et al, p 681. McMillan et al, pp 200-201. Rudolph et al, pp 82, 99, 105, 168, 207.*) There is loss of body weight of 1.5% to 2% per day for the first 5 days of life for a normal newborn infant as excessive fluid is excreted. One might think this would tend to cause hemoconcentration and produce an increase in hematocrit, but, to the contrary, the hematocrit falls as an adaptation to an environment of higher oxygen. Infants usually have several meconium stools during the first day or two of life, changing to soft yellow stools after 1 to 2 days of life. As the hematocrit falls, there is a corresponding increase in serum bilirubin that peaks around 3 to 5 days of life. Temperature should not change; temperature instability in a term infant is frequently a sign of serious infection.

154. The answer is c. *(Hay et al, pp 46, 1044. Kliegman et al, pp 685-686. McMillan et al, pp 191-192, 373 1850. Rudolph et al, pp 78, 191, 1639.)* It is generally presumed that duodenal atresia and tracheoesophageal fistula lead to hydramnios (polyhydramnios) by interference with reabsorption of swallowed amniotic fluid. Hydramnios is also associated with approximately 80% of infants who have trisomy 18. Approximately 50% of women with anencephalic fetuses have polyhydramnios. Oligohydramnios occurs in association with congenital abnormalities of the fetal kidneys or other parts of the genitourinary tract, such as renal agenesis or obstruction, that impede normal formation or excretion of fetal urine.

155. The answer is b. *(Hay et al, pp 49-58. Kliegman et al, pp 794-811. McMillan et al, pp 482-492. Rudolph et al, pp 86, 106-107.)* Although hypothyroid neonates may develop hyperbilirubinemia, the patient described most likely has a congenital or acquired infection requiring immediate diagnosis and, if possible, treatment. Among the important causes of neonatal sepsis are prenatal infections, including congenital syphilis, toxoplasmosis, cytomegalic inclusion disease, and rubella. Useful diagnostic studies, in addition to cultures for bacteria, include specific serologic tests for pathogens, viral cultures, lumbar puncture, and x-rays of the chest and long bones. Longitudinal striations in the metaphyses are characteristic of congenital rubella, whereas osteochondritis or periostitis usually indicates congenital syphilis. Congenital syphilis, cytomegalovirus, and rubella can be highly contagious. Urine can contain rubella virus for more than 6 months and is, therefore, a special hazard to nonimmune pregnant women.

156-159. The answers are 156-c, 157-e, 158-a, 159-d. *(Hay et al, pp 53-55. Kliegman et al, pp 1340, 1361, 1377-1379, 1486-1496. McMillan et al, pp 511-520, 528-532. Rudolph et al, pp 169-173, 1033, 1077-1079, 1147.)*

Congenital rubella infection affects all organ systems. Infants will be small, with intrauterine growth retardation. They may also manifest cataracts, microphthalmia, myocarditis, and a red or purple macular rash ("blueberry muffin" rash). Structural heart defects (such as a patent ductus arteriosis, pulmonary artery stenosis, and septal defects) are typical of congenital rubella, but not in the other TORCH infections. Laboratory anomalies may include a hemolytic anemia with thrombocytopenia, elevated liver functions, and pleocytosis in the spinal fluid. Affected children do not have a good prognosis. Congenital rubella is not commonly seen in developed countries with high immunization rates.

Transmission of HSV from mother to newborn can happen *in utero*, intrapartum, and postnatally. Intrapartum transmission is most common. Infants born vaginally to a mother with a primary genital herpes infection are at highest risk for disease, with up to 50% risk of perinatal transmission. About half the infants of congenital HSV are born to mothers who are unaware of their infection. Infants can display isolated CNS involvement, isolated cutaneous infection, or systemic generalized infection. Treatment usually is with acyclovir; even with therapy, morbidity is high in infants with CNS involvement.

Toxoplasmosis can cause symptoms similar to other congenital infections, but the combination of hydrocephalus, chorioretinitis, and intracranial calcifications are considered the "classic triad" of toxoplasma infection in a neonate. Infection usually occurs during primary infection of the mother or as a reactivation of infection in an immune-compromised host. These infants may also display symptoms similar to other congenital infections, such as anemia, a petechial rash, organomegaly, jaundice, and seizures.

Congenital cytomegalovirus is the most common sort of congenital infection, with infection estimates ranging from 0.4% to 2.4% of all live births. Many cases are asymptomatic; others may develop cytomegalic inclusion disease, a multiorgan manifestation of disease including intrauterine growth restriction (IUGR), hepatosplenomegaly, jaundice, petechiae or purpura, microcephaly, chorioretinitis, and intracranial calcifications. More than half of infants with this congenital infection develop sensorineural hearing loss.

160-163. The answers are 160-i, 161-f, 162-e, 163-d. *(Hay, pp 23, 506-507, 536, 1106-1108, 1044. Kliegman et al, pp 721, 726, 750-752, 1773-1777, 1783-1784. McMillan et al, pp 212, 313-314, 699-700, 1391-1394, 2492. Rudolph et al, pp 89, 148-151, 186, 191, 1984-1985.)* Infants with upper brachial plexus injury (cervical nerves 3, 4, 5) can also have ipsilateral phrenic nerve paralysis. These infants can present with labored, irregular breathings and cyanosis; the injury is usually unilateral. Confirmation of the diagnosis is made with ultrasound or fluoroscopy which confirms "seesaw" movements during respiration of the two sides of the diaphragm.

Pneumothorax occurs with a frequency of about 1% to 2% of births, but they are rarely symptomatic. Incidence is higher in infants born with meconium-stained fluid, and the chest radiograph is as that described. Transillumination may assist in the diagnosis while awaiting radiograph; immediate treatment for infants with significant distress is with a 23-guage butterfly needle attached to a stopcock and removal of the air. For those without significant distress and who are not on high levels of ambient oxygen, 100% oxygen therapy can assist in nitrogen washout.

Primary pulmonary hypoplasia (Potter sequence) includes a dysmorphic child (widely spaced eyes, low set ears, broad nose, receding chin, limb abnormalities) and bilateral renal agenesis, which leads to oligohydramnios. These infants have immediate respiratory distress; the condition is not compatible with life.

Bronchiolitis is a very common viral infection most often caused by respiratory syncytial virus. It is most often seen in the winter months with symptoms of wheezing, hypoxia, and respiratory distress seen in younger children; often an older sibling has milder, upper respiratory symptoms. Premature infants, infants with congenital heart disease, infants with a variety of lung disorders, and infants with immune system defects are at higher risk of severe complications. Diagnosis is made by clinical history and/or detection of the viral antigen in nasal secretions; treatment is supportive.

164-167. The answers are 164-a, 165-a, 166-c, 167-b. *(Hay et al, pp 996-997. McMillan et al, pp 2126-2127, 2153-2154, 2171-2172, 2187-2188. Rudolph et al, pp 609-611, 626, 640-641, 1486, 2065-2070.)* In galactosemia, an enzyme deficiency (galactose-l-phosphate uridyl transferase) results in a block in the metabolic pathway of galactose and leads to the accumulation of galactose-l-phosphate in the tissues. Infants with this condition develop serious damage to liver, brain, and eyes after being fed milk containing lactose (a disaccharide compound of glucose and galactose). Clinical manifestations include lethargy, vomiting and diarrhea, hypotonia, hepatomegaly and jaundice, failure to thrive, and cataracts. The course of the disease in untreated patients is variable; death from liver failure and inanition can occur; most untreated patients develop physical and mental retardation. Treatment consists of prompt elimination of lactose-containing milk from the diet in infancy and, as a more varied diet is introduced, exclusion of foods that contain casein, dry milk solids, whey, or curds.

Phenylketonuria, a genetically determined disorder with an autosomal recessive pattern of inheritance, is caused by the absence of an enzyme that metabolizes phenylalanine to tyrosine. The resultant accumulation of phenylalanine and its metabolites in the blood leads to severe mental retardation in untreated patients. Treatment consists of a diet that maintains phenylalanine at levels low enough to prevent brain damage but adequate to support normal physical and mental development. Careful supervision of the low-phenylalanine diet and monitoring of blood levels are necessary. Special formulas are available for the infant; older children have difficulty following the diet. It is not clear when and if the diet can be discontinued.

Biotinidase is the enzyme responsible for breakdown of biocytin (the lysyl precursor of biotin) to free biotin. Deficiency of the enzyme, which is inherited as an autosomal recessive trait, results in malfunctioning of the biotin-dependent mitochondrial enzymes and in organic acidemia. Clinical problems related to the deficiency appear several months or years after birth and include dermatitis, alopecia, ataxia, hypotonia, seizures, developmental delay, deafness, immunodeficiency, and metabolic acidosis. The treatment is lifelong administration of free biotin.

The treatment of congenital hypothyroidism with oral levothyroxine sodium should begin as early as possible to prevent psychomotor retardation. Periodic measurement of T3, T4, and TSH is necessary to assess the response to therapy and the need for adjustment of the dose of thyroxine. Careful evaluation of somatic growth by plotting sequential measurements and monitoring bone age is essential.

168-171. The answers are 168-c, 169-a, 170-b, 171-b. (*Hay et al, pp 435, 474, 750-751, 903-905. Kliegman et al, pp 2140-2143, 2484-2487 2621. McMillan et al, pp 1775-1777, 2385-2387, 2659-2660. Rudolph et al, pp 770-772, 1185, 1614-1616, 2347-2348.*) Aniridia is found in 1% to 2% of children with Wilms tumor. Genitourinary anomalies are found in 4% to 5%, and hemihypertrophy is associated with this tumor in 2% to 3% of patients. Wilms tumor is the most common primary renal malignancy in childhood. Presentation is usually an abdominal mass, sometimes with hypertension, hematuria, abdominal pain, and fever. Prognosis is generally good.

Waardenburg syndrome is inherited as an autosomal dominant trait with variable penetrance. It includes, in decreasing order of frequency, the following anomalies: lateral displacement of the medial canthi, broad nasal bridge, medial hyperplasia of the eyebrows, partial albinism commonly expressed by a white forelock or heterochromia (or both), and deafness in 20% of cases. A flat capillary vascular malformation in the distribution of the trigeminal nerve is the basic lesion in the Sturge-Weber syndrome. The malformation also involves the meninges and results in atrophy to the underlying cerebral cortex. The damage is manifested clinically by grand mal seizures, mental deficiency, and hemiparesis or hemianopsia on the contralateral side. The cause is unknown.

Infants who have tuberous sclerosis are often born with hypopigmented oval or irregularly shaped skin macules (ash leaf). Cerebral sclerotic tubers also present from birth and become visible radiographically by the third to fourth year of life. Myoclonic seizures, present in infancy, can convert to grand mal seizures later in childhood. Adenoma sebaceum appears at 4 to 7 years of age. The disease, which also affects the eyes, kidneys, heart, bones, and lungs, is inherited as an autosomal dominant trait with variable expression; new mutations are very common.

172-174. The answers are 172-e, 173-c, 174-a. *(Hay et al, pp 5, 23, 39-41, 63, 428. Kliegman et al, pp 171-178, 405, 714-717. McMillan et al, pp 150-152, 197, 271-276. Rudolph et al, pp 144, 186-187, 2242.)* A subgaleal or subaponeurotic hemorrhage can be life threatening; infants may lose a third or more of their blood volume into this potential space, leading to hypovolemic shock. A subgaleal hemorrhage will feel like a cephalohematoma that crosses the midline. Careful monitoring is essential.

Subdural hematomas are commonly seen as part of the shaken baby syndrome. This lesion occurs when the bridging cortical veins that drain the cerebral cortex have been ruptured, leading to a collection of blood between the dura and the cerebral mantle. Repeated trauma can lead to additional collections of blood. In many children, additional findings of abuse such as broken bones, bruises, and retinal hemorrhages are found.

Caput succedaneum is soft-tissue swelling of the scalp involving the presenting delivery portion of the head. This lesion is sometimes ecchymotic and can extend across the suture lines. The edema resolves in the first few days of life.

Intraventricular hemorrhage (IVH) is commonly seen in very small, preterm infants. The incidence of IVH increases with smaller-size infants and in those with perinatal complications. It occurs in the gelatinous subependymal germinal matrix of the brain and can lead to progressive posthemorrhagic hydrocephalus. Hydrocephalus in these children can present with enlarging head circumference, apnea and bradycardia, lethargy, bulging fontanelle, widely split sutures, or no signs at all. Therapy can include ventricular-peritoneal shunting.

Cephalohematomas do not cross the suture line, since they are subperiosteal hemorrhages. No discoloration of the scalp is seen, and the swelling usually progresses over the first few hours of life. Occasionally, skull fractures are present as well. Most cephalhematomas resolve within the first few weeks or months of life without residual findings.

The Cardiovascular System

Questions

175. A 14-year-old girl, angry at her mother for taking away her MP3 player, takes an unknown quantity of a friend's pills. Within the first hour she is sleepy, but in the emergency center she develops a widened QRS complex on her electrocardiogram (ECG), hypotension, and right bundle branch block. The therapy you would initiate for this ingestion is which of the following?

a. *N*-acetylcysteine (Mucomyst)
b. Naloxone
c. Intensive care unit (ICU) admission, close monitoring, and possible Fab antibody fragments
d. Ethanol
e. Deferoxamine

176. A 10-year-old boy, the star pitcher for the Salt Lake City Little League baseball team, had a sore throat about 2 weeks ago but did not tell anyone because he was afraid he would miss the play-offs. Since several children have been diagnosed with rheumatic fever in the area, his mother is worried that he may be at risk as well. You tell her that several criteria must be met to make the diagnosis but the most common finding is which of the following?

a. Carditis
b. Arthralgia
c. Erythema marginatum
d. Chorea
e. Subcutaneous nodules

177. You are seeing a 2-year-old boy for the first time. His father denies any past medical or surgical history, but does note that the child's day care recently sent a note home asking about several episodes, usually after the child does not get what he wants, when he "breathes funny" and sits in a corner with his knees under his chin for a few minutes. The day-care staffers think this "self-imposed time-out" is a good thing, but they worry about the breathing. One teacher even thought he once looked blue, but decided that it was probably because of the finger paints he had been using. On examination, you identify a right ventricular impulse, a systolic thrill along the left sternal border, and a harsh systolic murmur (loudest at the left sternal border but radiating through the lung fields). His chest radiograph and ECG are shown. Which of the following congenital cardiac lesions would you expect to find in this child?

a. Patent ductus arteriosus
b. Right ventricular outflow obstruction
c. Atrial septal defect (ASD)
d. Transposition of the great vessels with a patent foramen ovale
e. Hypoplastic left heart

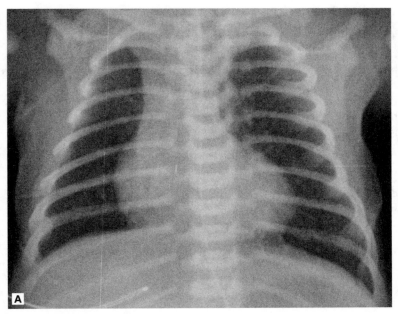

(Courtesy of Susan John, MD.)

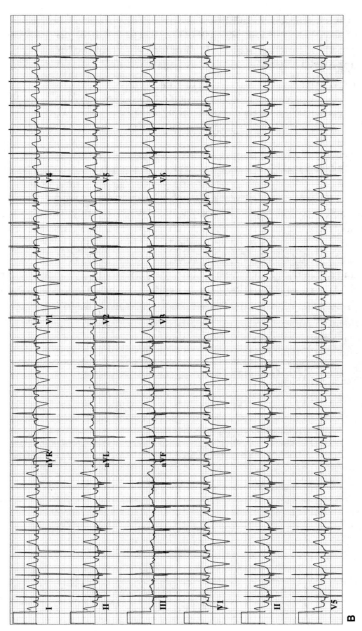

B

(Courtesy of Steven Lorch, MD.)

178. The parents of a 2-month-old baby boy are concerned about his risk of coronary artery disease because of the recent death of his 40-year-old maternal uncle from a myocardial infarction. Which of the following is the most appropriate management in this situation?

a. Screen the parents for total cholesterol.
b. Counsel the parents regarding appropriate dietary practices for a 2-month-old infant and test him for total cholesterol at 6 months of age.
c. Reduce the infant's dietary fat to less than 30% of his calories by giving him skim milk.
d. Initiate lipid-lowering agents.
e. Recommend yearly ECGs for the patient.

179. For the past year, a 12-year-old boy has had recurrent episodes of swelling of his hands and feet, which has been getting worse recently. These episodes occur following exercise and emotional stress, last for 2 to 3 days, and resolve spontaneously. The last episode was accompanied by abdominal pain, vomiting, and diarrhea. The results of routine laboratory workup are normal. An older sister and a maternal uncle have had similar episodes, but they were not given a diagnosis. He presents today with another episode as shown in the photographs on the next page. Which of the following is the most likely diagnosis?

a. Systemic lupus erythematosus
b. Focal glomerulosclerosis
c. Congenital nephrotic syndrome
d. Hereditary angioedema
e. Henoch-Schönlein purpura

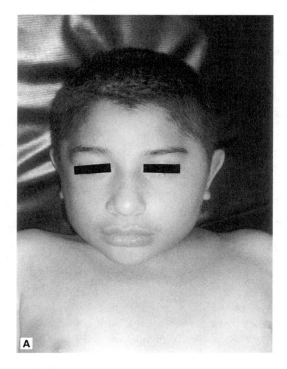

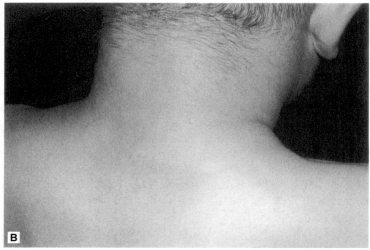

(Courtesy of Adelaide Hebert, MD.)

180. A 15-year-old girl with short stature, neck webbing, and sexual infantilism is found to have coarctation of the aorta. A chromosomal analysis likely would demonstrate which of the following?

a. Mutation at chromosome 15q21.1
b. Trisomy 21
c. XO karyotype
d. Defect at chromosome 4p16
e. Normal chromosome analysis

181. A newborn is diagnosed with congenital heart disease. You counsel the family that the incidence of heart disease in future children is which of the following?

a. 1%
b. 2% to 6%
c. 8% to 10%
d. 15% to 20%
e. 25% to 30%

182. During a regular checkup of an 8-year-old child, you note a loud first heart sound with a fixed and widely split second heart sound at the upper left sternal border that does not change with respirations. The patient is otherwise active and healthy. Which of the following heart lesions most likely explains these findings?

a. Atrial septal defect (ASD)
b. Ventricular septal defect (VSD)
c. Isolated tricuspid regurgitation
d. Tetralogy of Fallot
e. Mitral valve prolapse

183. A 2-year-old boy is brought into the emergency room with a complaint of fever for 6 days and the development of a limp. On examination, he is found to have an erythematous macular exanthem over his body as shown in image A, ocular conjunctivitis, dry and cracked lips, a red throat, and cervical lymphadenopathy. There is a grade 2/6 vibratory systolic ejection murmur at the lower left sternal border. A white blood cell (WBC) count and differential show predominant neutrophils with increased platelets on smear. Later, he develops the findings as seen in image B. Which of the following is the most likely diagnosis?

a. Scarlet fever
b. Rheumatic fever
c. Kawasaki disease
d. Juvenile rheumatoid arthritis
e. Infectious mononucleosis

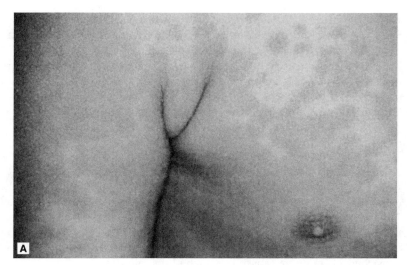

(Reproduced with permission from Wolff K, Johnson RA, Suurmond D. Fitzpatick's Color Atlas & Synopsis of Clinical Dermatology. 5th ed. New York, NY: McGraw-Hill; 2005.)

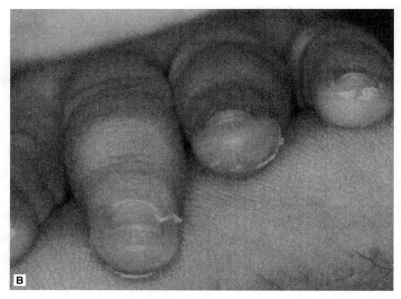

(Reproduced with permission from Wolff K, Goldsmith LA, Katz SI, et al. Fitzpatick's Dermatology in General Medicine. 7th ed. New York, NY: McGraw-Hill; 2007.)

184. An ill-appearing 2-week-old baby girl is brought to the emergency room. She is pale and dyspneic with a respiratory rate of 80 breaths per minute. Heart rate is 195 beats per minute, heart sounds are distant, a gallop is heard, and she has cardiomegaly on x-ray. An echocardiogram demonstrates poor ventricular function, dilated ventricles, and dilation of the left atrium. An ECG shows ventricular depolarization complexes that have low voltage. Which of the following is the most likely diagnosis based on this clinical picture?

a. Myocarditis
b. Endocardial fibroelastosis
c. Pericarditis
d. Aberrant left coronary artery arising from pulmonary artery
e. Glycogen storage disease of the heart

185. A newborn infant has mild cyanosis, diaphoresis, poor peripheral pulses, hepatomegaly, and cardiomegaly. Respiratory rate is 60 breaths per minute, and heart rate is 250 beats per minute. The child most likely has congestive heart failure caused by which of the following?

a. Large ASD and valvular pulmonic stenosis
b. VSD and transposition of the great vessels
c. Total anomalous pulmonary venous return
d. Hypoplastic left heart syndrome
e. Paroxysmal atrial tachycardia

186. A 3-month-old infant is brought to your office for pallor and listlessness. Your physical examination reveals tachycardia that is constant and does not vary with crying. He has no hepatomegaly and the lungs are clear. His ECG is shown. Which of the following is the most appropriate initial management of this patient?

a. Rapid verapamil infusion
b. Transthoracic pacing of the heart
c. Carotid massage
d. DC cardioversion
e. Precordial thump

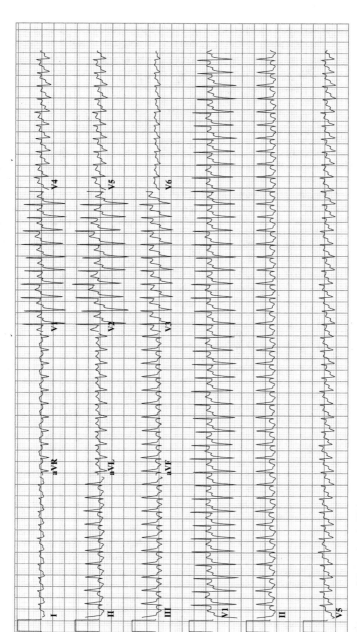

121

187. A 2-year-old child with minimal cyanosis has an S_3 and S_4 (a quadruple rhythm), a systolic murmur in the pulmonic area, and a middiastolic murmur along the lower left sternal border. An ECG shows right atrial hypertrophy and a ventricular block pattern in the right chest leads. Which of the following is the most likely diagnosis?

a. Tricuspid regurgitation and pulmonic stenosis
b. Pulmonic stenosis and a VSD (tetralogy of Fallot)
c. Atrioventricular canal
d. Ebstein anomaly
e. Wolff-Parkinson-White syndrome

188. A 4-year-old girl is brought to the pediatrician's office. Her father reports that she suddenly became pale and stopped running while he had been playfully chasing her and her pet Chihuahua. After 30 minutes, she was no longer pale and wanted to resume the game. She has never had a previous episode and has never been cyanotic. Her physical examination was normal, as were her chest x-ray and echocardiogram. An ECG showed the pattern seen on the next page, which indicates which of the following?

a. Paroxysmal ventricular tachycardia
b. Paroxysmal supraventricular tachycardia
c. Wolff-Parkinson-White syndrome
d. Stokes-Adams pattern
e. Excessive stress during play

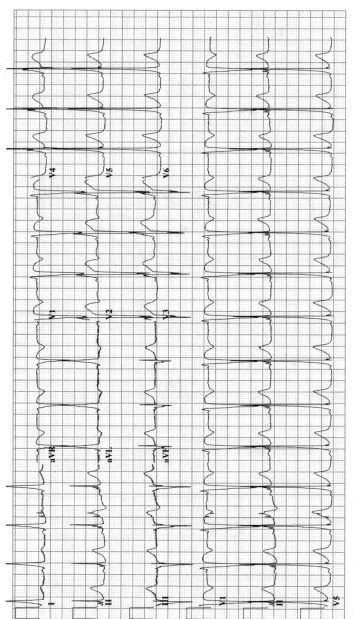

123

189. A child has a 2-week history of spiking fevers, which have been as high as 40°C (104°F). She has spindle-shaped swelling of finger joints and complains of upper sternal pain. When she has fever, the parents note a faint salmon-colored rash that resolves with the resolution of the fever. She has had no conjunctivitis or mucositis, but her heart sounds are muffled and she has increased pulsus paradoxus. Which of the following is the most likely diagnosis?

a. Rheumatic fever
b. Juvenile rheumatoid arthritis
c. Toxic synovitis
d. Septic arthritis
e. Osteoarthritis

190. A cyanotic newborn is suspected of having congenital heart disease. He has an increased left ventricular impulse and a holosystolic murmur along the left sternal border. The ECG shows left-axis deviation and left ventricular hypertrophy (LVH). Which of the following is the most likely diagnosis?

a. Transposition of the great arteries
b. Truncus arteriosus
c. Tricuspid atresia
d. Tetralogy of Fallot
e. Persistent fetal circulation

191. A 3-day-old infant with a single second heart sound has had progressively deepening cyanosis since birth but no respiratory distress. Chest radiography demonstrates no cardiomegaly and normal pulmonary vasculature. An ECG shows an axis of 120° and right ventricular prominence. Which of the following congenital cardiac malformations is most likely responsible for the cyanosis?

a. Tetralogy of Fallot
b. Transposition of the great vessels
c. Tricuspid atresia
d. Pulmonary atresia with intact ventricular septum
e. Total anomalous pulmonary venous return below the diaphragm

192. During a physical examination for participation in a sport, a 16-year-old girl is noted to have a late apical systolic murmur, which is preceded by a click. The rest of the cardiac examination is normal. She states that her mother also has some type of heart "murmur" but knows nothing else about it. Which of the following is the most likely diagnosis?

a. ASD
b. Aortic stenosis
c. Tricuspid regurgitation
d. Mitral valve prolapse
e. VSD

193. A previously normal newborn infant in a community hospital nursery is noted to be cyanotic at 14 hours of life. She is placed on a face mask with oxygen flowing at 10 L/min. She remains cyanotic, and her pulse oximetry reading does not change. An arterial blood gas shows her PaO_2 to be 23 mm Hg. Bilateral breath sounds are present, and she has no murmur. She is breathing deeply and quickly, but she is not retracting. While you are waiting for the transport team from the nearby children's hospital, you should initiate which of the following?

a. Indomethacin infusion
b. Saline infusion
c. Adenosine infusion
d. Prostaglandin E_1 infusion
e. Digoxin infusion

Questions 194 to 196

For each case presented, select the cardiovascular defect with which the examination findings are most likely to be associated. Each lettered option may be used once, more than once, or not at all.

a. Coarctation of the aorta
b. ASD
c. Mitral valve prolapse
d. Pulmonic stenosis
e. Patent ductus arteriosis

194. An infant in the neonatal intensive care unit (NICU) has shortened lower distal arms but with thumbs. Her platelet count is profoundly low.

195. A 15-year-old boy comes to your office for a Special Olympics sports physical. His height is in the 3rd to 5th percentile and his weight is in the 50th percentile. Physical examination reveals a young man with shieldlike chest, cryptorchidism, low-set and malformed ears, ptosis, and pectus excavatum.

196. A new patient to your practice, a happy 10-year-old girl has a history of hyperextensible skin and easy bruising. She often has sprains and joint dislocations when she exercises.

Questions 197 to 200

For each of the cases presented below, choose the most likely cardiac diagnosis based on the patient's presentation. Each lettered option may be used once, more than once, or not at all.

a. Congenital heart block
b. Hypertrophic cardiomyopathy
c. Prolonged QT syndrome
d. Congestive heart failure
e. Cor pulmonale

197. A 15-year-old adolescent male presents to the office for a sports physical. In his screening questionnaire, he notes that he occasionally gets short of breath and dizzy during exercise, with occasional chest pain. He lost consciousness once last summer during football practice, but attributed it to the heat. His grandfather died suddenly at the age of 35 of unknown etiology, but otherwise the family is healthy.

198. A 15-year-old adolescent female comes to be evaluated for syncopal episodes. Her only other medical problem is congenital deafness. She notes through a signing interpreter that syncopal episodes happen during stressful or emotional situations and that they started only within the past year or so. Her mother and father are from the same small farming town and are second cousins.

199. You are called to the nursery to evaluate a newborn. The mother has a history of systemic lupus erythematosus and gestational diabetes. The nurses are concerned because the baby has developed petechiae and bruising after his bath. Vital signs have been stable, with a heart rate in the 60 beats per minute range and a respiratory rate in the 40 breaths per minute range. You note a large liver, scattered petechiae, and an erythematous rash on the cheeks and on the bridge of the nose.

200. An infant previously diagnosed with a large muscular VSD comes to the office with complaints from the mother of fatigue and poor feeding over the past month. You note the child has not gained weight since the previous visit 2 months ago. The child is apathetic, tachypneic, and has wheezes and crackles on lung auscultation.

The Cardiovascular System

Answers

175. The answer is c. *(Hay et al, pp 339, 346-347, 349-352. Kleigman et al, pp 345-351. McMillan et al, pp 749, 751-754, 759-764. Rudolph et al, pp 360-361, 364-365, 367-368, 371.)* The clinical presentation is that of a tricyclic antidepressant ingestion. In smaller children the central nervous system (CNS) symptoms of drowsiness, lethargy, coma, and seizures are more commonly seen than the cardiac effects of tachycardia, initial hypertension followed by hypotension, and a variety of cardiac effects such as widening of the QRS complex and bundle branch blocks which are often seen in adolescents. Close monitoring in the ICU and tricyclic antidepressant Fab antibody fragments (if available) are administered.

Acetaminophen ingestion results initially in nausea, vomiting, and diaphoresis. These early symptoms often resolve in about 24 to 48 hours progressing to right upper quadrant abdominal pain and liver function enzyme elevation. By 2 to 3 days after the ingestion the peak liver function abnormalities are noted and by 4 days to about 2 weeks either recovery of liver function is noted or complete liver failure ensues. Therapy is with N-acetylcysteine. Narcotic ingestions result in respiratory depression as a major symptom during an acute ingestion as described; naloxone (repeated doses may be necessary) is the therapeutic choice. Ethanol is used to compete with methanol (not a pill); methanol ingestion causes mild inebriation, visual disturbances, nausea and vomiting, drowsiness, and profound acidosis. Iron overdose (treated with deferoxamine) leads to early nausea, vomiting, diarrhea, abdominal pain, bloody stools, hypotension, and ultimately gastric scarring.

176. The answer is b. *(Hay et al, pp 580-582. Kleigman et al, pp 1141-1145. McMillan et al, pp 1662-1669. Rudolph et al, pp 1901-1904.)* The diagnosis of rheumatic fever can be difficult because no single clinical manifestation or laboratory test is confirmatory. However, an accurate diagnosis must be made since treatment of the acute problems promptly and effectively is required and long-term antibiotic prophylaxis to prevent recurrences must be instituted.

To assist in diagnosis, the American Heart Association identified a set of major and minor standards relating to the manifestations of the disease, called the *Jones criteria* (modified), and recommends these criteria be applied in the diagnosis of every patient with possible rheumatic fever. The major criteria are carditis, arthritis, erythema marginatum, chorea, and subcutaneous nodules. The minor criteria are arthralgia (joint pain with no objective findings), fever or history of rheumatic fever, increased erythrocyte sedimentation rate (ESR), positive C-reactive protein, increased WBC and anemia, and prolonged PR and QT intervals on ECG. To make the diagnosis of rheumatic fever, the following criteria should be met: two major manifestations, one major and two minor manifestations plus strong evidence of a preceding group A β-hemolytic streptococcal infection (culture, rapid antigen-antibody rise, or elevation), or scarlet fever.

177. The answer is b. (*Hay et al, pp 570-572. Kleigman et al, pp 1906-1911. McMillan et al, pp 1547-1549. Rudolph et al, pp 1820-1823.*) This child has tetralogy of Fallot, which consists of right ventricular outflow obstruction (pulmonary stenosis), VSD, dextroposition of the aorta, and right ventricular hypertrophy. The radiograph shows the typical "boot-shaped" heart, while the ECG demonstrates the increased right ventricular forces. Children with tetralogy of Fallot may have cyanotic episodes ("tet spells") associated with acute reduction in pulmonary blood flow. Typically, these spells are self-limited, lasting no more than 30 minutes. Assuming the knee-chest position is thought to increase peripheral resistance, decreasing the amount of right-to-left shunting and thus increasing pulmonary blood flow. Alternative therapies include morphine sulfate and propranolol. Prolonged hypoxia can lead to acidosis; correction may require infusion of sodium bicarbonate.

Patent ductus arteriosus is likely to present in this aged child with a constant, machine-like murmur, and if the flow is big enough, with evidence of progressive congestive heart failure. An ASD will have a fixed split-second heart sound and a pulmonic stenosis murmur; it can also present with progressive evidence of heart failure if the flow across the ASD is large enough. Transposition of the great vessels with a patent foramen ovale and hypoplastic left heart syndrome are neonatal conditions; presentations are in the newborn period.

178. The answer is a. (*Hay et al, p 233. Kleigman et al, p 585. McMillan et al, p 2194. Rudolph et al, pp 696-698.*) Identification of those with a genetic predisposition to hypercholesterolemia and of the factors that increase the risk of the condition is recommended so that dietary and other measures to reduce serum lipids can be introduced if indicated. Children with a first- or second-degree relative with early onset of coronary heart disease should be evaluated early in life but after 2 years of age. Other known risk factors include obesity, diabetes, hypertension, and smoking. No change in current infant dietary practice is recommended for children under 2 years of age. The high total fat content of the infant diet is considered to be biologically sound, given the need for lipid for a developing nervous system and the infant's limited capacity for an intake of high volume during this period of rapid growth. It is generally agreed that a dietary fat intake of 40% of calories is excessive over the age of 2 years. There is, however, concern about the potential loss of minerals such as iron, zinc, and calcium when dietary fat is reduced below 30% of calories in children 2 to 18 years of age. Principal sources of fat in the American diet are meat and milk, which are also sources of minerals such as iron and calcium. Simple modifications in the current US diet of children of these ages (trimming excess fat from meat and drinking 1% fat milk) would effect a reduction of fat intake by 5% of calories without the risk of lowering mineral intake. It would be helpful in this situation to determine whether the uncle had hypercholesterolemia. Yearly ECGs and lipid-lowering agents are not indicated in this situation.

179. The answer is d. *(Hay et al, p 931. Kleigman et al, pp 979-982. McMillan et al, pp 2413-2416. Rudolph et al, p 1196.)* The picture shows edema around the neck. This condition often worsens in adolescents. Although hereditary angioedema is relatively rare as a cause of edema, the recurrent episodes in late childhood, the normal laboratory results, and the family history make the other choices less likely. Hereditary angioedema, transmitted as an autosomal dominant trait, is a result of inadequate function (owing to either deficient quantity or quality) of an inhibitor of the first step in the complement cascade, which results in the excessive production of a vasoactive kinin. In addition to otherwise asymptomatic subcutaneous edema, edema can occur in the gastrointestinal tract and produce the symptoms mentioned in the question. Laryngeal edema with airway obstruction can also occur.

180. The answer is c. *(Hay et al, pp 569, 1032. Kleigman et al, pp 2386-2389. McMillan et al, p 2635-2336. Rudolph et al, pp 2087-2089.)* Short stature, neck webbing, sexual infantilism, and a shieldlike chest with widely spaced nipples are signs of Turner syndrome, which is usually associated with an XO karyotype. Aortic coarctation occurs in about 15% to 20% of those with this disorder. Down syndrome is most commonly associated with endocardial cushion defects or VSD. Marfan syndrome (mutation 15q21.1) is associated with dilatation of the aorta and mitral and aortic regurgitation. Ellis-van Creveld syndrome (defect 4p16) is associated with ASD.

181. The answer is b. *(Kleigman et al, pp 1878-1881. McMillan et al, pp 335-338. Rudolph et al, p 1781.)* The incidence of congenital heart disease in the population is about 1%. The risk of congenital heart disease in a family with one child born with heart disease varies depending on the type of lesion the first child had but, overall, the rate averages from about 2% to 6% if the heart disease is not associated with a diagnosable syndrome. The risk of congenital heart disease for an infant is increased if there is a history of congenital heart disease in the mother. If two children with congenital heart disease are diagnosed, the risk escalates to 20% to 30%.

182. The answer is a. *(Kleigman et al, pp 1883-1885. McMillan et al, pp 287, 1329-1332, 1346-1350, 1354-1357, 1378-1380. Rudolph et al, pp 1788-1794, 1797-1798, 1820-1823.)* Most children with an ASD are asymptomatic; the lesion is found during a routine examination. In older children, exercise intolerance can be noted if the lesion is of significant size. On examination, the pulses are normal, a right ventricular systolic lift at the left sternal border is palpable, and a fixed splitting of the second heart sound is audible. For lesser degrees of ASD, surgical treatment is more controversial.

VSD commonly present as a harsh or blowing holosystolic murmur best heard along the left lower sternum, often with radiation throughout the precordium. Tricuspid regurgitation is a middiastolic rumble at the lower left sternal border; a history of birth asphyxia or findings of other cardiac lesions often is present. Tetralogy of Fallot is a common form of congenital heart disease. The four abnormalities include right ventricular outflow obstruction, VSD, dextroposition of the aorta, and right ventricular hypertrophy; the cyanosis presents in infants and in young children. Mitral valve prolapse occurs with the billowing into the atria of one or both mitral valve leaflets at the end of systole. It is a congenital abnormality that frequently manifests only during adolescence or later. It is more common in girls than in boys and seems to be inherited in an autosomal dominant fashion. On clinical examination, an apical murmur is noted late in systole, which can be preceded by a midsystolic click. The diagnosis is confirmed with an echocardiogram that shows prolapse of the mitral leaflets during mid to late systole.

183. The answer is c. *(Hay et al, pp 582-583. Kleigman et al, pp 1036-1042. McMillan et al, pp 1015-1023. Rudolph et al, pp 844-845.)* Many conditions can be associated with prolonged fever, a limp caused by arthralgia, exanthem, adenopathy, and pharyngitis. Conjunctivitis, however, is suggestive of Kawasaki disease. The fissured lips, although common in Kawasaki disease, could occur after a long period of fever from any cause if the child became dehydrated. The predominance of neutrophils and high ESR are common to all. An increase in platelets within this constellation of symptoms, however, is found typically in Kawasaki disease. Kawasaki disease presents as a picture of prolonged fever, rash, epidermal peeling on the hands and feet (especially around the fingertips), conjunctivitis, lymphadenopathy, fissured lips, oropharyngeal mucosal erythema, and arthralgia or arthritis. The diagnosis is still possible in the absence of one or two of these physical findings. Coronary artery aneurysms can develop, as can aneurysms in other areas. Initial treatment is typically intravenous immunoglobulin (IVIG) and high-dose aspirin. The child will usually defervesce shortly after the infusion. Aspirin is typically kept at a higher dose until the platelet count begins to decrease, and then is continued at a lower dose for several weeks. While bacterial infection is in the differential diagnosis for this patient's presentation and blood cultures are usually part of the evaluation, IV vancomycin should be reserved for a culture-proven susceptible organism resistant to other antibiotics, or as empiric therapy in a critically ill patient.

184. The answer is a. *(Hay et al, pp 587-588. Kleigman et al, pp 1970-1971. McMillan et al, pp 1614-1624. Rudolph et al, pp 1860-1861.)* The findings of pallor, dyspnea, tachypnea, tachycardia, and cardiomegaly are common in congestive heart failure regardless of the cause. The most common causes of myocarditis include adenovirus and coxsackievirus B, although many other viruses can cause this condition. The constellation of findings in the question point to myocarditis as the etiology of this patient's condition.

The echocardiogram in the question shows ventricular and left atrial dilatation as well as poor ventricular function. With glycogen storage disease of the heart muscle thickening would be expected and with pericarditis a pericardial effusion would be seen. The echocardiogram findings in this case are not consistent with an aberrant origin of the left coronary artery, although the origin of the coronary arteries can be difficult to visualize. On ECG, the voltages of the ventricular complexes seen with aberrant origin of the left coronary artery are not diminished, and a pattern of myocardial infarction can be seen. Voltages from the left ventricle are usually high in endocardial fibroelastosis, and both right and left ventricular forces are high in glycogen storage disease of the heart.

185. The answer is e. (*Hay et al, pp 597-600. Kleigman et al, pp 1945-1947. McMillan et al, pp 1679-1681. Rudolph et al, pp 1854-1856.*) Congestive heart failure from any cause can result in mild cyanosis, even in the absence of a right-to-left shunt, and in poor peripheral pulses when cardiac output is low. Congestive heart failure from many causes can be associated with a rapid pulse rate (up to 200 beats per minute). A pulse rate greater than 250 beats per minute, however, should suggest the presence of a tachyarrhythmia. Common causes for supraventricular tachycardia include Wolff-Parkinson-White (WPW) syndrome, congenital heart disease, and sympathomimetic drugs. In this patient, evaluation for WPW syndrome and cardiac abnormalities must be accomplished after the congestive heart failure from the increased heart rate is under control.

186. The answer is c. (*Hay et al, pp 597-600. Kleigman et al, pp 1945-1947. McMillan et al, pp 1679-1681. Rudolph et al, pp 1854-1856.*) Supraventricular tachycardia, as shown on the ECG, is characterized by rapid heart rate (in this case about 250 beats per minute), little rate variability, and a consistent P wave for each QRS complex. Prolonged SVT can lead to heart failure with hepatomegaly and respiratory compromise. Fetal SVT can lead to hydrops fetalis. The first-line treatment is to stimulate the vagus nerve using techniques such as carotid massage, immersion of the face in cold water, or voluntary straining. Rapid infusion of IV adenosine can affect resolution if the maneuvers are not successful. Verapamil is contraindicated in this age group, as it may cause acute hypotension and cardiac arrest. Synchronized DC cardioversion may be performed in patients in shock or with heart failure; it must, however, be synchronized to the QRS complex. Transthoracic pacing is typically useful in bradyarrhythmias. A precordial thump might help individuals with an acute arrest from ventricular fibrillation, but does not resolve SVT.

187. The answer is d. (*Hay et al, pp 563-564. Kleigman et al, pp 1915-1918. Rudolph et al, pp 1817-1818.*) A quadruple rhythm associated with the murmur of tricuspid regurgitation and a middiastolic murmur at the lower left sternum suggests the diagnosis of Ebstein anomaly (downward displacement of the tricuspid valve). The presence of right atrial hypertrophy and right ventricular conduction defects confirms the diagnosis. Both tricuspid regurgitation with pulmonic stenosis and tetralogy of Fallot give ECG evidence of right ventricular enlargement. The WPW syndrome, which frequently accompanies Ebstein malformation, is not associated with murmurs or cyanosis as an isolated entity, but also includes supraventricular tachycardia.

188. The answer is c. (*Hay et al, p 598. Kleigman et al, p 1945-1947. McMillan et al, p 1677. Rudolph et al, pp 1452-1453.*) The child described in the question has no cyanosis or murmur, no cardiac or pulmonary vascular abnormalities by chest x-ray, and no evidence of structural anomalies by echocardiogram, and therefore is unlikely to have an underlying gross anatomic defect. The ECG pattern in the figure shows the configuration of preexcitation, the pattern seen in the WPW syndrome. These patients have an aberrant atrioventricular conduction pathway, which causes the early ventricular depolarization appearing on the ECG as a shortened PR interval. The initial slow ventricular depolarization wave is referred to as the *delta wave.* Seventy percent of patients with WPW syndrome have single or repeated episodes of paroxysmal supraventricular tachycardia, which can cause the symptoms described in the question. The preexcitation ECG pattern and WPW syndrome can occur in Ebstein malformation, but this is unlikely in the absence of cyanosis and with a normal echocardiogram. If ventricular tachycardia were present, the symptoms would likely be more profound. Active play and exposure to over-the-counter medications containing sympathomimetics in a healthy 4-year-old child can cause symptoms such as those described in the question in children with WPW syndrome by precipitating paroxysmal supraventricular tachycardia.

189. The answer is b. (*Hay et al, pp 822-824. Kleigman et al, pp 1001-1010. McMillan et al, pp 2538-2543. Rudolph et al, pp 836-839.*) Juvenile rheumatoid arthritis (JRA, or Still disease) frequently causes spindle-shaped swelling of finger joints and can involve unusual joints such as the sternoclavicular joint. Presentation of JRA occurs as either polyarthritis (five or more joints, systemic symptoms not so severe or persistent), pauciarticular (four or fewer joints, lower-extremity joints, extra-articular disease unusual), or systemic disease (severe constitutional disease, systemic symptoms prior to arthritis, rheumatoid rash, high spiking fevers, variable joint involvement). This disorder can be associated with spiking high fevers and diffuse rash, which are not a feature of rheumatic fever, toxic synovitis, or osteoarthritis. Although septic arthritis can affect any joint, it would not be likely to affect finger joints by causing spindle-shaped swellings. Toxic synovitis usually involves larger joints, such as the hip, and osteoarthritis is not a disease of childhood.

190. The answer is c. (*Hay et al, pp 573-574. Kleigman et al, pp 1913-1915. McMillan et al, pp 1543-1546. Rudolph et al, pp 1816-1817.*) Patients with tricuspid atresia typically have a hypoplastic right ventricle, and therefore the ECG shows left-axis deviation and left ventricular hypertrophy; this translates to a left ventricular impulse on physical examination. Almost all other forms of cyanotic congenital heart disease are associated with elevated pressures in the right ventricle and increased right ventricular impulse. In those conditions, therefore, the ECG will show right-axis deviation and right ventricular hypertrophy.

191. The answer is b. (*Hay et al, pp 575-577. Kleigman et al, pp 1918-1922. McMillan et al, pp 1537-1539. Rudolph et al, pp 1823-1826.*) Transposition of the great vessels with an intact ventricular septum presents with early cyanosis, a normal-sized heart (classic "egg on a string" radiographic pattern in one-third of cases), normal or slightly increased pulmonary vascular markings, and an ECG showing right-axis deviation and right ventricular hypertrophy. In tetralogy of Fallot, cyanosis is often not seen in the first few days of life. Tricuspid atresia, a cause of early cyanosis, causes diminished pulmonary arterial blood flow; the pulmonary fields on x-ray demonstrate a diminution of pulmonary vascularity, and left-axis and left ventricular hypertrophy are shown by ECG. Total anomalous pulmonary venous return below the diaphragm is associated with obstruction to pulmonary venous return and a classic radiographic finding of marked, fluffy-appearing venous congestion ("snowman"). In pulmonic atresia with an intact ventricular septum, cyanosis appears early, the lung markings are normal to diminished, and the heart is large.

192. The answer is d. (*Hay et al, pp 567-568. Kleigman et al, p 1905. McMillan et al, pp 1603-1605. Rudolph et al, pp 1797-1798.*) Mitral valve prolapse occurs with the billowing into the atria of one or both mitral valve leaflets at the end of systole. It is a congenital abnormality that frequently manifests only during adolescence or later. It is more common in girls than in boys and seems to be inherited in an autosomal dominant fashion. On clinical examination, an apical murmur is noted late in systole, which can be preceded by a click. The diagnosis is confirmed with an echocardiogram that shows prolapse of the mitral leaflets during mid to late systole. The ECG and chest x-ray are usually normal. β-Blockers and digitalis are unlikely to be required, and penicillin prophylaxis for dental procedures for patients with mitral valve prolapse is no longer recommended by the American Heart Association.

193. The answer is d. *(Hay et al, pp 572-573, 575-577. Kleigman et al, pp 1912-1913, 1915. McMillan et al, p 355. Rudolph et al, pp 1818-1820.)* The vignette describes an infant with a ductal-dependant cyanotic congenital heart lesion. In this example, the child had pulmonary atresia without a corresponding VSD; another example would have been transposition of the great vessels without a septal defect to allow mixing of oxygenated and nonoxygenated blood. Cyanotic infants who do not improve their saturations with supplemental oxygen should be evaluated carefully for structural heart disease. The ductus arteriosis typically closes in the first few hours of life; thus, these children will develop their cyanosis in the same time frame. Prostaglandin E_1 will help keep the ductus patent until a surgical procedure can be performed. PGE_1 does have the tendency to cause hypoventilation, so arrangements must be made for a potential artificial airway if necessary. Indomethacin closes a patent ductus arteriosis. Adenosine is used for supraventricular tachycardia.

194 to 196. The answers are 194-b, 195-d, 196-c. *(Hay et al, pp 567-568, 861, 871-872. Kleigman et al, pp 514, 2085, 2717-1718. McMillan et al, pp 2645, 2650, 2656. Rudolph et al, pp 738, 764-768, 2089.)* Thrombocytopenia-absent radius syndrome (TAR) is diagnosed in the newborn who demonstrates profound thrombocytopenia, bilateral absence of radius, and abnormally shaped thumbs. Cardiac lesions include TOF and ASD. About 40% of patients die in the newborn period as a result of low-platelet-induced bleeding.

Noonan syndrome, the "male Turner syndrome," occurs in both sexes. The most common features include short stature, downslanting palpebral fissures, ptosis, low set and malformed ears, webbed neck, shieldlike chest, pulmonic stenosis, and cryptorchidism. Mental retardation is seen in one-forth of affected individuals. It is associated with advanced paternal age.

Mitral valve prolapse is seen in patients with Ehlers-Danlos syndrome. Patients with Ehlers-Danlos syndrome have hyperextensibility and easy bruising, joint hypermobility (leading to joint dislocations and sprains), skin that is velvety to touch, and tissue fragility. Six different kinds are described with "classic" and "hypermobility" forms predominating.

197 to 200. The answers are 197-b, 198-c, 199-a, 200-d. *(Hay et al, pp 556-558, 585-586. Kleigman et al, pp 1019, 1888-1891, 1967-1969, 2477. McMillan et al, pp 466-467, 1575-1578, 1638-1641, 1681-1682. Rudolph et al, pp 847, 1858, 1860-1862, 1869-1877.)* Hypertrophic cardiomyopathy (HCM), also called idiopathic hypertrophic subaortic stenosis, is often inherited in autosomal dominant fashion with variable penetrance. Many children are completely asymptomatic, while others may have complaints of weakness, fatigue, chest pain, and syncope. A midsystolic ejection murmur and a left ventricular lift sometimes can be appreciated on physical examination. The diagnosis is confirmed by echocardiography. HCM can be a cause of arrhythmia and death in young athletes.

Prolonged QT syndrome occurs in 1:10,000 to 1:15,000 children, usually first causing syncopal episodes in late childhood or adolescence. During the syncope episode arrhythmias may be noted, including ventricular fibrillation. These episodes may result in death. QT intervals are elongated on ECG. An autosomal recessive form associated with deafness (Jervell-Lange-Nielsen syndrome) and an autosomal dominant form (Romano-Ward syndrome) has been described.

Neonatal lupus is a rare manifestation of transferred maternal IgG autoantibodies. Infants can have thrombocytopenia, neutropenia, rash, liver dysfunction, and a congenital heart block. Most manifestations are self-resolved; however, the congenital heart block is permanent and frequently requires pacing.

Congestive heart failure can result from a number of causes, including congenital heart disease, Kawasaki disease, metabolic cardiomyopathies, arrhythmias, and viral myocarditis. The case presented is typical of an infant with heart failure. Such infants are weak, diaphoretic, have poor weight gain, and may be tachypneic with retractions. Lung findings can include crackles, wheezes, or both. Prompt evaluation by a pediatric cardiologist is imperative.

The Respiratory System

Questions

201. You are asked to evaluate an infant born vaginally 3 hours previously to a mother whose only pregnancy complication was poorly controlled gestational diabetes. The nursing staff noticed that the infant was breathing abnormally. On examination, you find that the infant is cyanotic, has irregular, labored breathing, and has decreased breath sounds on the right side. You also note decreased tone in the right arm. You provide oxygen and order a stat portable chest radiograph, which is normal. Which of the following studies is most likely to confirm your diagnosis?

a. Nasal wash for viral culture
b. Fiberoptic bronchoscopy
c. Chest CT
d. Chest ultrasound
e. Induced sputum culture

202. A 10-month-old infant has poor weight gain, a persistent cough, and a history of several bouts of pneumonitis. The mother describes the child as having very large, foul-smelling stools for months. Which of the following diagnostic maneuvers is likely to result in the correct diagnosis of this child?

a. CT of the chest
b. Serum immunoglobulins
c. TB skin test
d. Inspiratory and expiratory chest x-ray
e. Sweat chloride test

203. A previously well 1-year-old infant has had a runny nose and has been sneezing and coughing for 2 days. Two other members of the family had similar symptoms. Four hours ago, his cough became much worse. On physical examination, he is in moderate respiratory distress with nasal flaring, hyperexpansion of the chest, and easily audible wheezing without rales. His chest radiographs are shown. Which of the following is the appropriate next course of action?

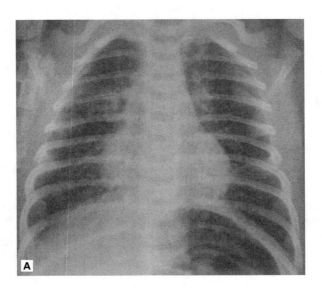

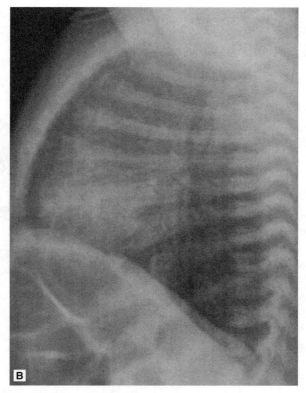

(Courtesy of Susan John, MD.)

a. Monitoring oxygenation and fluid status alone
b. Inhaled epinephrine and a single dose of steroids
c. Acute-acting bronchodilators and a short course of oral steroids
d. Emergent intubation and antibiotics
e. Chest tube placement

204. A 6-year-old girl presents with a 2-day history of cough and fever. At your office she has a temperature of 39.4°C (103°F), a respiratory rate of 45 breaths per minute, and decreased breath sounds on the left side. Her chest x-ray is shown below. Which of the following is the most appropriate initial treatment?

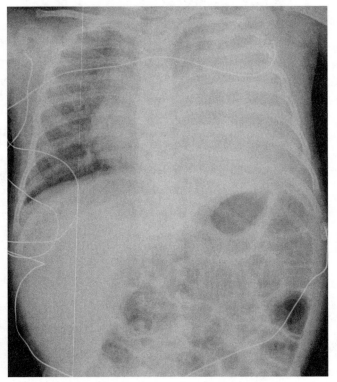

(Courtesy of Susan John, MD.)

a. *N*-acetylcysteine chest physiotherapy
b. Vancomycin
c. Partial lobectomy
d. Postural drainage
e. Placement of tuberculosis skin test

205. A 2-year-old girl is playing in the garage with her Chihuahua, only partially supervised by her father, who is weed-whacking around the garden gnomes in the front yard. He finds her in the garage, gagging and vomiting. She smells of gasoline. In a few minutes she stops vomiting, but later that day she develops cough, tachypnea, and subcostal retractions. She is brought to your emergency center. Which of the following is the most appropriate first step in management?

a. Administer charcoal
b. Begin nasogastric lavage
c. Administer ipecac
d. Perform pulse oximetry and arterial blood gas
e. Administer gasoline-binding agent intravenously

206. A 3-year-old girl is admitted with the x-ray shown below. The child lives with her parents and a 6-week-old brother. Her grandfather stayed with the family for 2 months before his return to the West Indies 1 month ago. The grandfather had a 3-month history of weight loss, fever, and hemoptysis. Appropriate management of this problem includes which of the following?

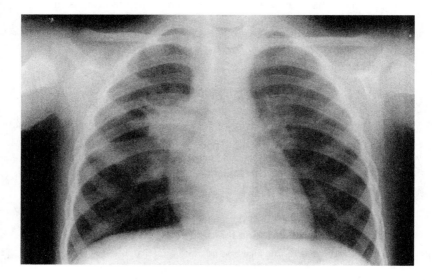

a. Bronchoscopy and culture of washings for all family members
b. Placement of a Mantoux test on the 6-week-old sibling
c. Isolating the 3-year-old patient for 1 month
d. Treating the 3-year-old patient with isoniazid (INH) and rifampin
e. HIV testing for all family members

207. You are asked to evaluate a 4-year-old boy admitted to your local children's hospital with a diagnosis of pneumonia. The parents state that the child has had multiple, intermittent episodes of fever and respiratory difficulty over the past 2 years, including cyanosis, wheezing, and dyspnea; each episode lasts for about 3 days. During each event he has a small amount of hemoptysis, is diagnosed with left lower lobe pneumonia, and improves upon treatment. Repeat radiographs done several days after each event are reportedly normal. His examination on the current admission is significant for findings similar to those described above, as well as digital clubbing. Which of the following is the most appropriate primary recommendation?

a. Intravenous cephalosporin and oral macrolide therapy
b. Modified barium swallow study to evaluate for aspiration
c. Nasal swab for viral culture
d. Incentive spirometry
e. Bronchoalveolar lavage

208. A previously healthy, active, 18-month-old African American child presents with unilateral nasal obstruction and foul-smelling discharge. The child's examination is otherwise unremarkable. Which of the following is the most likely diagnosis?

a. Foreign body
b. Nasal polyps
c. Frontal sinusitis
d. Deviated septum
e. Choanal atresia

209. A 7-year-old child is brought by his mother for a school physical. His growth parameters show his height to be 50th percentile and his weight to be significantly higher than 95th percentile. His mother complains that he always seems sleepy during the day and that he has started complaining of headaches. His second-grade teacher has commented that he has difficulty staying awake in class. His mother complains that he wakes up the whole house with his snoring at night. Which of the following is the most appropriate next step in evaluating and managing this condition?

a. Try steroids to decrease tonsillar and adenoid hypertrophy.
b. Refer to an otolaryngologist for tonsillectomy and adenoidectomy.
c. Arrange for continuous positive airway pressure (CPAP) at home.
d. Arrange for home oxygen therapy for use at night.
e. Arrange for polysomnography.

210. You admitted to the hospital the previous evening a 1-year-old boy who presented with cough, fever, and mild hypoxia. At the time of his admission, he had evidence of a right upper lobe consolidation on his chest radiograph. A blood culture has become positive in less than 24 hours for *Staphylococcus aureus*. Approximately 20 hours into his hospitalization, the nurse calls you because the child has acutely worsened over the previous few minutes, with markedly increased work in breathing, increasing oxygen requirement, and hypotension. As you move swiftly to the child's hospital room, you tell the nurse to order which of the following?

a. A second chest radiograph to evaluate for pneumatocele formation
b. A large-bore needle and chest tube kit for aspiration of a probable tension pneumothorax
c. A change in antibiotics to include gentamicin
d. A sedative to treat the child's attack of severe anxiety
e. A thoracentesis kit to drain his probable pleural effusion

211. A fully immunized 2-year-old presents to the emergency room with several days of low-grade fever, barking cough, and noisy breathing. Over the past few hours he has developed a fever of 40°C (104°F) and looks toxic. He has inspiratory and expiratory stridor. The family has not noticed drooling, and he seems to be drinking without pain. Direct laryngoscopy reveals a normal epiglottis. The management of this disease process includes which of the following?

a. Intubation and intravenous antibiotics
b. Inhaled epinephrine and oral steroids
c. Inhaled steroids
d. Observation in a cool mist tent
e. Oral antibiotics and outpatient follow-up

212. A 6-year-old, fully immunized boy is brought to the emergency room with a 3-hour history of fever to 39.5°C (103.1°F) and sore throat. The child appears alert, but anxious and toxic. He has mild inspiratory stridor and is drooling. He is sitting on the examination table leaning forward with his neck extended. A lateral radiograph of his neck is shown below. Which of the following is the most appropriate immediate management of this patient?

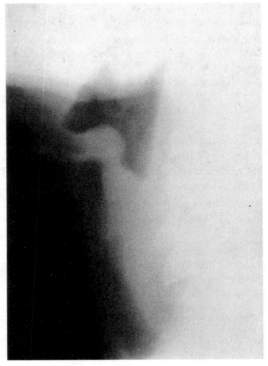

(Courtesy of Susan John, MD.)

a. Examine the throat and obtain a culture.
b. Obtain an arterial blood gas and start an IV line.
c. Administer a dose of nebulized epinephrine.
d. Prepare to establish an airway in the operating room.
e. Admit the child and place him in a mist tent.

213. A 4-year-old boy was admitted to the hospital last night with the complaint of "difficulty breathing." He has no past history of lung infection, no recent travel, and no day-care exposure; he does, however, have an annoying tendency to eat dirt. In the emergency center he was noted to be wheezing and to have hepatomegaly. He is able to talk, relaying his concern about his 6-week-old Chihuahua being left alone at home. Laboratory studies revealed marked eosinophilia (60% eosinophils). Which of the following tests is most likely to produce a specific diagnosis?

a. Tuberculin skin test
b. Histoplasmin test
c. ELISA for *Toxocara*
d. Silver stain of gastric aspirate
e. Stool examination for ova and parasites

214. A 10-year-old girl has had a "cold" for 14 days. In the 2 days prior to the visit to your office, she has developed a fever of 39°C (102.2°F), purulent nasal discharge, facial pain, and a daytime cough. Examination of the nose after topical decongestants shows pus in the middle meatus. Which of the following is the most likely diagnosis?

a. Brain abscess
b. Maxillary sinusitis
c. Streptococcal throat infection
d. Sphenoid sinusitis
e. Middle-ear infection

215. You are awakened in the night by your 2-year-old son, who has developed noisy breathing on inspiration, marked retractions of the chest wall, flaring of the nostrils, and a barking cough. He has had a mild upper respiratory infection (URI) for 2 days. Which of the following therapies is indicated?

a. Short-acting bronchodilators and a 5-day course of steroids
b. Intubation and antibiotics
c. Observation for hypoxia and dehydration alone
d. Inhaled epinephrine and a dose of steroids
e. Rigid bronchoscopy

216. An 8-year-old girl presents with well-controlled, moderately persistent asthma. Her therapies consist of occasional use of short-acting β-agonists, daily inhaled steroids, and a leukotriene inhibitor. She presents with white patches on her buccal mucosa. You recommend which of the following?

a. HIV testing
b. Tuberculosis skin testing
c. Measurement of serum immunoglobulins
d. Discontinuation of all her asthma medications
e. Rinse her mouth after use of her inhaled medications

217. A 13-year-old develops fever, malaise, sore throat, and a dry, hacking cough over several days. He does not appear to be particularly sick, but his chest examination is significant for diffuse rales and rhonchi. The chest radiograph is shown below. Which of the following is the most likely pathogen?

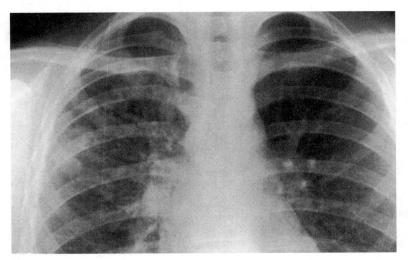

(Courtesy of Susan John, MD.)

a. *Staphylococcus aureus*
b. *Mycobacterium tuberculosis*
c. *Haemophilus influenzae*
d. *Streptococcus pneumoniae*
e. *Mycoplasma pneumoniae*

218. You have just given a 10-year-old boy an injection of pollen extract as prescribed by his allergist. You are about to move on to the next patient when the boy starts to complain about nausea and a funny feeling in his chest. You note that his face is flushed and his voice sounds muffled and strained. Which of the following is the first priority in managing this episode of anaphylaxis?

a. Preparation for endotracheal intubation
b. Intramuscular injection of diphenhydramine
c. Administration of oxygen
d. Subcutaneous injection of 1:1000 epinephrine
e. Administration of corticosteroids

219. A previously healthy 18-month-old has been in a separate room from his family. The family notices the sudden onset of coughing, which resolves in a few minutes. Subsequently, the patient appears to be normal except for increased amounts of drooling and refusal to take foods orally. Which of the following is the most likely explanation for this toddler's condition?

a. Severe gastroesophageal reflux
b. Foreign body in the airway
c. Croup
d. Epiglottitis
e. Foreign body in the esophagus

220. You receive a telephone call from the mother of a 4-year-old child with sickle-cell anemia. She tells you that the child is breathing fast, coughing, and has a temperature of 40°C (104°F). Which of the following is the most conservative, prudent course of action?

a. Prescribe aspirin and ask her to call back if the fever does not respond.
b. Make an office appointment for the next available opening.
c. Make an office appointment for the next day.
d. Refer the child to the laboratory for an immediate hematocrit, white blood cell count, and differential.
e. Admit the child to the hospital.

221. You are asked by a colleague to evaluate a 5-year-old boy as a second opinion. He has a history of chronic and recurrent upper respiratory tract infections, several admissions to the hospital for pneumonia, and three surgeries for PE tubes for chronic otitis media. Of note is a right-sided heart on repeated radiographs. Convinced you know the diagnosis based on history alone, you confirm your diagnosis with a biopsy of the nasal mucosa. You expect to find which of the following?

a. Eosinophilic infiltrate
b. *Bordetella pertussis*
c. Absence of nasal mucous glands
d. Random orientation of cilia
e. Nasal polyps

222. A 13-year-old patient with sickle-cell anemia presents with respiratory distress; she has an infiltrate on chest radiograph. The laboratory workup of the patient reveals the following: hemoglobin 5 g/dL; hematocrit 16%; white blood cell count 30,000/μL; and arterial blood (room air) pH 7.1, Po$_2$ 35 mm Hg, and Paco$_2$ 28 mm Hg. These values indicate which of the following?

a. Acidemia, metabolic acidosis, respiratory alkalosis, and hypoxia
b. Alkalemia, respiratory acidosis, metabolic alkalosis, and hypoxia
c. Acidosis with compensatory hypoventilation
d. Long-term metabolic compensation for respiratory alkalosis
e. Primary respiratory alkalosis

223. A 24-year-old woman arrives in the emergency center in active labor. She is at term, but received no prenatal care after 16 weeks of gestation when she lost her insurance coverage. The mother has an uncomplicated vaginal delivery. You are paged shortly after birth when the baby is noted to have respiratory distress. The infant has diminished breath sounds on the left, and the PMI is shifted toward the right. A chest radiograph is shown. The NG tube you placed earlier reveals the stomach to be below the diaphragm. Which of the following is the most likely diagnosis at this point?

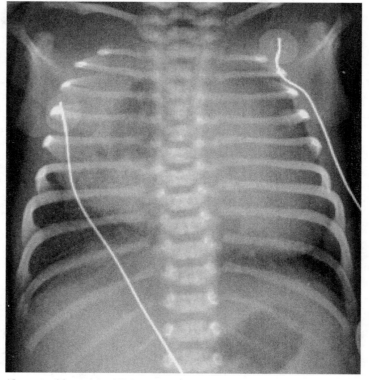

(Courtesy of Susan John, MD.)

a. Congenital cystic adenomatoid malformation
b. Congenital diaphragmatic hernia
c. Bronchogenic cysts
d. Congenital lobar emphysema
e. Congenital pneumonia

224. A 13-year-old boy has a 3-day history of low-grade fever, symptoms of upper respiratory infection, and a sore throat. A few hours before his presentation to the emergency room, he has an abrupt onset of high fever, difficulty swallowing, and poor handling of his secretions. He indicates that he has a marked worsening in the severity of his sore throat. His pharynx has a fluctuant bulge in the posterior wall. A soft tissue radiograph of his neck is shown. Which of the following is the most appropriate initial therapy for this patient?

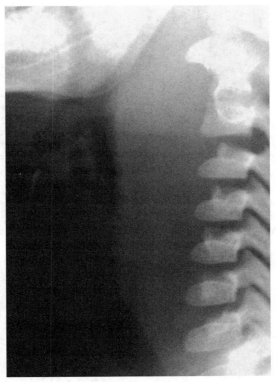

(Courtesy of Susan John, MD.)

a. Narcotic analgesics
b. Trial of oral penicillin V
c. Surgical consultation for incision and drainage under general anesthesia
d. Rapid streptococcal screen
e. Monospot test

225. A 6-week-old child arrives with a complaint of "breathing fast" and a cough. On examination you note the child to have no temperature elevation, a respiratory rate of 65 breaths per minute, and her oxygen saturation to be 94%. Physical examination also is significant for rales and rhonchi. The past medical history for the child is positive for an eye discharge at 3 weeks of age, which was treated with a topical antibiotic drug. Which of the following organisms is the most likely cause of this child's condition?

a. *Neisseria gonorrhoeae*
b. *Staphylococcus aureus*
c. Group B streptococcus
d. *Chlamydia trachomatis*
e. Herpesvirus

226. One of your asthmatic patients arrives for a checkup. The mother reports that the child seems to need albuterol daily, especially when exercising, and she has coughing fits that awaken her from sleep about twice a week. Her grandmother had recommended a Chihuahua as a "cure" for her asthma, but her mother has seen no difference since the arrival of the pet. Appropriate treatment measures would include which of the following?

a. Short-acting, inhaled β-agonists, as needed
b. Daily leukotriene modifier with short-acting β-agonist
c. Inhaled nedocromil with short-acting β-agonists
d. Medium-dose, inhaled corticosteroids with short-acting β-agonists
e. High-dose, inhaled corticosteroids with theophylline and short-acting β-agonists

227. A previously healthy 2-year-old black child has developed a chronic cough during the previous 6 weeks. He has been seen in different emergency rooms on two occasions during this period and has been placed on antibiotics for pneumonia. Upon auscultation, you hear normal breath sounds on the left. On the right side, you hear decreased air movement during inspiration but none upon expiration. Inspiratory (A) and expiratory (B) radiographs of the chest are shown below. Which of the following is the most appropriate next step in making the diagnosis in this patient?

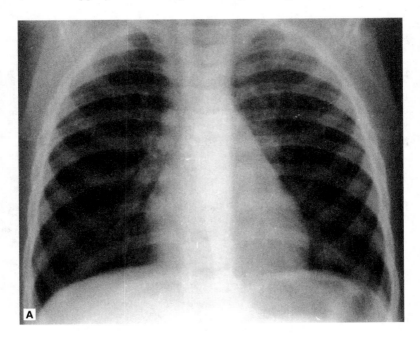

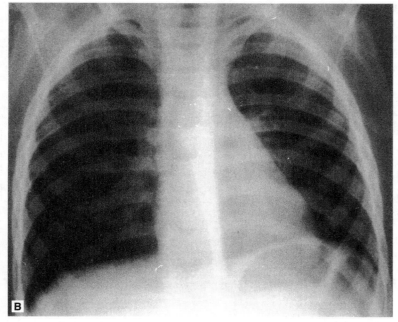

(Courtesy of Susan John, MD.)

a. Measure the patient's sweat chloride.
b. Consult pediatric surgery for bronchoscopy.
c. Prescribe broad-spectrum oral antibiotics.
d. Initiate a trial of inhaled β-agonists.
e. Prescribe appropriate doses of oral prednisone.

Questions 228 to 230

Match each management procedure below with the appropriate set of arterial blood gas results of patients spontaneously breathing room air. Each lettered option may be used once, more than once, or not at all.

Base	PCO_2 (mm Hg)	PO_2 (mm Hg)	Excess pH (mEq/L)
a. 7.20	28	95	16
b. 7.20	70	41	2
c. 7.64	18	94	1
d. 7.34	32	39	8

228. Have patient rebreathe in a paper bag.

229. Administer FIO_2 0.4.

230. Perform thoracentesis to remove air under pressure.

Questions 231 to 234

Match each management procedure below with the appropriate arterial blood gas results of patients spontaneously breathing room air. Each lettered option may be used once, more than once, or not at all.

Base	PCO_2 (mm Hg)	PO_2 (mm Hg)	Excess pH (mEq/L)
a. 6.92	101	19	15
b. 7.36	60	50	7
c. 7.50	46	76	11
d. 7.41	60	90	10

231. Place the patient on a ventilator with an FIO_2 of 1.0.

232. Discontinue diuretics, discontinue base, and increase KCI in IV fluids.

233. Perform tonsillectomy.

234. Repeat the test because of obvious laboratory error.

The Respiratory System

Answers

201. The answer is d. *(Hay et al, pp 22-23. Kliegman et al, pp 720-721. Rudolph et al, p 89.)* Infants born to mothers with gestational diabetes are at risk for being large for their gestational age and thus at increased risk for peripheral nerve injuries such as Erb-Duchenne and phrenic nerve paralysis. An ultrasound or fluoroscopy of the chest would reveal asymmetric diaphragmatic motion in a seesaw manner. With a negative chest radiograph, a chest CT would not be helpful at this point. Bronchoscopy would help delineate airway abnormalities and foreign bodies, but would not identify phrenic nerve paralysis.

202. The answer is e. *(Hay et al, pp 678-681. Kliegman et al, pp 1803-1816. McMillan et al, pp 1425-1437. Rudolph et al, pp 1967-1979.)* Cystic fibrosis (CF) is a multisystem disease caused by an abnormally functioning cystic fibrosis transmembrane regulator (CFTR) protein. Abnormal secretions are produced as a result of decreased permeability of ionized chloride in the secretory epithelium of a number of organs. Progressive lung failure is caused by accumulation of viscid secretions that obstruct the airway and lead to infection, bronchiectasis, and inflammatory changes. Survival has improved markedly during the past few decades as a result of prompt recognition of CF and aggressive treatment; the median age at death has increased from less than 10 years to more than 30 years. Therapeutic approaches have included inhalation therapy, chest physical therapy, aggressive antibiotic administration, bronchodilators, oxygen, and nutritional support. Heart–lung transplants have prolonged life and improved qualify of life for some terminal patients. Several new approaches to the treatment of CF have been proposed, namely, the use of amiloride, purified human plasma α_1-antitrypsin, recombinant DNAase, and gene therapy. The rationale for these therapeutic modalities is that they focus directly on ameliorating or correcting the basic deficit: amiloride by inhibiting sodium, and with it water reabsorption, thereby improving airway hydration; α_1-antitrypsin by counteracting the effects on the lungs of neutrophil elastase, a proteolytic enzyme released by neutrophils; DNAase by reacting with DNA released by dead leukocytes to reduce sputum viscosity; and gene therapy by altering genetic material. Lung cancer does not appear to be associated with cystic fibrosis.

Unlike many other tests, there is almost no overlap in chloride values in sweat between patients with cystic fibrosis and normal control participants. A chloride concentration of greater than 60 mEq/L is diagnostic, values less than 40 are normal, and values between 40 and 60 are intermediate. Genetic studies that assay for about 30 of the most common mutations known to cause CF are available. A number of states have included a test for immunoreactive trypsinogen in their newborn screening programs, and when combined with confirmatory testing, the sensitivity has been reported to be as high as 95%.

Conditions other than cystic fibrosis can manifest an elevated sweat chloride, including adrenal insufficiency, ectodermal dysplasia, nephrogenic diabetes insipidus, hypothyroidism, and malnutrition.

203. The answer is a. (*Hay et al, pp 506-507. Kliegman et al, pp 1773-1777. McMillan et al, pp 699-700, 1391-1394. Rudolph et al, pp 1984-1985.*) Of the choices given and with the findings on the radiograph (patchy infiltrates with flat diaphragms), monitoring oxygenation and hydration status is the most appropriate course of action as bronchiolitis is the most likely diagnosis. Bronchodilators and a short course of steroids are treatments for asthma, a less likely diagnosis in this patient without previous wheezing episodes and without a family history of atopy; a single dose of short-acting β-agonist might be tried in this patient but would be expected to be of limited benefit for a patient with bronchiolitis. Viral croup (a single dose of steroids) and epiglottitis (emergency intubation and antibiotics) are not reasonable choices because there are no signs of extrathoracic airway obstruction. Pneumothorax (chest tube placement) may be required if unilateral breath sounds were present or if the radiograph demonstrated collapse; neither is noted in this case.

The most likely cause of the illness is infection by respiratory syncytial virus, which causes outbreaks of bronchiolitis of varying severity, usually in the winter and spring. Other viruses, such as parainfluenza and the adenoviruses, have also been implicated in producing bronchiolitis. Treatment is generally supportive in this usually self-limited condition.

204. The answer is b. (*Hay et al, pp 517-521. Kliegman et al, pp 1795-1800. McMillan et al, pp 1407-1411. Rudolph et al, pp 1980-1982.*) The x-ray reveals a lung empyema on the left side, characterized by nearly complete white out of that side by the pleural or extrapleural fluid collection. Lung abscesses are usually caused by *S aureus, S pneumoniae, or S pyogenes*. These organisms, previously sensitive to penicillin, now have a variety of resistance patterns requiring extended spectrum antibiotics or vancomycin. Patients who do not improve quickly with antibiotic therapy alone are also surgical candidates.

205. The answer is d. (*Hay et al, p 349. Kliegman et al, pp 1789-1790. McMillan et al, p 753. Rudolph et al, pp 366-367.*) Hydrocarbons with low viscosity and high volatility are the most likely agents to cause respiratory symptoms. Gasoline, kerosene, and furniture polish (which contain hydrocarbons) are common agents responsible for hydrocarbon aspiration. Hydrocarbon aspiration can produce dyspnea, cyanosis, and respiratory failure. Treatment is symptomatic, sometimes requiring intubation and mechanical ventilation. Induction of emesis is contraindicated, as this may cause further aspiration. Placement of a nasogastric tube is used only in high-volume ingestions or when the hydrocarbon is mixed with another toxin. Charcoal is not useful, and no intravenous binding agent is available.

206. The answer is d. (*Hay et al, pp 521-523, 1197-1200. Kliegman et al, pp 1240-1254. McMillan et al, pp 1142-1155. Rudolph et al, pp 949-959.*) The key to controlling tuberculosis in children and eradicating the disease is early detection and appropriate treatment of adult cases; the child, once infected, is at lifelong risk for the development of the disease and for infecting others, unless given appropriate prophylaxis. The usual source of the disease is an infected adult, since smaller children are not infectious because they typically are unable to produce enough intrathoracic pressure with a cough to spread the disease. Household contacts of a person with newly diagnosed active disease have a considerable risk of developing active tuberculosis, and the risk is greatest for infants and children. Therefore, when tuberculosis is diagnosed in a child, the immediate family and close contacts should be tested with tuberculin skin tests and chest radiographs and treated appropriately when indicated. Bronchoscopy would be indicated only in unusual circumstances. Three to eight weeks is required after exposure before hypersensitivity to tuberculin develops. This means that the tuberculin test must be repeated in exposed persons if there is a negative reaction at the time that contact with the source of infection is broken. TB skin tests are usually negative in infants of this age, even when active disease is ongoing. A logical preventive measure is the administration of isoniazid to the 6-week-old baby for 3 months when a Mantoux (purified protein derivative, PPD) can then be placed. Transmission of tuberculosis occurs when bacilli-laden, small-sized droplets are dispersed into the air by the cough or sneeze of an infected adult. Small children with primary pulmonary tuberculosis are not considered infectious to others, and they are not capable of coughing up and producing sputum. Sputum, when produced in child of this age, is promptly swallowed, and for this reason specimens for microbial confirmation can be obtained by means of gastric lavage from smaller children.

In the child described in the case, the chest film is abnormal, suggesting active TB disease. While the medications listed in the answer are part of the treatment for TB disease, they are typically used with several other medications.

207. The answer is e. *(Hay et al, pp 529-530. Kliegman et al, pp 1824-1826. McMillan et al, pp 1438-1440. Rudolph et al, pp 1997-1999.)* This child likely has idiopathic pulmonary hemosiderosis (IPH). While fever, respiratory distress, and localized chest radiograph findings should point initially toward an acute pneumonia, the history of recurrence, the rapid clearing of radiographic findings, and the hemoptysis suggest pulmonary hemorrhage. The examination finding of digital clubbing suggests a chronic process. Other typical findings would include microcytic and hypochromic anemia, low serum iron levels, and occult blood in the stool (from swallowed pulmonary secretions). Bronchoalveolar lavage will reveal hemosiderin-laden macrophages and would be most likely to make the diagnosis. A distinct subset of patients with pulmonary hemosiderosis have hypersensitivity to cow's milk (the association is called Heiner syndrome) and may improve with a diet free of cow's milk products.

208. The answer is a. *(Hay et al, p 481. Kliegman et al, pp 1744-1775. Rudolph et al, p 1265.)* Small children frequently introduce any number of small objects into their noses, ranging from food to small toys. Initially, only local irritation occurs. Later, as prolonged obstruction is seen, symptoms increase to include worsening of pain, and a purulent, malodorous, bloody discharge can be seen. Unilateral nasal discharge in the presence of obstruction suggests the need to examine the patient for a nasal foreign body.

Polyps are a possible cause of unilateral nasal obstruction, but at 18 months of age they are unusual and would suggest a diagnosis of cystic fibrosis. While not impossible, cystic fibrosis is rare in a black child. Frontal sinusitis usually does not cause unilateral symptoms, and sinusitis in an 18-month-old child is rare owing to poor sinus development. Similarly, deviated septum is not found in small children. Choanal atresia would present in the newborn period with periods of respiratory distress at rest with improvement with crying.

209. The answer is e. *(Hay et al, pp 487-489, 536-537. Kliegman et al, pp 94-97. McMillan et al, pp 1441-1443. Rudolph et al, pp 1937-1941.)* A nasopharyngeal airway, the use of nasal CPAP, and tonsillectomy and adenoidectomy can be effective treatments for obstructive sleep apnea (OSA). However, the diagnosis of OSA should first be made by polysomnography (sleep study) to exclude other causes of snoring. Administering oxygen may decrease the respiratory drive in severe OSA, and thus should be used only with caution. Untreated OSA can lead to *cor pulmonale*, as well as growth and developmental abnormalities.

210. The answer is b. *(Hay et al, pp 324, 536. Kliegman et al, pp 1835-1837. McMillan et al, pp 1456-1457. Rudolph et al, pp 149-150, 1981.)* Tension pneumothorax, a recognized complication of staphylococcal (and other) pneumonia is caused by toxin production by the bacteria leading to rupture of the alveoli into the pleural space. Tension pneumothorax can be quickly lethal if not recognized and treated; this makes a high index of suspicion and prompt diagnosis mandatory. The other complications can also occur but do not require so prompt a response. Immediate action to relieve the tension is mandatory, usually accomplished by inserting a needle or catheter into the second or third intercostal spaces in the midclavicular line, with the patient supine.

211. The answer is a. *(Hay et al, p 502. Kliegman et al, pp 1766-1767, McMillan et al, pp 1506-1507, Rudolph et al, p 1944.)* Bacterial tracheitis is an uncommon, but severe and life-threatening sequelae of a viral laryngotracheobronchitis. The typical story is that presented in the case, with several days of viral upper respiratory symptoms, followed by an acute elevation of temperature and an increase in respiratory distress. Inspiratory stridor is typical in croup; the biphasic stridor and high fever in this patient should be a clue to consider alternative diagnoses. Children may also present acutely and without the initial viral symptoms. The differential must include epiglottitis; the lack of drooling and dysphagia (and the rarity of epiglottitis) help make this a case of tracheitis. Management for tracheitis includes establishing an airway with endotracheal intubation and IV antibiotics. Special attention is focused on preservation of the airway, as even intubated children with tracheitis can have secretions thick and copious enough to occlude the airway.

Oral antibiotics and outpatient follow-up for a patient with respiratory distress and toxic appearance is never appropriate. Inhaled epinephrine and oral steroids as well as observation in a cool mist tent suggest a diagnosis of croup, a disease that presents without high fever but with stridor a few days after an upper respiratory infection. In the case presentation, the fever and toxic appearance differentiate this condition from viral croup. Inhaled steroids suggest asthma, a diagnosis unlikely in a patient with high fever as outlined.

212. The answer is d. (*Hay et al, pp 501-502. Kliegman et al, pp 1763-1766. McMillan et al, pp 695-696. Rudolph et al, p 1276.*) In the past, epiglottitis was most commonly caused by invasive *H influenzae* type B. Due to the widespread use of the Hib vaccine, this condition is now more commonly caused by group A β-hemolytic streptococcus, *Moraxella catarrhalis,* or *S pneumoniae*. The radiography shows the typical "thumb" sign of a swollen epiglottis. Epiglottitis is a life-threatening form of infection-produced upper airway obstruction. The course of the illness is brief and prodromal symptoms are lacking. The patient experiences a sudden onset of sore throat, high fever, and prostration that is out of proportion to the duration of the illness. Drooling and difficulty in swallowing, a muffled voice, and preference for a characteristic sitting posture with the neck hyperextended may be noted. Radiography of the neck, which may delay definitive treatment, is often avoided. Rather, preparations are made for immediate intubation by skilled personnel, and any attempt to visualize the epiglottis should be avoided. Morbidity and mortality are usually related to a delay in establishing an airway early in the disease.

213. The answer is c. (*Hay et al, pp 1233-1234. Kliegman et al, pp 1506-1507. McMillan et al, pp 1370-1373. Rudolph et al, pp 1110-1111.*) The presentation described is characteristic of visceral larva migrans from infestation with a common parasite of dogs, *Toxocara canis*. Dirt-eating children ingest the infectious ova. The larvae penetrate the intestine and migrate to visceral sites, such as the liver, lung, and brain, but do not return to the intestine, so the stools do not contain the ova or parasites. The diagnosis can be made by a specific enzyme-linked immunosorbent assay (ELISA) for *Toxocara*.

214. The answer is b. (*Hay et al, pp 476-479. Kliegman et al, pp 1749-1752. McMillan et al, pp 1470-1476. Rudolph et al, pp 1263-1264.*) Maxillary and ethmoid sinuses are large enough to harbor infections from infancy. Frontal sinuses are rarely large enough to harbor infections until the sixth to tenth year of life. Sphenoid sinuses do not become large until about the third to fifth year of life. In general, a "cold" lasting longer than 10 to 14 days with fever and facial pain is indicative of sinusitis. Examination of the nose can reveal pus draining from the middle meatus in maxillary, frontal, or anterior ethmoid sinusitis. Pus in the superior meatus indicates sphenoid or posterior ethmoid sinuses. Diagnosis is on clinical grounds and can be difficult. Positive findings on plain sinus films in a symptomatic child are supportive of sinusitis. CT scans are more sensitive, but are usually reserved for the more complicated cases. The treatment is usually oral antibiotics for 10 to 14 days. Decongestants and antihistamines have not been shown to be helpful or necessary.

Brain abscess is unlikely in this patient who demonstrates no neurologic symptoms. A streptococcal throat infection should present with acute onset of sore throat without other signs and symptoms of upper respiratory infection. Sphenoid sinusitis usually does not cause facial pain or drainage from the middle meatus. The child might have a middle-ear infection simultaneous with a sinusitis, but her lack of ear pain suggests otherwise.

215. The answer is d. (*Hay et al, pp 500-502. Kliegman et al, pp 1762-1766. McMillan et al, pp 694-695, 1505-1508. Rudolph et al, pp 1275-1276.*) The signs of illness described are those involving the airway above the point at which the trachea enters the neck and leaves the thorax, resulting in inspiratory stridor such as in croup. The extrathoracic airway tends to collapse on inspiration, producing the characteristic findings this patient demonstrates; therapy usually is with a single dose of steroids. Agents causing croup include parainfluenza types 1 and 3, influenza A and B, RSV, and occasionally other viruses. Treatment is usually supportive, but racemic epinephrine and corticosteroids reduce the length of time in the emergency room and hospitalizations.

Intrathoracic airway diseases, such as asthma (bronchodilators and short course of steroids) or bronchiolitis (supportive therapy including observation for hypoxia or dehydration alone), produce breathing difficulty on expiration, with expiratory wheezing, prolonged expiration, and signs of air trapping due to the increased narrowing during expiration as the airways are exposed to the same intrathoracic pressure changes as the alveoli.

Acute airway foreign body (rigid bronchoscopy) should result in differential air movement between the two lungs. The typical case of epiglottis (intubation and antibiotics) presents acutely and the child is toxic in appearance; it is now a rare disease with the widespread use of vaccines.

216. The answer is e. (*Hay et al, pp 1049-1060. Kliegman et al, pp 953-970. McMillan et al, pp 2404-2410. Rudolph et al, pp 1956, 1959.*) The patient in the question has well-controlled, moderately persistent asthma; this suggests that she is likely on inhaled steroids. Failure to rinse her mouth after administration of this medication can result in localized candida infection (thrush). Discontinuation of her asthma medications is contraindicated. While it is possible she has an immune dysfunction, simply rinsing her mouth is more likely to be both diagnostic and therapeutic.

217. The answer is e. *(Hay et al, pp 520-521. Kliegman et al, pp 1278-1281. McMillan et al, pp 1395-1400. Rudolph et al, pp 949-959, 965-967, 1980-1982.)* The radiograph shown has reticulonodular opacities in the right upper lobe and prominence of the right hilum (lymphadenopathy) consistent with *M pneumoniae*. Infections with *M pneumoniae* are common in older children and young adults. Although the infection typically produces an interstitial infiltrate, its effects are characteristically nonspecific, and it can produce lobar pneumonia as well. It can produce upper respiratory infection, pharyngitis, otitis media and externa, bronchiolitis, hemolytic anemia, and Guillain-Barré syndrome. Treatment of choice is a macrolide antibiotic.

S aureus traditionally is seen in infants less than 6 months of age; *H influenzae* is rarely seen because of the widespread use of *H influenzae* B vaccine. At this age, a child with *M tuberculosis* presents most typically with hilar adenopathy and localized lobar pneumonia in the upper lobe, and *S pneumoniae* causes the sudden onset of high fever and a lobar pneumonia, often with pleural effusion. A TB skin test for this patient would be reasonable.

218. The answer is a. *(Hay et al, pp 1069-1071. Kliegman et al, pp 983-984. McMillan et al, p 2398. Rudolph et al, pp 821-822.)* Anaphylaxis is a medical emergency that must be recognized and managed promptly. The onset of symptoms is usually dramatic. In the case presented, the change in voice suggests impending airway compromise, making airway stabilization is your top priority. The other choices are all important in managing anaphylaxis and, in reality, may be occurring concurrently; of those listed, subcutaneous epinephrine would be the first medication used. Additional treatment can include plasma expanders, diphenhydramine, and cimetidine, as indicated by the clinical course of the patient. Additional treatment such as administration of corticosteroids should be started early, but the effect will be delayed.

219. The answer is e. *(Hay et al, pp 504-506. Kliegman et al, pp 1769-1770. McMillan et al, pp 693-694. Rudolph et al, pp 1397-1398.)* Many types of objects produce esophageal obstruction in young children, including small toys, coins, and food. Most are lodged below the cricopharyngeal muscle at the level of the aortic arch. Initially, the foreign body may cause a cough, drooling, and choking. Later, pain, avoidance of food (liquids are tolerated better), and shortness of breath can develop. Diagnosis is by history (as outlined in the question) and by radiographs (especially if the object is radiopaque). The usual treatment is removal of the object via esophagoscopy.

Severe gastroesophageal reflux would likely not present with acute findings as those outlined in the question, but rather with ongoing respiratory symptoms (asthma or pneumonia) or failure to thrive. Symptoms of foreign body in the airway may present acutely as described with resolution as the offending object settles in the lung, but the symptoms of failure to drink and to begin drooling would not be expected. Croup causes a barking cough, often at night, several days after an acute upper respiratory infection. Epiglottitis can be diagnosed in a toxic-appearing, febrile child with stridor.

220. The answer is e. (*Hay et al, pp 845-848. Kliegman et al, pp 2026-2031. McMillan et al, pp 1696-1700. Rudolph et al, pp 1531-1534.*) Fever, cough, and tachypnea in a patient with sickle cell anemia can be manifestations of pneumonia, pulmonary thromboemboli, or sepsis. Aside from being relatively common in patients with sickle-cell anemia, these diseases can be rapidly progressive and quickly fatal. It is therefore important for the patient to be evaluated and treated on an emergency basis. The treatment requires hospitalization, because it will almost certainly include systemic antibiotics, intravenous fluids, oxygen, and perhaps blood transfusion.

221. The answer is d. (*Hay et al, p 509. Kliegman et al, pp 1817-1819. McMillan et al, pp 1422-1424. Rudolph et al, p 1949.*) Patients with primary ciliary dyskinesia (immotile cilia syndrome) have dysfunctional cilia and, as such, have abnormal airway clearance. Described structural aberrations include abnormal cytoskeletal proteins and defects in the dynein arms. Kartagener syndrome (the triad of situs inversus, chronic sinusitis and otitis media, and airway disease) is associated with primary ciliary dyskinesia; approximately 50% of patients with the latter also have the former. Although it is a chronic disease, patients with PCD can have a normal life span.

Allergic rhinitis can cause polyps and eosinophilia on a nasal smear, but the story is not an allergic one. *B pertussis* infection is not commonly found in immunized children, but it can be found in adults. Pertussis does not cause the chronic and recurrent findings in the vignette.

222. The answer is a. (*Hay et al, pp 495-496. Kliegman et al, pp 1726-1727. McMillan et al, pp 2582-2587. Rudolph et al, pp 1656-1657.*) The low pH in the arterial blood can be called *acidemia*. In this context, it is likely that the hydrogen ions come from lactic acid produced by anaerobic metabolism in tissues with inadequate oxygen delivery. Inadequate oxygenation is caused by the low PO_2, the low oxygen-carrying capacity of the blood (Hgb 5 g/dL), and circulatory inadequacy due to the sickling itself and to the vascular disease it produces. The low PCO_2 reflects the hyperventilation, which is secondary to the respiratory difficulty, and to the anemia, and is also respiratory compensation for the metabolic acidosis.

223. The answer is a. *(Hay et al, pp 516-517. Kliegman et al, p 1784. McMillan et al, p 1453. Rudolph et al, pp 190, 202.)* Congenital cystic adenomatoid malformation (CCAM) is thought to arise from an embryonic disruption before the thirty-fifth day that causes improper development of bronchioles. The cystic mass is usually identified on prenatal ultrasound around the 20th week. Large lesions (as that noted on the radiograph on the right side) may compress the affected lung and cause pulmonary hypoplasia, which may cause midline shift away from the lesion (note the heart is shifted toward the left on the radiograph). Treatment is typically surgical excision of the affected lobe. Some patients may be at risk for primary pulmonary malignancy.

224. The answer is c. *(Hay et al, p 485. Kliegman et al, pp 1754-1756. McMillan et al, pp 1493-1494. Rudolph et al, p 1944.)* Suppurative infection of the chain of lymph nodes between the posterior pharyngeal wall and the prevertebral fascia leads to retropharyngeal abscesses. The most common causative organisms are *S aureus,* group A β-hemolytic streptococci, and oral anaerobes. Presenting signs and symptoms include a history of pharyngitis, abrupt onset of fever with severe sore throat, refusal of food, drooling, and muffled or noisy breathing. A bulge in the posterior pharyngeal wall is diagnostic, as are radiographs of the lateral neck that reveal the retropharyngeal mass (the radiograph in the question demonstrates thickening of the prevertebral space). Palpation (with adequate provision for emergency control of the airway in case of rupture) reveals a fluctuant mass. Treatment should include incision and drainage if fluctuance is present. All of the wrong answers listed would delay definitive treatment and/or might be life threatening.

225. The answer is d. *(Hay et al, p 520. Kliegman et al, pp 1285-1287. McMillan et al, pp 984-985. Rudolph et al, p 930.)* Chlamydiae organisms, sexually transmitted among adults, are spread to infants during birth from genitally infected mothers. The sites of infection in infants are the conjunctivae and the lungs, where chlamydiae cause inclusion conjunctivitis and afebrile pneumonia, respectively, in infants between 2 and 12 weeks of age. Diagnosis is confirmed by culture of secretions and by antibody titers. In adolescents, chlamydial infections may be a cause of cervicitis, salpingitis, endometritis, and epididymitis and appear to be an important cause of tubal infertility. The most common treatment for this condition includes macrolide antibiotics orally, which clears both the nasopharyngeal secretions when conjunctivitis is present and prevents the pneumonia that can occur later. Topical treatment for chlamydia conjunctivitis is not effective in clearing the nasopharynx. Early treatment with oral macrolides is, however, associated with an increased incidence in the development of idiopathic hypertrophic pyloric stenosis; their use in a neonate is with caution.

N gonorrhoeae can cause a sepsis syndrome in children (and not just respiratory symptoms), but its presentation would be in the first days of life and not at 6 weeks; the child would be toxic. S aureus, and more unusually Group B streptococcus (which more likely would occur in the first days of life), can cause pneumonia in a child of this age, but the presentation would more likely be of a toxic, febrile child. Herpesvirus, when it causes pneumonia, does so more likely in a child in the first days of life; the child is toxic.

226. The answer is d. (*Hay et al, pp 1049-1060. Kliegman et al, pp 953-970. McMillan et al, pp 2404-2410. Rudolph et al, p 1953.*) Asthma may be classified by severity based on the frequency of symptoms. Patients with *mild intermittent* asthma have symptoms less than two times a week and have less than two nighttime episodes a month. These patients do not require daily medication and only short-acting β-agonists are needed. The second classification is *mild persistent* asthma; these children have symptoms more than two times a week, and have 3 to 4 nights a month with symptoms. These patients may be managed with a number of anti-inflammatory choices, including low-dose, inhaled corticosteroids, cromolyn, or a leukotriene inhibitor, and use short-acting β-agonists for rescue. Our patient has *moderate persistent* asthma; she has daily symptoms and difficulty at night more than once a week. Her treatment should consist of medium-dose corticosteroids, or a combination of low-dose corticosteroids and a long-acting β-agonist; alternatives include a leukotriene modifier or sustained release theophylline. Patients with *severe persistent* asthma have continual symptoms and frequent nighttime symptoms. This group requires daily high-dose glucocorticoids as well as long-acting β-agonists; they may require oral steroids as well.

227. The answer is b. *(Hay et al, pp 504-506. Kliegman et al, pp 1769-1770. McMillan et al, pp 693-694. Rudolph et al, pp 1277-1278.)* Recurrent pneumonias in an otherwise healthy child should suggest the potential for anatomic blockage of an airway. In the patient in this question, the findings on clinical examination suggest a foreign body in the airway. Inspiratory and expiratory films can be helpful. Routine inspiratory films are likely to appear normal or near normal (as outlined in the question and noted in the first radiograph). Expiratory films will identify air trapping behind the foreign body (as noted on the second radiograph). It is uncommon for the foreign body to be visible on the plain radiograph; a high index of suspicion is necessary to make the diagnosis. Suspected foreign bodies in the airway are potentially diagnosed with fluoroscopy, but rigid bronchoscopy is not only diagnostic but also the treatment of choice for removal of the foreign body.

228-230. The answers are 228-c, 229-d, 230-b. *(Hay et al, pp 495-496. Kliegman et al, pp 1726-1727. McMillan et al, pp 2582-2587. Rudolph et al, pp 278-284, 1656-1657.)* The laboratory results of row C indicate a striking respiratory alkalosis. This could be secondary to voluntary hyperventilation or inappropriate respirator settings for a patient on a ventilator. The findings are also typical of acute hyperventilation syndrome secondary to anxiety; such a patient can complain of dyspnea, chest pain, tingling, and dizziness, and can even have generalized convulsions secondary to low ionized calcium levels. Rebreathing into a paper bag can be both therapeutic and diagnostic.

The blood gases of row D are the only ones shown that are relatively normal, except for a low-oxygen partial pressure. The mild respiratory alkalosis and metabolic acidosis can be a consequence of the hypoxia. These results could be obtained in a patient with moderately severe pneumonia, bronchiolitis or asthma, or secondary to ventilation-perfusion inequality with some areas of the lung underventilated with respect to perfusion. This cause of hypoxia can be easily corrected by giving the patient relatively small increases in oxygen concentration to breathe. These results would also be typical of findings in patients with right-to-left shunting of blood, as in tetralogy of Fallot, in which case giving oxygen would not help.

The results in row A show fairly severe metabolic acidosis with respiratory compensation and without hypoxia. These would be typical for someone in early shock and would most commonly be seen in children with diarrhea. Treatment of this type of acidosis is hydration.

The blood gases of row B demonstrate an uncompensated respiratory acidosis with hypoxia but with no metabolic acidosis. This is compatible with acute hypoventilation, which could be produced by a tension pneumothorax, for example. This can be treated easily by placing a needle or catheter in the pleural space and evacuating the air.

231-234. The answers are 231-a, 232-c, 233-b, 234-d. *(Hay et al, pp 495-496. Kliegman et al, pp 1726-1727. McMillan et al, pp 2582-2587. Rudolph et al, pp 278-284, 1656-1657.)* The data on row A indicate severe acidemia and severe hypoxia with a marked respiratory acidosis and metabolic acidosis. These are manifestations of severe ventilatory failure, probably accompanied by circulatory failure or cardiac arrest. This mandates the most aggressive therapy, including assisted ventilation with administration of high oxygen levels. Other measures to restore circulation and improve the acidemia are also indicated.

The results of row C show metabolic alkalosis. The high P_{CO_2} and low P_{O_2} result from compensatory hypoventilation. This can all be secondary to excessive body potassium losses from diuretics.

The results in row B indicate respiratory acidosis with metabolic compensation, indicating chronic upper airway obstruction. A common cause of chronic hypoventilation in children is hypertrophied tonsils and adenoids, which may be an indication for tonsillectomy or adenoidectomy (or both).

The blood gases of row D are impossible in a patient breathing room air. The P_{CO_2} cannot go up without the P_{O_2} dropping roughly proportionately. An increase in P_{CO_2} of 20 mm Hg, from 40 to 60 mm Hg, should therefore produce a fall in P_{O_2} from 90 to 70 mm Hg. The test should be repeated after the blood gas equipment has been checked and recalibrated.

The Gastrointestinal Tract

Questions

235. A 4-year-old boy presents with a history of constipation since the age of 6 months. His stools, produced every 3 to 4 days, are described as large and hard. Physical examination is normal; rectal examination reveals a large ampulla, poor sphincter tone but present anal wink, and stool in the rectal vault. The plain film of his abdomen is shown. Which of the following is the most appropriate next step in the management of this child?

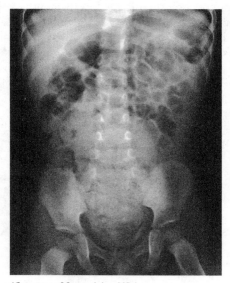

(Courtesy of Susan John, MD.)

a. Lower gastrointestinal (GI) barium study
b. Parental reassurance and dietary counseling
c. Serum electrolyte measurement
d. Upper GI barium study
e. Initiation of thyroid-replacement hormone

236. A 10-year-old boy has been having "bellyaches" for about 2 years. They occur at night as well as during the day. Occasionally, he vomits after the onset of pain. Occult blood has been found in his stool. His father also gets frequent, nonspecific stomachaches. Which of the following is the most likely diagnosis?

a. Peptic ulcer
b. Appendicitis
c. Meckel diverticulum
d. Functional abdominal pain
e. Pinworm infestation

237. An 8-year-old boy presents to your office for a second opinion. He has a 2-year history of intermittent vomiting, dysphagia, and epigastric pain. His father reports he occasionally gets food "stuck" in his throat. He has been on a proton pump inhibitor for 18 months without symptom relief. His past history is significant only for eczema and a peanut allergy. Endoscopy was performed 6 months ago; no erosive lesions were noted and a biopsy was not performed. You arrange for a repeat endoscopy with biopsy. Microscopy on the biopsy sample reveals many eosinophils. Treatment of this condition should include which of the following?

a. Corticosteroids
b. Prolonged acid blockade
c. Treatment for *Candida* sp.
d. Treatment for *Aspergillus* sp.
e. Observation

238. A 1-week-old previously healthy infant presents to the emergency room with the acute onset of bilious vomiting. The abdominal plain film in the emergency department (A) and the barium enema done after admission (B) are shown. Which of the following is the most likely diagnosis for this patient?

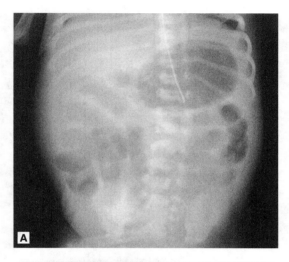

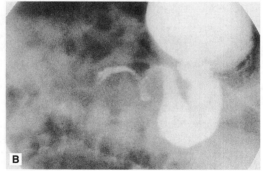

(Courtesy of Susan John, MD.)

a. Jejunal atresia
b. Hypertrophic pyloric stenosis
c. Malrotation with volvulus
d. Acute appendicitis
e. Intussusception

239. The newborn nursery calls to notify you that a 1-day-old baby boy has developed abdominal distension and bilious emesis. Prenatal history was significant for areas of echogenic bowel seen on ultrasound. You order an abdominal radiograph; based on the results you order a contrast enema. Both are shown here. This infant is most likely to have which of the following?

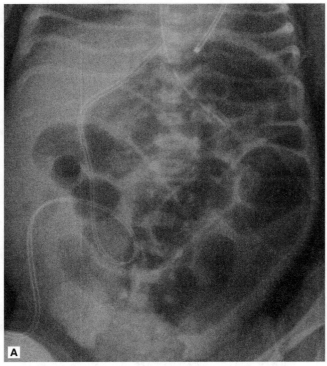

(Courtesy of Susan John, MD.)

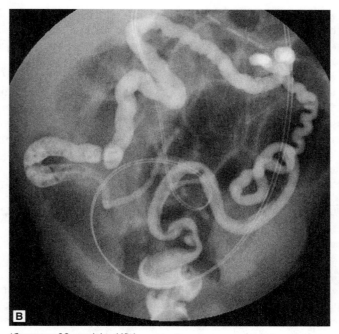

(Courtesy of Susan John, MD.)

a. Duodenal atresia
b. Cystic fibrosis
c. Gastroenteritis
d. Malrotation with volvulus
e. Hirschsprung disease

240. A 15-year-old girl is admitted to the hospital with a 6-kg weight loss, bloody diarrhea, and fever that have occurred intermittently over the previous 6 months. She reports cramping abdominal pain with bowel movements. She also reports secondary amenorrhea during this time. Stool cultures in her physician's office have shown only normal intestinal flora. A urine pregnancy test was negative, while an erythrocyte sedimentation rate (ESR) was elevated. Her examination is significant for the lack of oral mucosal ulcerations and a normal perianal examination. Anti-*Saccharomyces cerevisiae* antibodies (ASCA) are negative, while anti-neutrophil cytoplasm antibodies (p-ANCA) are positive. You confirm your presumptive diagnosis with a rectal biopsy. In counseling her about her disease, which of the following statements would be true?

a. Inheritance is autosomal dominant.
b. Her risk of colon cancer is minimally elevated over the general population.
c. Intestinal strictures are common.
d. The most serious complication of her disease is toxic megacolon.
e. The intestinal involvement is separated by areas of normal bowel.

241. A 3-year-old child presents to your office for an evaluation of constipation. The mother notes that since birth, and despite frequent use of stool softeners, the child has only about one stool per week. He does not have fecal soiling or diarrhea. He was born at term and without pregnancy complications. The child stayed an extra day in the hospital at birth because he did not pass stool for 48 hours, but has not been in the hospital since. Initial evaluation of this child should include which of the following?

a. A child psychiatry evaluation for stool retention and parenting assistance
b. A barium enema and rectal manometry
c. Plain films of the abdomen
d. Dietary log and observation
e. Beginning oral antispasmodic medication

242. A 4-week-old boy presents with a 10-day history of vomiting that has increased in frequency and forcefulness. The vomitus is not bile stained. The child feeds avidly and looks well, but he has been losing weight. An ultrasound of the abdomen is shown. Which of the following is the most likely diagnosis?

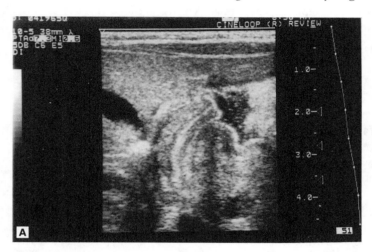

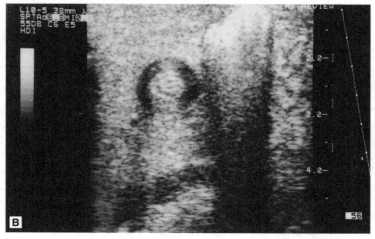

a. Surgical consultation for pyloromyotomy
b. Upper GI with small-bowel follow through
c. Intravenous (IV) fluids alone to maintain hydration
d. Air contrast enema
e. Computed tomography (CT) of the brain

243. A 17-year-old adolescent female is 6 weeks postpartum. She presents to the emergency room with the complaints of increased jaundice, abdominal pain, nausea, vomiting, and fever. Her examination is remarkable for jaundice, pain of the right upper quadrant with guarding, and a clear chest. Chest radiographs appear normal. Which of the following tests is most likely to reveal the cause of this pain?

a. Serum chemistries
b. Complete blood count (CBC) with platelets and differential
c. Ultrasound of the right upper quadrant
d. Upper GI series
e. Hepatitis panel

244. An 8-year-old is accidentally hit in the abdomen by a baseball bat. After several minutes of discomfort, he seems to be fine. Over the ensuing 24 hours, however, he develops a fever, abdominal pain radiating to the back, and persistent vomiting. On examination, the child appears quite uncomfortable. The abdomen is tender, with decreased bowel sounds throughout, but especially painful in the midepigastric region with guarding. Which of the following tests is most likely to confirm the diagnosis?

a. Serum amylase levels
b. CBC with differential and platelets
c. Serum total and direct bilirubin levels
d. Abdominal radiograph
e. Electrolyte panel

245. A 10-month-old baby boy, recently adopted from Guyana, has a 5-hour history of crying, with intermittent drawing up of his knees to his chest. On the way to the emergency room he passes a loose, bloody stool. He has had no vomiting and has refused his bottle since the crying began. Physical examination is noteworthy for an irritable infant whose abdomen is very difficult to examine because of constant crying. His temperature is 38.8°C (101.8°F). The rectal ampulla is empty, but there is some gross blood on the examining finger. Which of the following studies would be most helpful in the immediate management of this patient?

a. Stool culture
b. Examination of the stool for ova and parasites
c. Air contrast enema
d. Examination of the blood smear
e. Coagulation studies

246. A 12-month-old girl has been spitting up her meals since 1 month of age. Her growth is at the 95th percentile, and she is otherwise asymptomatic and without findings on physical examination. Which of the following is the most likely diagnosis?

a. Pyloric stenosis
b. Partial duodenal atresia
c. Hypothyroidism
d. Gastroesophageal reflux
e. Tracheoesophageal fistula

247. A 14-year-old girl has a 9-month history of diarrhea, abdominal pain (usually periumbilical and postprandial), fever, and weight loss. She has had several episodes of blood in her stools. Which of the following is the most likely diagnosis?

a. Chronic appendicitis
b. Chronic pancreatitis
c. Crohn disease
d. Bulimia
e. Gallstones

248. A 4-year-old boy, recently adopted through an international adoption service, is noted to have intermittent watery diarrhea, nausea, belching, and abdominal pain. His weight is less than the fifth percentile for his age. Which of the following studies would be most helpful in making the diagnosis?

a. CBC and differential
b. ESR
c. Abdominal ultrasound
d. Liver function studies
e. Stool microscopy for ova and parasites

249. A 5-month-old child regularly regurgitates a large portion of her feeds. A pH probe study showed significant periods of low esophageal pH. The child has normal growth and no other significant past medical history. Which of the following is the best management at this point?

a. Barium swallow and upper GI series
b. Oral reflux medications
c. Esophageal manometry
d. Close observation only
e. Surgical correction with fundoplication

250. A 2-year-old presents to the emergency center with several days of rectal bleeding. The mother first noticed reddish-colored stools 2 days prior to arrival and has since changed several diapers with just blood. The child is afebrile, alert, and playful, and is eating well without emesis. He is slightly tachycardic, and his abdominal examination is normal. Which of the following is the best diagnostic study to order to confirm the diagnosis?

a. Exploratory laparotomy
b. Barium enema
c. Ultrasound of the abdomen
d. Radionucleotide scan
e. Stool culture

251. A 15-year-old otherwise healthy boy presents with a complaint of intermittent abdominal distention, crampy abdominal pain, and excessive flatulence. He first started noticing these symptoms when he moved into his father's house, and his stepmother insisted on milk at dinner every night. He has normal growth, has not lost weight, and has no travel history. Which of the following is the most appropriate study to diagnose his condition?

a. Barium swallow and upper GI
b. Hydrogen excretion in breath after oral administration of lactose
c. Esophageal manometry
d. Stool pH after one to 2 weeks of a lactose-free diet
e. Fasting serum lactose levels

252. A 6-week-old infant is admitted to the hospital with jaundice. Her outpatient blood work demonstrated a total bilirubin of 12 mg/dL with a direct portion of 3.5 mg/dL. Which of the following disorders is most likely to be responsible?

a. ABO incompatibility
b. Choledochal cyst
c. Rh incompatibility
d. Gilbert disease
e. Crigler-Najjar syndrome

253. A 2-year-old arrives in the emergency center after having swallowed a button battery from one of her toys. She is breathing comfortably, without stridor. Radiographs show the battery to be lodged in the esophagus. Which of the following is the correct next step?

a. Induce emesis with syrup of ipecac.
b. Admit for observation, and obtain serial radiographs to document movement of the battery.
c. Discharge home with instructions to monitor the stool for the battery.
d. Immediate removal of the battery via endoscopy.
e. Encourage oral intake to assist in passage of the battery.

254. An awake, alert infant with a 2-day history of diarrhea presents with a depressed fontanelle, tachycardia, sunken eyes, and the loss of skin elasticity. Which of the following is the correct percentage of dehydration?

a. Less than 1%
b. 1% to 5%
c. 5% to 9%
d. 10% to 15%
e. More than 20%

255. A 9-month-old is brought to the emergency center by ambulance. The child had been having emesis and diarrhea with decreased urine output for several days, and the parents noted that she was hard to wake up this morning. Her weight is 9 kg, down from 11 kg the week prior at her 9-month checkup. You note her heart rate and blood pressure to be normal. She is lethargic, and her skin is noted to be "doughy." After confirming that her respiratory status is stable, you send electrolytes, which you expect to be abnormal. You start an IV. Which of the following is the best solution for an initial IV bolus?

a. One-fourth normal saline (38.5 mEq sodium/L)
b. D10 water (100 g glucose/L)
c. Normal saline (154 mEq sodium/L)
d. 3% saline (513 mEq sodium/L)
e. Fresh-frozen plasma

256. You are admitting to the hospital a 3-month-old infant who has been having poor feeding, emesis, and diarrhea for 3 days. In the emergency center, her electrolytes were found to be: sodium 157 mEq/L, potassium 2.6 mEq/L, chloride 120 mEq/L, bicarbonate 14 mEq/L, creatinine 1.8 mEq/L, blood urea nitrogen (BUN) 68 mEq/L, and glucose 195 mEq/L. She was given a fluid bolus in the emergency center and has subsequently produced urine. Which of the following is the most appropriate next step in her management?

a. Slow rehydration over 48 hours
b. Continued rapid volume expansion with ¼ normal saline
c. Packed red blood cells (RBCs)
d. Rehydration with free water
e. Urinary electrolytes

257. The mother of a 6-month-old infant is concerned that her baby may be teething. You explain to her that the first teeth to erupt in most children are which of the following?

a. Mandibular central incisors
b. Maxillary lateral incisors
c. Maxillary first molars
d. Mandibular cuspids (canines)
e. First premolars (bicuspids)

258. An 8-year-old boy is brought to your office with the complaint of abdominal pain. The pain is worse during the week and seems to be less prominent during the weekends and during the summer. The patient's growth and development are normal. The physical examination is unremarkable. Laboratory screening, including stool for occult blood, CBC, urinalysis, and chemistry panel, yields normal results. Which of the following is the best next step in the care of this patient?

a. Perform an upper GI series
b. Perform CT of the abdomen
c. Administer a trial of H₂ blockers
d. Observe the patient and reassure the patient and family
e. Recommend a lactose-free diet

259. The 4-year-old child pictured below is noted to have the tooth decay as shown. This characteristic pattern of tooth decay is caused by which of the following?

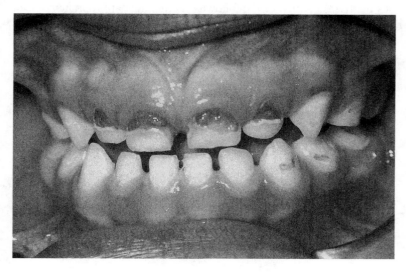

a. Excessive use of fluoride
b. Tetracycline
c. Use of bottled water that lacks fluoride
d. Prolonged use of a baby bottle
e. Consumption of too much candy

260. A 12-year-old girl was hit in the face by a baseball 15 minutes earlier and has had her mandibular incisors knocked out. Which of the following represents the best plan of action?

a. The teeth should be rinsed in hot water then carefully dried.
b. Foreign matter adhering to the teeth should be immediately scrubbed off.
c. The teeth may be transported in tea, juice, or cola.
d. Avulsed teeth can be transported in the mouth of the parent or a cooperative patient.
e. A dental appointment should be made within 48 to 72 hours.

261. A 55-day-old infant born prematurely at 27 weeks of gestation is shown below. The swelling is not tender, firm, hot, or red, and it does not transilluminate. It seems to resolve with pressure, but returns when the infant cries or strains. Which of the following is the most appropriate course of action at this point?

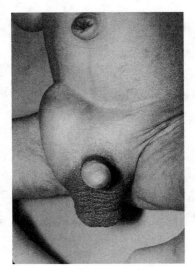

a. Obtain a surgical consultation
b. Perform a needle aspiration
c. Order a barium enema
d. Order a KUB (plain radiographs of kidney, ureter, and bladder)
e. Observe the patient and reassure the patient and family

262. An 18-month-old infant is found with the contents of a bottle of drain cleaner in his mouth. Which of the following treatment options is most appropriate?

a. Immediate emesis
b. Endoscopic examination within the first 12 to 24 hours
c. Decontamination by activated charcoal
d. Neutralization by drinking a solution of the opposite pH
e. Have the patient drink copious amounts of milk or water

263. A 16-year-old male, despondent over a recent breakup, tries to commit suicide by taking an unknown quantity of an unknown material he found at home. He is brought to the emergency center by his parents within 30 minutes of the ingestion. For which of the following household materials and medications should he be given activated charcoal as part of his emergency center treatment?

a. Drain cleaner
b. Ethylene glycol
c. Bleach
d. Phenobarbital
e. Lithium

Questions 264 to 268

For each of the patient descriptions below, choose the best initial diagnostic step in the evaluation of the patient's apparent GI hemorrhage. Each lettered option may be used once, more than once, or not at all.

a. Abdominal series
b. Fiberoptic endoscopy
c. Apt test
d. Routine stool culture
e. Barium enema
f. No immediate intervention
g. Meckel scan
h. Stool culture on sorbitol-MacConkey medium

264. A newborn infant, the product of an emergency cesarean section, is 24 hours old and has a grossly bloody stool. She looks well otherwise.

265. A 7-day-old premature infant born at 26 weeks of gestation now has a grossly bloody stool, abdominal distention, and increasing oxygen requirements.

266. A 2-year-old has crampy abdominal pain and grossly bloody diarrheal stool, but no fever. His abdominal examination reveals no masses. A family member, who ate at the same local hamburger shop the night prior, has the same symptoms.

267. A 7-year-old has been vomiting for 2 days and has had diarrhea for 1 day. He now notes that he has small streaks of blood in his emesis. The rest of his family has had similar symptoms.

268. A 10-year-old has complained for 1 month of intermittent epigastric pain that awakens him from sleep. He notes that eating food sometimes helps. He reports black stools during the prior week, and also admits that he has occasionally vomited frank blood.

Questions 269 to 274

For each presented child, choose the one most appropriate vitamin or trace element—replacement therapy to treat the described condition. Each lettered option may be used once, more than once, or not at all.

a. Vitamin A
b. Vitamin B_6
c. Vitamin C
d. Vitamin D
e. Vitamin E
f. Iron
g. Vitamin K
h. Folate
i. Niacin

269. A 15-year-old vegetarian being treated for tuberculosis develops peripheral neuropathy.

270. A 9-month-old infant, who has been fed cow's milk exclusively for 4 months, is tachycardic and pale.

271. A 3-day-old infant born at home is brought to the emergency center with bloody stools, hematemesis, and purpura. His circumcision is oozing blood.

272. A 17-month-old toddler has been irritable over the past month. She now refuses to walk and seems to have tenderness in both of her legs. She has had a low-grade fever, and she has petechiae on her skin and mucous membranes. She has a small cut that has not healed well. Radiographs of the legs reveal generalized bony atrophy with epiphyseal separation.

273. A 4-year-old whose diet consists mostly of cheese puffs and cola begins to have problems walking at night, complaining that he cannot see well. In addition, his skin has become dry and scaly, and he has complained of headache for a month.

274. An exclusively breast-fed 2-year-old is brought to the emergency center with pain in his right leg after a fall. Physical examination reveals a small child with a 3-cm anterior fontanelle, a flattened occiput, a prominent forehead, significant dental caries, bumpy ribs, and bowed extremities. Radiographs reveal a greenstick fracture at the site of pain, along with fraying at the distal ends of the femur.

Questions 275 to 277

For each description of symptoms below, select the study which is most likely to be diagnostic. Each lettered option may be used once, more than once, or not at all.

a. Esophageal manometry
b. 24-hour pH probe
c. Upper GI endoscopy
d. Upper GI fluoroscopy (upper GI series)
e. Modified barium swallow

275. A 3-week-old child currently admitted to the hospital for pneumonia who gags and chokes during feedings

276. A 12-year-old who has several weeks of abdominal pain and black stools

277. A newborn with arching of the back temporally related to feeds but no emesis

The Gastrointestinal Tract

Answers

235. The answer is b. *(Hay et al, pp 612-613, 629-630. Kliegman et al, pp 1565-1567. McMillan et al, pp 373-375, 1920-1923. Rudolph et al, pp 1368-1370, 1461-1463.)* The radiograph demonstrates a stool-filled megacolon. Finding a dilated, stool-filled anal canal with poor tone on the physical examination of a well-grown child supports the diagnosis of functional constipation. Hirschsprung disease is usually suspected in the chronically constipated child despite 98% of such children having functional constipation. The difficulty in treating functional constipation, once it has been established as the diagnosis, emphasizes the need for prompt identification and treatment of problems with defecation and for counseling of parents regarding proper toileting behavior. An extensive workup of this patient would likely be negative and expensive, and is not indicated. Hirschsprung usually presents in infancy with increasingly difficult defecation in the first few weeks of life. Typically no stool is found in the rectum, and anal sphincter tone is abnormal. Diagnosis of Hirschsprung disease may be made with rectal manometry and rectal biopsy.

236. The answer is a. *(Hay et al, pp 608-609. Kliegman et al, pp 1572-1574. McMillan et al, pp 1932-1937. Rudolph et al, pp 1433-1434.)* The presence of nocturnal abdominal pain and GI bleeding in a patient with a positive family history support a diagnosis of peptic ulcer disease (PUD). Pain is the most common symptom. Symptoms often persist for several years before diagnosis. The increased incidence of peptic ulcer disease in families (25%-50%) and concordance in monozygotic twins suggest a genetic basis for the disease. Diagnosis may be made conclusively with endoscopy; stains and cultures obtained during endoscopy can diagnose PUD caused by *Helicobacter pylori*. Serum testing for *H pylori* is controversial, and typically does not distinguish between acute and past infection; the urea breath test may turn out to be more reliable than the serum assay, and is becoming more available. The mainstay of treatment is acid blockade. Antibiotic treatment for *H pylori* can cure this disease in infected patients, although the optimal combination of medications is still unclear. Appendicitis is an acute event. Pinworms produce perianal pruritus but do not commonly cause abdominal pain or other serious problems. Meckel diverticulum causes painless rectal bleeding, usually during early childhood. Functional, or recurrent, abdominal pain is a benign, self-limited diagnosis of exclusion; GI bleeding is not a typical finding.

237. The answer is a. *(Kliegman et al, pp 1550-1551. McMillan et al, pp 1986-1988. Rudolph et al, pp 1396-1397.)* Information about eosinophilic esophagitis continues to evolve, but it appears to be an allergic response. Males are affected more than females. The history usually includes atopy or food allergy. Symptoms are similar to those seen in gastroesophageal reflex disease, but are not relieved with acid blockade. Some have elevated IgE levels or peripheral eosinophilia (hinted at by his history of eczema and peanut allergy). Endoscopy reveals mucosal furrowing; strictures can develop as well. Biopsy reveals many eosinophils (normal mucosa does not have eosinophils). Treatment includes avoidance of specific food allergens. Inhaled or systemic steroids have been helpful. Candidal or *Aspergillus* esophagitis is usually seen in immunocompromised individuals, and thus would be unlikely in this patient. Observation would not be helpful in this case.

238. The answer is c. *(Hay et al, pp 610-611. Kliegman et al, pp 1561-1562. McMillan et al, p 372. Rudolph et al, pp 1400-1402.)* The plain films demonstrate dilated stomach and proximal loops of bowel. The cross-table upper GI demonstrates a "curly Q" twist of barium as it passes through the malrotated portion of bowel. Malrotation results when incomplete rotation of the intestines occurs during embryologic development. The most common type of malrotation is failure of the cecum to move to its correct location in the right lower quadrant. Most patients present in the first weeks of life with bili-ous vomiting indicative of bowel obstruction and/or intermittent abdominal pain. Acute presentation, similar to that in the question, is caused by a volvulus of the intestines. The diagnosis is confirmed by radiographs; barium contrast studies (upper GI and/or enema) demonstrate malposition of the cecum in the vast majority of cases. Treatment is surgical. Appendicitis is rare at this age and presents as an acute, rigid abdomen and signs of sepsis. Pyloric stenosis usually does not occur until after 3 weeks of life and presents with nonbilious vomiting. If the child were 6 months or older, intussusception would be higher on the differential, but it is an unusual condition for this age. Jejunal atresia would have been noted on the first day of life, as the patient would not have tolerated any feeds prior to newborn discharge.

239. The answer is b. *(Hay et al, pp 507-508. Kliegman et al, p 754. McMillan et al, p 1428. Rudolph et al, pp 1968, 1977-1978.)* The radiographs are consistent with meconium ileus, a condition virtually pathognomonic for cystic fibrosis (CF). Approximately 15% of children with CF will present with meconium ileus. Echogenic bowel on prenatal ultrasound can be an early hint. Inspissated meconium obstructs the small bowel, usually at the level of the terminal ileum. Radiographs show dilated loops of bowel, and usually reveal a bubbly or granular pattern at the level of obstruction. The enema shows microcolon from disuse. Complications of meconium ileus may include perforation and meconium peritonitis. Meconium ileus should be distinguished from meconium plug, which is more commonly seen and is not as predictive of CF.

240. The answer is a. *(Hay et al, pp 633-637. Kliegman et al, pp 1575-1585. McMillan et al, pp 1954-1972. Rudolph et al, pp 1435-1444.)* The patient in the vignette has ulcerative colitis, a chronic inflammatory condition usually involving the entire colon. While there does seem to be some genetic predisposition (twin concordance is 16%, while twin concordance for Crohn disease is 36%), inheritance is not clearly dominant or recessive. Patients usually have intermittent symptoms of bloody diarrhea, and can have abdominal pain and growth failure. Perianal disease is uncommon, as are mouth ulcerations. So-called skip areas, portions of the intestine free of disease, are common in Crohn disease, but are not seen in ulcerative colitis. ASCA is positive in about 55% of those with Crohn disease, but are uncommon in ulcerative colitis; conversely, p-ANCA is positive in about 70% of patients with ulcerative colitis, but in less than 20% of patients with Crohn disease. The most serious complication of ulcerative colitis is toxic megacolon, a medical and surgical emergency in which patients develop fever, tachycardia, dehydration, leukocytosis, and electrolyte abnormalities associated with a markedly dilated colon. This complication comes with a high risk of intestinal perforation. Patients with ulcerative colitis have a markedly elevated risk of colonic carcinoma; after 10 years of disease, the annual cumulative risk is 0.5% to 1% a year. Strictures are more common in Crohn disease and are unusual in ulcerative colitis.

241. The answer is b. *(Hay et al, pp 612-613. Kliegman et al, pp 1565-1567. McMillan et al, pp 373-375. Rudolph et al, pp 1461-1463.)* The diagnosis of

Hirschsprung disease should be suspected in a child with intractable chronic constipation without fecal soiling (although approximately 3% do have soiling). In contrast, overflow diarrhea caused by leakage of the unformed fecal stream around a rectal impaction is common in functional constipation. A neonatal history of delayed passage of meconium is often obtained, and the infant can continue to be constipated and to have bouts of abdominal distention and vomiting. The infant is also at risk of developing enterocolitis, a life-threatening consequence of the partial obstruction. Radiologic study by barium enema and rectal manometry are accurate diagnostic tools. Identification of an aganglionic segment of bowel by punch or suction biopsy can establish the diagnosis. Histochemical tissue examination showing increased amounts of acetylcholinesterase and an absence of ganglia cells is confirmatory. Rectal manometric studies have shown that in aganglionic megacolon, the usual relaxation of the internal rectal sphincter in response to balloon inflation does not occur. Surgery is indicated as soon as the diagnosis is made. Antispasmodic agents and dietary changes are not helpful, and a plain film of the abdomen would not confirm the diagnosis.

242. The answer is a. (*Hay et al, pp 607-608. Kliegman et al, pp 1555-1557. McMillan et al, pp 371-372. Rudolph et al, p 1402.*) A history of nonbilious vomiting for 10 days in a child of this age who does not look ill points to infantile hypertrophic pyloric stenosis as the most likely diagnosis; surgical consultation for a likely pyloromyotomy is indicated. The ultrasound in the question demonstrates the thickened pylorus. The incidence of this condition in infants is between 1:200 and 1:750, with males affected more often than females. Although there is no specific pattern of inheritance, a familial incidence has been observed in about 15% of patients. Information about predisposing ancestry is conflicting, as are data concerning the assertion of a firstborn predilection. Metabolic alkalosis with low serum potassium and chloride levels is frequently seen in pyloric stenosis as a result of loss of gastric contents from vomiting. A child with a small-bowel obstruction (who may require an upper GI with small-bowel follow through to help diagnose the point of obstruction) should develop bilious emesis and should not look well 10 days into the illness; similarly, a child with intussusception (who requires an air contrast enema, which is both diagnostic and perhaps therapeutic) would be markedly ill at this point. Gastroenteritis (IV fluids alone to maintain hydration) does not usually last for 10 days. A brain tumor causing increased intracranial pressure could present with isolated emesis, but should show other symptoms such as irritability and somnolence.

243. The answer is c. *(Hay et al, pp 670-671. Kliegman et al, pp 1708-1709. McMillan et al, pp 2042-2045. Rudolph et al, pp 1507-1508.)* Cholecystitis and cholelithiasis are unusual diseases in children and are almost always associated with predisposing disorders such as hemolytic anemia, pregnancy, cystic fibrosis, Crohn disease, obesity, rapid weight loss, or prior ileal resection. Pain of the right upper quadrant, nausea, vomiting, fever, and jaundice are symptoms of acute cholecystitis. The diagnosis is confirmed with an ultrasound of the gallbladder. While some of the other answers listed might result in abnormalities, the findings would be neither sensitive nor specific for cholecystitis. Thus, the diagnostic test of choice is an ultrasound.

244. The answer is a. *(Hay et al, pp 676-677. Kliegman et al, pp 1653-1655. McMillan et al, pp 1210-1211. Rudolph et al, pp 1466-1467.)* While no diagnostic test is completely accurate, an elevated total serum amylase with the correct clinical history and signs and symptoms of pancreatitis is the best diagnostic tool. The causes of pancreatitis in children are varied, with about one-fourth of cases without predisposing etiology and about one-third of cases as a feature of another systemic disease. Traumatic cases are usually due to blunt trauma to the abdomen. Acute pancreatitis is difficult to diagnose; a high index of suspicion is necessary. Common clinical features include severe pain with nausea and vomiting. Tenderness, guarding or rebound pain, abdominal distention, and a paralytic ileus are often seen. Plain films of the abdomen may exclude other diagnoses; ultrasonography of the pancreas can reveal enlargement of the pancreas, gallstones, cysts, and pseudocysts. Supportive care is indicated until the condition resolves.

245. The answer is c. *(Hay et al, pp 616-617. Kliegman et al, pp 1569-1570. McMillan et al, pp 1938-1940. Rudolph et al, pp 1407-1408.)* The usual presentation of intussusception is that of an infant between 4 and 10 months of age who has a sudden onset of intermittent colicky abdominal pain. The child can appear normal when the pain abates, but as it recurs with increasing frequency, the child can begin to vomit and become progressively more obtunded. The passage of stool containing blood and mucus, frequently described as resembling currant jelly, is often observed. Early examination of the abdomen can be unremarkable, but as the problem persists, a sausage-shaped mass in the right upper quadrant is frequently palpated. An air, barium, or saline enema examination under fluoroscopic or ultrasound control can be therapeutic as well as diagnostic when the hydrostatic effects of the contrast serve to reduce the intussusception, but should be performed with surgical backup, as a complication of attempted reduction is intestinal perforation. Rates of intestinal perforation are lowest with air reduction. Early diagnosis prevents bowel ischemia. The cause of most intussusceptions is unknown, but a Meckel diverticulum or polyp can serve as a lead point. None of the other choices would result in a correct diagnosis (and potential therapy) for the child with a classic presentation for intussusception.

246. The answer is d. (*Hay et al, pp 605-606. Kliegman et al, pp 1547-1550. McMillan et al, pp 382-384. Rudolph et al, pp 1389-1393.*) Gastroesophageal reflux is a common pediatric complaint, often seen in the first 1 to 2 months of life and resolving by 1 to 2 years of age. Occasional episodes of gastroesophageal reflux in infancy are physiologic; gastroesophageal reflux disease is the pathologic form, involving respiratory symptoms, esophagitis, related apnea, or weight loss. About 7% of children have reflux severe enough to require medical attention, and only 2% of that group requires investigation. For children who are growing well and do not have respiratory symptoms attributed to reflux, conservative treatment (small feeds, thickened formula, avoiding high-fat meals and overfeeding, etc) suffices. A small number need pharmacologic therapy. Medications to treat GERD include acid blockade with H_2 blockers or proton pump inhibitors, resulting in decreased esophagitis. Prokinetic agents are frequently used in conjunction with acid blockade for this illness, but have not been consistently shown to decrease symptoms.

Pyloric stenosis presents with nonbilious vomiting in the first weeks of life and not at 12 months of age. Similarly, a patient with a partial duodenal atresia would be noted in the newborn period, likely with bilious vomiting. Hypothyroidism can cause constipation, among other findings, but a presentation with isolated vomiting would be distinctly unusual. A 12-month-old patient with a tracheoesophageal fistula would likely have an "H-type" fistula, which presents with ongoing respiratory issues and not emesis.

247. The answer is c. (*Hay et al, pp 633-637. Kliegman et al, pp 1580-1585. McMillan et al, pp 1962-1972. Rudolph et al, pp 1441-1444.*) The presentation of Crohn disease depends on the location and extent of lesions. Onset of the GI or extraintestinal symptoms is insidious. The common presentation is as described. Crohn disease (granulomatous colitis) characteristically is associated with transmural, granulomatous intestinal lesions that are discontinuous and can appear in both the small and large intestines. Although Crohn disease can first appear as a rectal fissure or fistula, the rectum is often spared. Arthritis/arthralgia occurs in a minority (11%) of affected children.

Other extraintestinal symptoms include erythema nodosum or pyoderma gangrenosum, liver disease, renal calculi, uveitis, anemia, specific nutrient deficiency, and growth failure. In relation to the general population, the risk of colonic carcinoma in affected persons is increased, but not nearly to the degree associated with ulcerative colitis.

248. The answer is e. (*Hay et al, pp 1227-1229. Kliegman et al, pp 1083-1084, 1462-1464. McMillan et al, pp 680-684, 1329-1331. Rudolph et al, pp 521-522, 1131-1132.*) Parasites are a common medical problem, found in about 60% of international adoptees, in most cases related to tainted water ingestion; *Giardia* is the most frequent isolate. Patients with *Giardia* infection complain of recurrent abdominal pain, cramping, intermittent diarrhea, bloating, and weight loss. Although many cases are self-limited, symptoms can recur or become chronic. Identifying the *Giardia* cysts or trophozoites makes the diagnosis. Upper endoscopy and microscopic examination of duodenal biopsies can also be diagnostic. Although international adoptees may also have hepatitis, it is much less common than parasitic infection. Most patients with *Giardia* infection have normal CBCs. An upper GI series may reveal nonspecific changes associated with *Giardia* infection, but an ultrasound would not be helpful. An ESR is merely a nonspecific marker for inflammation, and would not help make the diagnosis.

249. The answer is d. (*Hay et al, pp 605-606. Kliegman et al, pp 1547-1550. McMillan et al, pp 382-383. Rudolph et al, pp 1390-1393.*) Barium swallow and upper GI series are helpful in detecting anatomic abnormalities such as antral web, pyloric stenosis, malrotation, and annular pancreas. To confirm the presence of gastroesophageal reflux (GER), the best test is the esophageal pH probe, which measures the frequency and duration of falls in pH, thereby indicating acid reflux. Esophageal manometry is used to identify poor tone of the lower esophageal sphincter. In this child, who is growing well and developing properly and has no other medical problems such as reflux-induced apnea or bradycardia or aspiration pneumonia, pharmacologic treatment is not necessary, as most infants will outgrow this common problem of esophageal reflux. Surgical correction is reserved for infants with poor weight gain or reflux-associated apnea and bradycardia who have failed pharmacologic therapy.

250. The answer is d. (*Hay et al, pp 611-612. Kliegman et al, p 1563. McMillan et al, pp 372-373. Rudolph et al, pp 1405-1406.*) The child described has a typical presentation for Meckel diverticulum. The embryonic duct connecting the yolk sac to the intestine can fail to regress completely and persist as a diverticulum attached to the ileum. It is common, occurring in 1.5% of the population; however, it rarely causes symptoms. Children symptomatic with this condition usually present with painless rectal bleeding in the first 2 years of life, but they can have symptoms throughout the first decade. The lining of the Meckel diverticulum usually contains acid-secreting gastric mucosa that can produce ulcerations of the diverticulum itself or the adjacent ileum. Bleeding, perforation, or diverticulitis can occur. More seriously, the diverticulum can lead to volvulus of itself and of the small intestine, and it can also undergo eversion and intussusception. Diagnosis can be made by technetium scan that labels gastric mucosa, and treatment is surgical excision. Barium studies do not readily reveal the diverticulum, nor do plain films.

251. The answer is b. (*Hay et al, pp 626-627. Kliegman et al, p 1598. McMillan et al, p 1978. Rudolph et al, p 1424.*) Lactase is a disaccharidase localized in the brush border of the intestinal villous cells. It hydrolyzes lactose to its constituent monosaccharides, glucose, and galactose. Intestinal lactase levels are usually normal at birth in all populations; however, lactase deficiency is a common, genetically predetermined condition. Lactase activity is not readily increased by the oral administration of substrate or the inclusion of lactose in the diet. The clinical symptoms of lactose malabsorption are due to the presence of osmotically active, undigested lactose, which may act to increase intestinal fluid volume, alter transit time, and produce the symptoms of abdominal cramps, distention, and occasionally, watery diarrhea. Bacterial metabolism of the nonabsorbed carbohydrates in the colon into carbon dioxide and hydrogen may contribute to the clinical symptoms. Acquired lactase deficiency is often associated with conditions of the GI tract that cause intestinal mucosal injury (eg, sprue and regional enteritis). Diagnostic techniques for lactose intolerance include removal of the offending sugar, with a reproduction of symptoms upon reintroduction. Although the ingestion of even small amounts of lactose can be diagnostic if GI symptoms occur, the measurement of breath hydrogen is more specific, as it is not affected by glucose metabolism or gastric emptying. Similarly, an acidic stool pH in the presence of reducing substances would be diagnostic.

252. The answer is b. (*Hay et al, p 648. Kliegman et al, p 1705. McMillan et al, pp 2034-2035. Rudolph et al, p 1482.*) Obstructive jaundice (ie, direct-reacting bilirubin greater than 20% of the total) requires investigation in all infants. Cystic fibrosis and α_1-antitrypsin deficiency should be considered in the diagnostic evaluation of any child with obstructive jaundice. Other diseases to be excluded are galactosemia, tyrosinemia, and urinary tract or other infections (including toxoplasmosis, cytomegalovirus, rubella, syphilis, and herpesvirus). Ultrasound examination to rule out choledochal cyst may be included with a technetium ^{99m}Tc hepatic iminodiacetic acid (HIDA) scan to assess the patency of the biliary tree. Liver biopsy can assist in the diagnosis by providing a histologic diagnosis (eg, hepatitis, biliary atresia), tissue for enzyme activity (ie, inborn error of metabolism), or tissue for microscopic determination of storage diseases. ABO and Rh incompatibility occasionally cause direct hyperbilirubinemia if there were brisk hemolysis at birth, which would then lead to inspissated bile syndrome. All of the other causes listed typically lead to indirect hyperbilirubinemia.

253. The answer is d. *(Hay et al, p 617. Kliegman et al, p 1552. Rudolph et al, pp 1397-1398.)* In patients without respiratory symptoms, observation for 24 hours of some foreign bodies in the esophagus can be effected; the foreign body usually passes uneventfully into the stomach. However, button batteries that lodge in the esophagus must be removed urgently via endoscopy as they carry a high risk of esophageal perforation in as little as 1 hour. Patients who have stridor associated with external compression of the airway also need emergent intervention. Some advocate removing esophageal foreign bodies using a balloon catheter (passing the catheter past the foreign body, inflating the balloon, and pulling both the catheter and the object out). However, this does not allow direct visualization of the mucosa to determine the extent of the injury and also carries the risk of aspiration; it should be performed only by experienced personnel.

254. The answer is c. *(Hay et al, p 1278. Kliegman et al, p 313. McMillan et al, p 63. Rudolph et al, p 1645.)* A moribund state is characteristic of a loss of greater than 10% of body weight from dehydration. The other findings are characteristic of a loss of body weight of 5% to 9% when there is no hypernatremia. Additional findings at this level of dehydration can be restlessness, absent or reduced tears, weak radial pulses, and possibly orthostatic hypotension.

255. The answer is c. *(Hay et al, pp 1279-1280. Kliegman et al, pp 313-316. McMillan et al, pp 63-66. Rudolph et al, pp 1644-1646, 1650-1652.)* The description is that of a child with hypernatremia (in this case, the child's sodium was 170 mEq/dL); the "doughy" skin is often seen in hypernatremia. The extracellular fluid and circulating blood volumes tend to be preserved with hypernatremic dehydration at the expense of the intracellular volume. Therefore, hypotension may not be observed, nor may the other signs of circulatory inadequacy that are typical of isotonic or hypotonic dehydration. Signs suggesting involvement of the central nervous system (such as irritability or lethargy) are characteristic of hypotonic dehydration. Isotonic saline is the best fluid for an initial bolus in a patient such as the one described in the question.

Use of $\frac{1}{4}$ normal saline (38.5 mEq sodium/L) or D10 water (100 g glucose/L) in this dehydrated child would not expand the intravascular space and its hyponatremic nature might lead to cerebral edema. The child in the question is hypernatremic, so 3% saline (513 mEq sodium/L) would only exacerbate the problem; its use in dehydration might be considered for some patients with severe hyponatremia. Fresh-frozen plasma can be used in the situation described, but it is generally not rapidly available, is more expensive, can be associated with infectious agents, and offers no advantage to saline.

256. The answer is a. (*Hay et al, pp 1276-1280. Kliegman et al, pp 313-316. McMillan et al, pp 63-66. Rudolph et al, pp 1644-1646, 1650-1652.*) Initial bolus therapy in the emergency center should have been with isotonic fluid such as normal saline or lactated Ringer solution. Slow correction of this hypernatremia (more than 24-48 hours) prevents significant fluid shifts and increased intracranial pressure. Hyperglycemia may be seen in hypernatremic dehydration because of decreased insulin secretion and cell sensitivity to insulin; this is particularly important to recognize because increased serum glucose can cause the serum sodium to be falsely decreased. Blood products such as fresh-frozen plasma are not indicated, and rapid infusion of hypotonic solutions such as D10W and $\frac{1}{4}$ normal saline could cause rapid fluid shifts resulting in cerebral edema and death. Hypertonic (3%) saline is used only in the event of seizures caused by rapid rehydration (or in children with hyponatremic dehydration and associated central nervous system symptoms), along with other emergent measures typically used to reduce cerebral edema.

257. The answer is a. (*Hay et al, pp 451-453. Kliegman et al, p 1205. Rudolph et al, p 1285.*) In general, mandibular teeth erupt before maxillary teeth; teeth tend to erupt in girls before they do in boys. The first teeth to erupt usually are the mandibular central incisors at 5 to 7 months, followed by the maxillary central incisors at 6 to 8 months. Lateral incisors (mandibular then maxillary) erupt next at 7 to 11 months, followed by the first molars (10-16 months), the cuspids (16-20 months), and the second molars (20-30 months).

258. The answer is d. *(Hay et al, pp 631-633. Kliegman et al, pp 1627-1628. McMillan et al, pp 1977-1979. Rudolph et al, pp 1357-1363.)* Recurrent abdominal pain is a common complaint occurring in at least 10% of school-age children. In children older than 2 years, less than 10% of cases have an identifiable organic cause. Management of these children is difficult and frustrating for the physician and the family. Excessive testing and treatments are not typically useful. A thorough history and physical examination, including growth parameters, are frequently helpful in separating organic from nonorganic causes of abdominal pain. Any signs or symptoms of organic causes, such as growth failure, should be pursued. If nothing in the history or physical examination is found, as is likely in the case described, reassurance of the children and family members is indicated. Close follow-up for new or changing symptoms as well as further reassurance to the family is important.

259. The answer is d. *(Hay et al, pp 453-454. Kliegman et al, pp 1534-1536. McMillan et al, p 795. Rudolph et al, pp 1288-1290.)* The pattern of dental disease found with the use of bottles that contain high concentrations of sugars, which promotes dental disease, includes extensive maxillary decay (especially frontal) and posterior maxillary and mandibular decay, but essentially normal mandibular frontal teeth. Prevention of this disease is possible through counseling families to avoid the use of fruit juices in bottles or sweetened pacifiers. In addition, children should not be permitted to take a bottle to bed with them; weaning from the bottle should be discussed with the parents toward the end of the first year of life. Genetic predisposition seems to play a role as well.

260. The answer is d. *(Hay et al, pp 455-456. Kliegman et al, pp 1537-1538. McMillan et al, p 798. Rudolph et al, pp 1303-1304.)* The earlier that permanent teeth are replanted, the greater the rate of success, decreasing from 90% in the first 30 minutes to 5% after 2 hours. The rate of success is a function of the integrity of the periodontal ligament. The teeth can be rinsed in cold water, but not brushed (to avoid damaging the root and periodontal ligament). Milk or saline are good transport media if the child is uncooperative or for some other reason the teeth cannot be reinserted at the scene. Teeth may also be transported in the mouth of the older, cooperative patient or the parent. The immediate application of acrylic splints is needed to keep the teeth in place, so immediate dental attention is required. The need for full tetanus immunization should be evaluated. Unless the tooth is available, patients who are suspected of having a total avulsion should be evaluated for partial avulsion or total intrusion with a radiograph. A completely avulsed primary tooth is generally not replaced, to avoid damage to the underlying permanent tooth.

261. The answer is a. (*Hay et al, p 618. Kliegman et al, pp 1644-1650. McMillan et al, pp 1925-1927. Rudolph et al, p 1742.*) A congenital indirect inguinal hernia is the result of a patent processus vaginalis. This is in contrast to the less common acquired direct inguinal hernia, caused by weakness in the musculature of the inguinal canal. Inguinal hernias are commonly seen in premature infants (16%-25%). Incarceration is common; elective repair is often considered prior to hospital discharge. The diagnosis is so common that diagnostic tests are performed infrequently.

262. The answer is b. (*Hay et al, pp 344-345, 607. Kliegman et al, pp 352-353. McMillan et al, p 750. Rudolph et al, pp 1395-1396.*) Endoscopic examination of the esophagus and stomach is a diagnostic method of determining the extent of the mucosal injury. Vomiting is to be avoided since it would expose the mucosal surfaces to the caustic agent a second time. The child can be given small amounts of milk or water, but large amounts, which might cause vomiting, are unwise. Neutralization of the caustic can result in an exothermic reaction and produce a thermal burn. The use of steroids after endoscopy in second-degree chemical burns of the esophagus has been effective in diminishing the inflammatory response in some patients. Optimal treatment is still controversial and requires expert consultation or review of the most current literature. Charcoal, however, does not absorb the alkaline agent in drain cleaner.

263. The answer is d. (*Hay et al, p 338. Kliegman et al, p 344. McMillan et al, p 750. Rudolph et al, p 359.*) The absorption of certain toxins from the GI tract is diminished by the use of activated charcoal administered during the first few hours after the ingestion in the minimum dose of 10 to 30 g for a child or 30 to 100 g for an adult. Activated charcoal exerts its effect by adsorbing particles of toxin on its surface. Compounds not adsorbed include alcohols, acids, ferrous sulfate, strong bases (such as drain cleaners and oven cleaners), cyanide, lithium, and potassium. For drugs with an enterohepatic circulation (eg, phenobarbital and tricyclic antidepressants), or those with prolonged absorption (eg, sustained-release theophylline), the use of multiple-dose activated charcoal can be effective in decreasing the half-life and increasing the total body clearance of the toxic substance.

264 to 268.   The answers are 264-c, 265-a, 266-h, 267-f, 268-b. (*Hay et al, pp 38-39, 48, 608-609, 1178-1180. Kliegman et al, pp 755-756, 774 1195, 1527-1528, 1572-1574. McMillan et al, pp 389-397, 443, 1066-1067, 1930, 1932-1937. Rudolph et al, pp 140-143, 987, 1372, 1432-1434.*) Swallowed maternal blood can be differentiated from neonatal hemorrhage by the Apt test, which distinguishes fetal hemoglobin from adult hemoglobin based on the specimen's reaction to alkali (fetal hemoglobin is unchanged, whereas adult hemoglobin changes to hematin). Infants may swallow blood during delivery or from a cracked nipple during breast-feeding.

Necrotizing enterocolitis is a life-threatening condition seen mostly in premature infants. Although the precise etiology is unknown, contributing factors include GI tract ischemia, impaired host immunity, the presence of bacterial or viral pathogens, and the presence of breast milk or formula in the gut. Findings include bloody stools, abdominal distension, hypoxia, acidosis, and emesis. The initial diagnostic test of choice is plain film radiographs. The characteristic finding in necrotizing enterocolitis (NEC) is pneumatosis intestinalis; free air in the peritoneum may also be seen. Perforation is a surgical emergency, otherwise observation and antibiotics are indicated.

Enterohemorrhagic *Escherichia coli* are pathogens found in poorly cooked beef, and some have been responsible for outbreaks of bloody diarrhea that were well-publicized in the media. These organisms secrete shiga toxin. Routine stool cultures do not isolate this particular pathogen; the laboratory must use sorbitol-MacConkey agar to isolate the bacteria. Enzyme assays for shiga toxin are becoming available as well.

Forceful emesis can result in small tears in the esophagus, termed Mallory-Weiss syndrome. This is usually a benign condition, only occasionally resulting in significant blood loss. In a patient who is otherwise stable, diagnostic procedures are not indicated.

Peptic ulcer disease can result in hematemesis and melena, along with the typically epigastric abdominal pain. Children can have both chronic and acute blood loss associated with ulceration. Fiberoptic endoscopy is the diagnostic method of choice. An upper GI series can sometimes reveal an ulcer as well. While *H pylori* serum assays are available, they have limited usefulness in children.

269 to 274. The answers are 269-b, 270-f, 271-g, 272-c, 273-a, 274-d. *(Hay et al, pp 294-299. Kliegman et al, pp 242-264. McMillan et al, pp 113-114. Rudolph et al, pp 1322-1326.)* Treatment for tuberculosis usually includes the medication isoniazid (INH), and INH competitively inhibits pyridoxine utilization. In most children, this does not result in clinical manifestations, but in individuals with a poor dietary intake of pyridoxine (eg, teenagers, vegetarians, and exclusively breast-fed infants) numbness and tingling of the hands and feet may develop. Treatment is replacement of pyridoxine.

Cow's milk contains an insufficient quantity of iron to sustain normal RBC production. Therefore, children whose primary caloric source is cow's milk are likely to develop iron-deficiency anemia, characterized by microcytosis and hypochromia on the peripheral smear.

Hemorrhagic disease of the newborn is now rare, as the vast majority of newborns receive a vitamin K injection shortly after birth. Classic disease presents within the first week of life and is characterized by hematemesis, hematuria, umbilical stump and circumcision oozing, and purpura.

Vitamin C deficiency impairs wound healing. In its severe form, also termed *scurvy,* children can have diffuse tenderness, which is worse in the legs; evidence of hemorrhage; irritability; low-grade fever; swelling; tachypnea; and poor appetite. Diagnosis is based on clinical picture and radiographic findings; there are no definitive laboratory studies.

Vitamin A deficiency manifests first in visual changes, including night blindness. Deficiency can also cause drying of the conjunctivas and sclera. Skin is frequently dry. Poor growth and impaired cognition are also seen.

Vitamin D deficiency leads to rickets, a failure of bone mineralization, and the clinical picture described in the question. Vitamin D deficiency is usually not a problem in developed parts of the world. In addition to nutritional rickets, there are congenital forms of rickets. Despite vitamin D supplementation, these children can have permanent bony disfigurement.

275 to 277. The answers are 275-e, 276-c, 277-b. *(Hay et al, pp 496, 605, 608-609. Kliegman et al, pp, 1547, 1572-1574, 1732-1733. McMillan et al, pp 383, 721, 1932-1937. Rudolph et al, pp 1274, 1390, 1392, 1433-1434.)* An infant who gags and chokes while feeding may have an uncoordinated suck-swallow reflex, or may have significant gastroesophageal reflux. More rarely there may be an H-type tracheoesophageal fistula. A modified barium swallow with fluoroscopy allows direct visualization of the swallow reflex. In some situations during the modified barium swallow, the patient may be given different consistencies of food to document if thickened feeds decrease the dysphasia. A normal barium study does not, however, rule out a fistula.

The second patient's story is concerning for peptic ulcer disease. An upper GI series may show findings suggestive of the diagnosis, but endoscopy is the preferred diagnostic method, as it allows biopsy for microscopy and culture, and direct visualization.

The third child may have gastroesophageal reflux, causing Sandifer syndrome, a condition in which infants will arch and become tonic to protect their airway from the refluxing gastric contents. While an upper GI series can sometime diagnose gastroesophageal reflux, esophageal pH probe is currently the preferred diagnostic test.

The Urinary Tract

Questions

278. You are seeing a 4-year-old girl with the physical examination finding shown below. She has no significant past history. The most appropriate management is which of the following?

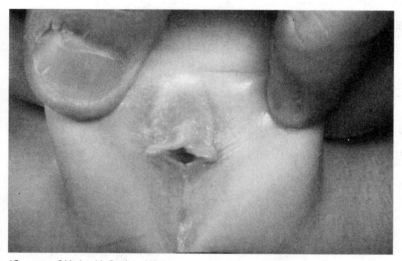

(Courtesy of Michael L. Ritchey, MD.)

a. Surgical consultation for correction
b. Topical estrogen cream daily for a week
c. Topical steroid cream for a week
d. Referral to social services for possible sexual abuse
e. Karyotype studies

279. At the 2-week checkup of a term female infant, the mother reports a grayish and sometimes bloody vaginal discharge since birth. The infant's mother and grandmother are the only caretakers. Examination of the external genitalia reveals an intact hymen with a thin grayish mucous discharge. Which of the following is the most appropriate next step?

a. Parental reassurance
b. MRI of the brain
c. Ultrasound of the abdomen
d. Gonorrhea and chlamydial swabs
e. Referral to social services for possible sexual abuse

280. The delivery of a newborn boy is remarkable for oligohydramnios. The infant (pictured) is also noted to have undescended testes and clubfeet, and to be in respiratory distress. Which of the following is the most likely diagnosis to explain these findings?

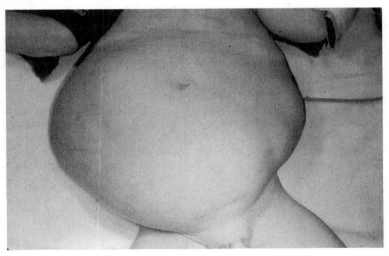

(Courtesy of Michael L. Ritchey, MD.)

a. Surfactant deficiency
b. Turner syndrome
c. Prune belly syndrome
d. Hermaphroditism
e. Congenital adrenal hyperplasia

281. A 17-year-old boy is brought to the emergency department by his parents with the complaint of coughing up blood. He is stabilized, and his hemoglobin and hematocrit levels are 11 mg/dL and 33%, respectively. During his hospitalization, he is noted to have systolic blood pressure persistently greater than 130 mm Hg and diastolic blood pressure greater than 90 mm Hg. His urinalysis is remarkable for hematuria and proteinuria. You are suspicious the patient has which of the following?

a. Hemolytic-uremic syndrome
b. Goodpasture syndrome
c. Nephrotic syndrome
d. Poststreptococcal glomerulonephritis
e. Renal vein thrombosis

282. A 1-year-old child presents with failure to thrive, frequent large voids of dilute urine, excessive thirst, and three episodes of dehydration not associated with vomiting or diarrhea. Over the years, other family members reportedly have had similar histories. Which of the following is the most likely diagnosis?

a. Water intoxication
b. Diabetes mellitus
c. Diabetes insipidus
d. Child abuse
e. Nephrotic syndrome

283. A 6-month-old infant has poor weight gain, vomiting, episodic fevers, and chronic constipation. Laboratory studies reveal a urinalysis with a pH of 8.0, specific gravity of 1.010, 1+ glucose, and 1+ protein. Urine anion gap is normal. Serum chemistries show a normal glucose and a normal albumin with a hyperchloremic metabolic acidosis. Serum phosphorus and calcium are low. What is the best diagnosis to explain these findings?

a. Renal tubular acidosis type 1
b. Renal tubular acidosis type 3
c. Renal tubular acidosis type 4
d. Hereditary Fanconi syndrome
e. Congenital nephrotic syndrome

284. The mother of a 2-year-old male child states that she has noticed white, cheeselike material arising from his foreskin and also that he cannot fully retract the foreskin behind the glans penis. Which of the following is the correct advice for this parent?

a. The child has phimosis and requires a circumcision.
b. The child has paraphimosis, and in addition to a circumcision, likely has an infection requiring topical antibiotics.
c. The child is normal.
d. The child likely has a previously undiagnosed hypospadias.
e. Ultrasound of kidneys, bladder, and ureters is indicated to check for unidentified associated defects.

285. After her first urinary tract infection, a 1-year-old has a voiding cystoure-throgram with findings shown below. Which of the following is the most appropriate treatment option?

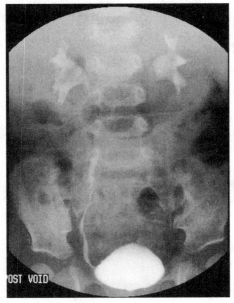

(Courtesy of Susan John, MD.)

a. Low-dose daily antibiotics
b. Immediate surgical reimplantation of the ureters
c. Weekly urinalyses and culture
d. Diet low in protein
e. Early toilet training

286. Physical examination of a baby boy shortly after birth reveals a large bladder and palpable kidneys. The nurses note that he produces a weak urinary stream. A voiding cystourethrogram is shown below. He appears to be otherwise normal. Which of the following is the most likely diagnosis?

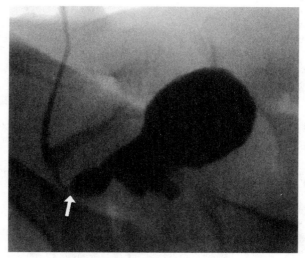

(Courtesy of Susan John, MD.)

a. Ureteropelvic junction obstruction
b. Posterior urethral valve
c. Prune belly syndrome
d. Duplication of the collecting system
e. Horseshoe kidney

287. A 5-year-old girl without past history of UTI is in the hospital on antibiotics for *Escherichia coli* pyelonephritis. She is still febrile after 4 days of appropriate antibiotics. A renal ultrasound revealed no abscess, but a focal enlargement of one of the lobes of the right kidney. CT of the abdomen reveals a wedge-shaped area in the right kidney distinct from the normal tissue with minimal contrast enhancement. Appropriate management of this patient includes which of the following interventions?

a. Prolonged antibiotic therapy
b. Routine treatment with 10 to 14 days of antibiotics for pyelonephritis
c. Surgical consultation
d. Dimercaptosuccinic acid (DMSA) scan
e. Renal biopsy

288. A 4-year-old boy, whose past medical history is positive for three urinary tract infections, presents with a blood pressure of 135/90 mm Hg. He is likely to exhibit which of the following symptoms or signs?

a. Multiple cranial nerve palsy
b. Headache
c. Hyporeflexia
d. Increased urine output
e. Right ventricular hypertrophy

289. The 1-year-old boy in the photograph below, who recently had a circumcision, requires an additional operation on his genitalia that will probably eliminate his risk of which of the following?

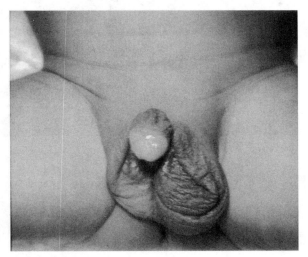

(Courtesy of Michael L. Ritchey, MD.)

a. Testicular malignancy
b. Decreased sperm count
c. Torsion of testes
d. Urinary tract infection
e. Epididymitis

290. A 6-week-old child is being evaluated for a fever of unknown etiology. As part of the laboratory evaluation, a urine specimen was obtained that grew *E coli* with a colony count of 2000/μL. These findings would be definite evidence of a urinary tract infection if which of the following is true about the sampled urine?

a. It has a specific gravity of 1.008.
b. It is from a bag attached to the perineum of an uncircumcised boy.
c. It is from an ileal-loop bag.
d. It is from a suprapubic tap.
e. It is the first morning sample.

291. A boy has returned home from visiting his grandmother in a rural area. He spent most of his time swimming, playing in the yard, helping in the gardens, and chasing his Chihuahua; his grandma says "he was generally dirty!" He was noted 2 weeks ago to have "infected mosquito bites" on his neck and chin for which the local doctor had him just scrub with soap; a few remain and are shown in the photograph below. His mother brings him into the office with the complaint of dark urine, swelling around his eyes, and shortness of breath. You also find him to have hypertension and hepatomegaly. Which of the following is the most likely cause of his problem?

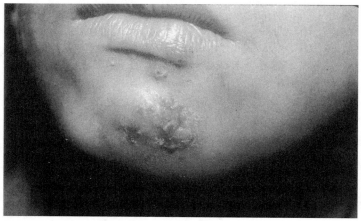

(Courtesy of Adelaide Hebert, MD.)

a. IgA nephropathy
b. Poststreptococcal glomerulonephritis
c. Idiopathic hypercalciuria
d. Pyelonephritis
e. Sexually transmitted disease

292. A 4-year-old boy and his family have recently visited a local amusement park. Several of the family members developed "gastroenteritis" with fever and diarrhea, but the 4-year-old's stool was slightly different, as it contained blood. His mother reports that in the past 24 hours he developed pallor and lethargy; she relates that his face looks swollen and that he has been urinating very little. Laboratory evaluation reveals a hematocrit of 28% and a platelet count of 72,000/μL. He has blood and protein in the urine. Which of the following diagnoses is most likely to explain these symptoms?

a. Henoch-Schönlein purpura
b. IgA nephropathy
c. Intussusception
d. Meckel diverticulum
e. Hemolytic-uremic syndrome

293. A 6-year-old girl is brought to the emergency room because her urine is red. She has been healthy her whole life, and has recently returned from an outing with her grandmother to a local amusement park. Her urine dip for heme is positive, suggesting which of the following is a possibility?

a. Ingestion of blackberries
b. Ingestion of beets
c. Phenolphthalein catharsis
d. Presence of myoglobin
e. Ingestion of Kool-Aid

294. The photomicrograph below is of a urine specimen from a 15-year-old girl. She has had intermittent fever, malaise, and weight loss over the previous several months. Recently she has developed swollen hands, wrists, and ankles, the pain of which seems out of proportion to the clinical findings. She also complains of cold extremities and has some ulceration of her distal digits. Which of the following laboratory tests is most likely to assist in the diagnosis of this condition?

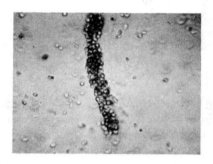

a. Antibodies to nDNA and Sm nuclear antigens
b. Throat culture for group A β-hemolytic streptococcus
c. Simultaneously acquired urine and serum bicarbonate levels
d. A urine culture
e. Erythrocyte sedimentation rate

295. A 12-year-old boy comes to the emergency department at midnight with a complaint of severe scrotal pain since 7 PM. There is no history of trauma. Which of the following is the most appropriate first step in management?

a. Order a surgical consult immediately.
b. Order a radioisotope scan as an emergency.
c. Order a urinalysis and Gram stain for bacteria.
d. Arrange for an ultrasound examination.
e. Order a Doppler examination.

296. The mother of a 2-year-old girl reports that her daughter complains of burning when she urinates and that she has foul-smelling discharge from her vagina. She has some slight staining on the front of her underwear, but denies fever, nausea, vomiting, or other constitutional signs. The child does not attend day care, and she has demonstrated no change in behavior. The physical examination is normal with an intact hymen, but the child's vulva is reddened and with a malodorous scent noted. Her urinalysis and culture are normal. Management of this condition includes which of the following?

a. Complete genitourinary (GU) examination under general anesthesia
b. Progesterone cream to the affected area for a week
c. Advice to stop taking prolonged bubble baths
d. Mebendazole to eradicate pinworm infestation
e. Referral to social services for possible sexual abuse

297. A 7-year-old boy has cramping abdominal pain and a rash mainly on the back of his legs and buttocks as well as on the extensor surfaces of his forearms. Laboratory analysis reveals proteinuria and microhematuria. You diagnose Henoch-Schönlein, or anaphylactoid, purpura. In addition to his rash and abdominal pain, what other finding is he likely to have?

a. Chronic renal failure
b. Arthritis or arthralgia
c. Seizures
d. Unilateral lymphadenopathy
e. Bulbar nonpurulent conjunctivitis

298. A 13-year-old boy's scrotum is shown below. He complains of several months of swelling but no pain just above his left testicle. He is sexually active but states that he uses condoms. On physical examination, the area in question feels like a "bag of worms." Which of the following is the most appropriate management for this condition?

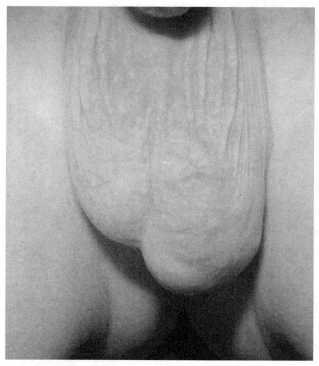

(Courtesy of Michael L. Ritchey, MD.)

  a. Doppler flow study of testes
  b. Radionuclide scan of testes
  c. Urinalysis and culture
  d. Ceftriaxone intramuscularly and doxycycline orally
  e. Reassurance and education only at this time

299. A 3-day-old infant's scrotum is shown below. Palpation reveals a tense, fluid-filled area surrounding the right testicle. The scrotum transilluminates well, and the amount of fluid does not vary with mild pressure. Which of the following is the most appropriate approach to this condition?

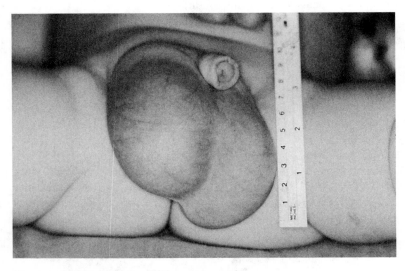

(Courtesy of Michael L. Ritchey, MD.)

a. Request a surgical consultation
b. Incision and drainage
c. Administer prophylactic antibiotics
d. Observe only
e. Perform a chromosome determination

300. A 2-year-old patient arrives late to your office with his father and a sign-language translator. They are very apologetic, but the father communicates that he had car trouble at his dialysis center and thus was late picking up the child from day care. The father is concerned about his child's having intermittent red, bloody-looking urine. A gross inspection of the child's urine in your office looks normal, but the dipstick demonstrates 3+ blood. Which of the following is the most likely cause of this child's hematuria?

a. Alport syndrome
b. Berger nephropathy (IgA nephropathy)
c. Idiopathic hypercalciuria
d. Membranous glomerulopathy
e. Goodpasture syndrome

301. A 9-year-old boy comes to the office for a pre-participation physical examination for summer camp. His parents report that he still has episodes of bed-wetting. The boy's father confides that he also had bed-wetting until he was 10. They are concerned about the bed-wetting, but they are more concerned about their son's upcoming week at summer camp and that the other boys may harass him for wetting the bed. Which of the following statements about nocturnal enuresis is correct?

a. The condition is three times more common in girls than boys.
b. Most patients with this condition have a psychiatric illness as the cause.
c. Spontaneous cure rates are high regardless of therapy.
d. Family history of this condition is uncommon.
e. Short courses of desmopressin acetate (DDAVP) lead to permanent cure in 50% of cases.

302. A 21-year-old woman presents to the emergency room in active labor. She has had no prenatal care, but her last menstrual period was approximately 9 months prior. Her membranes are artificially ruptured, yielding no amniotic fluid. She delivers an 1800-g (4-lb) term infant who develops significant respiratory distress immediately at birth. The first chest radiograph on this infant demonstrates hypoplastic lungs. After this infant is stabilized, which of the following is the most appropriate next step for this infant?

a. Cardiac catheterization
b. Renal ultrasound
c. MRI of the brain
d. Liver and spleen scan
e. Upper GI

Questions 303 to 306

For each condition listed below, match the category to which it belongs. Each lettered option may be used once, more than once, or not at all.

a. Nephrotic syndrome
b. Henoch-Schönlein purpura nephritis
c. Bartter syndrome
d. Acute glomerulonephritis
e. IgA nephropathy (Berger nephropathy)
f. Idiopathic hypercalciuria

303. An 8-year-old boy with the intermittent complaint of "burning" when he urinates and who has trace blood on his urine dip test.

304. A 6-year-old girl with a complaint of "dark urine"; she has a blood pressure of 120/80 mm Hg.

305. Elevated levels of cholesterol and triglycerides found in a 6-year-old boy whose mother reports that he has been awakening with puffy eyes each morning. On your physical examination you determine that he has had unexpected weight gain and has scrotal edema.

306. A 12-month-old girl whose height and weight are less than the fifth percentile; she has had several bouts of constipation and two previous admissions for dehydration. She is again admitted for dehydration and is noted to have serum potassium of 2.7 mEq/L.

The Urinary Tract

Answers

278. The answer is b. (*Kliegman et al, pp 2275-2276.*) The patient pictured has labial adhesions, a usually benign condition in which the labia minora are fused. Fusion ranges from a small area to the entire area between the clitoris and the fourchette. It is most common in young girls who are in the low-estrogen state of preadolescence. Sometimes urine pooling can cause an increased risk of urinary tract infection. Treatment can be merely observation, as the condition should resolve with the estrogenization that occurs with puberty. Nightly application of an estrogen cream for a week resolves this condition in the majority of patients. However, as recurrence is common, patients must be instructed to apply daily petrolatum for a month or two after separation.

279. The answer is a. (*Kliegman et al, p 2273. McMillan et al, p 197. Rudolph et al, p 90*). This patient has a physiologic discharge related to estrogen withdrawal. Examination can exclude vaginal trauma, and the history makes sexual abuse unlikely. Imaging is not indicated at this point. Parents should be reassured that it will resolve in a few weeks.

280. The answer is c. (*Hay et al, p 689. Kliegman et al, p 2240. McMillan et al, p 1834. Rudolph et al, pp 1737-1738.*) Prune belly syndrome, a malformation that occurs mostly in males, is characterized by a lax, wrinkled abdominal wall, a dilated urinary tract, and intra-abdominal testes. Additional urinary tract abnormalities include significant renal dysfunction or dysplasia. Oligohydramnios and commonly associated pulmonary complications, such as pulmonary hypoplasia and pneumothorax, are seen. Congenital hip dislocation, clubfeet, and intestinal malrotation with possible secondary volvulus can occur. There does not appear to be a genetic predisposition to prune belly syndrome.

281. The answer is b. (*Hay et al, pp 529-530. Kliegman et al, p 2180. McMillan et al, p 1439. Rudolph et al, p 1998.*) The patient in the question has a classic description of Goodpasture syndrome, a rare disease in children.

The pulmonary hemorrhage can be life threatening and the renal function progressive. Diagnosis is suggested by kidney biopsy and finding antibodies to the glomerular basement membrane.

Hemolytic-uremic syndrome presents in a child with fever, bloody diarrhea, and progression toward renal failure but not respiratory symptoms. Nephrotic syndrome presents with edema, hypertension, and proteinuria; respiratory symptoms related to congestive heart failure (and not pulmonary hemorrhage) might be seen. Poststreptococcal glomerulonephritis can result in hematuria, but the respiratory symptoms associated with the condition would be related to congestive heart failure and not to pulmonary hemorrhage. Renal vein thrombosis might result in hematuria but would not be expected to have pulmonary findings.

282. The answer is c. *(Hay et al, pp 703-704. Kliegman et al, pp 2200-2201, 2301. McMillan et al, pp 1901-1904. Rudolph et al, p 1714.)* Congenital nephrogenic diabetes insipidus is a hereditary disorder in which the urine is hypotonic and produced in large volumes because the kidneys fail to respond to antidiuretic hormone. Most North American patients thus involved are descendants of Ulster Scots who came to Nova Scotia in 1761 on the ship Hopewell. Males are primarily affected through an X-linked recessive inheritance causing inactivating mutation of the vasopressin V2 receptor; autosomal dominant and recessive forms are also known. The disorder is felt to result from primary unresponsiveness of the distal tubule and collecting duct to vasopressin. Although the condition is present at birth, the diagnosis is often not made until several months later, when excessive thirst, frequent voiding of large volumes of dilute urine, dehydration, and failure to thrive become obvious. Maintenance of adequate fluid intake and diet and use of saluretic medications (promoting the renal excretion of sodium) are the bases of therapy for this incurable disease. Acquired nephrogenic diabetes insipidus can be a result of lithium, methicillin, rifampin, and amphotericin. It may also be seen with hypokalemia, hypercalcemia, polycystic kidney disease, Sjögren syndrome, and sickle-cell disease.

Water intoxication would not present with episodes of dehydration; diabetes mellitus rarely presents with a protracted course in such a young child (it is usually a more acute illness and often with vomiting). Child abuse would be unlikely, especially with a family history as noted. Nephrotic syndrome would be expected to present with other signs such as edema and proteinuria.

283. The answer is d. *(Hay et al, pp 702-703. Kliegman et al, pp 2197-2198. McMillan et al, pp 1892-1897. Rudolph et al, pp 1709-1710.)* The nonspecific findings of anorexia, polydipsia and polyuria, vomiting, and unexplained fevers, along with the more specific laboratory abnormalities of glucosuria but normal blood sugar, abnormally high urine pH in the face of mild or moderate serum hyperchloremic metabolic acidosis, and mild albuminuria in the presence of normal serum protein and albumin, suggest Fanconi syndrome (FS, also called global proximal tubular dysfunction). FS can be hereditary or acquired; hereditary forms are usually secondary to a genetic abnormality such as cystinosis, galactosemia, Wilson disease, and some mitochondrial abnormalities. A number of agents can cause FS, including gentamicin (or other aminoglycosides), outdated tetracycline, cephalothin, cidofovir, valproic acid, streptozocin, 6-mercaptopurine, azathioprine, cisplatin, ifosfamide, heavy metals (eg, lead, mercury, cadmium, uranium, platinum), paraquat, maleic acid, and glue sniffing (toluene). The mechanism of action of these agents is through acute tubular necrosis, alteration of renal blood flow, intratubular obstruction, or allergic reactions within the kidney itself. Many of these toxic effects are reduced or eliminated with removal of the offending agent. Renal tubular acidosis (RTA) type 1 is a distal RTA, and has a positive urine anion gap, as does RTA type 4. Type 3 is not a recognized type of RTA. Congenital nephrotic syndrome is a rare version of nephrotic syndrome, characterized by edema early in infancy, with hypoalbuminemia.

284. The answer is c. *(Hay et al, pp 10-11. Kliegman et al, pp 2255-2256. McMillan et al, pp 200-201, 1830. Rudolph et al, p 1739.)* In about 90% of boys during their first 3 years of life, adhesions between the glans and the prepuce lyse and the distal portion of the foreskin loosens, thus allowing the glans to be exposed. The collection of cellular debris under the foreskin, extruded from under the foreskin, is sometimes deemed abnormal by parents; it requires no treatment. Phimosis (inability to retract the foreskin) is normal in the first years of life and is considered physiologic; inability to retract the foreskin after an age when it would be expected (about 3 years) is considered pathologic phimosis. Paraphimosis is a painful condition occurring when the foreskin gets retracted and trapped behind the glans and, because of edema and venous congestion, cannot be relocated into its normal position. Hypospadias is defined as a urethral opening on the ventral surface of the penile shaft, usually with an absent ventral portion of the prepuce. The general arguments in favor of circumcision include religious reasons; reduced risk of urinary tract infections and sexually transmitted diseases; and reduced rate of penile cancer, phimosis, and balanitis (inflammation of the glans). Phimosis is not associated with other abnormalities of the genitourinary system.

285. The answer is a. *(Hay et al, p 706. Kliegman et al, pp 2228-2234. McMillan et al, pp 1823-1824, 1839-1840. Rudolph et al, pp 1671-1673.)* The radiograph shows reflux into the ureters and into the kidney, with dilation of the renal pelvis, making the diagnosis of vesicoureteral reflux. The higher the reflux into the renal system, especially if the renal pelvis is dilated, the more likely it is for renal damage to occur; the grading system is based upon these radiographic observations. Grade I VUR is reflux of urine into an undilated ureter. Reflux into the ureter and collecting system without dilatation is called grade II. Grade III lesions have dilatation of the ureter and collecting system without blunting of the calyces. Grade IV lesions are characterized by blunting of the calyces, and grade V lesions demonstrate even more dilatation and tortuosity of the ureter. Low-grade lesions (grade I and grade II) are conservatively managed with close observation, daily low-dose antibiotics, and urinalyses and cultures every 3 to 4 months. Grade V lesions (and some grade IV lesions) require surgical reimplantation of a ureter if the findings persist. Lesions in between these two extremes are treatment dilemmas.

286. The answer is b. *(Kliegman, pp 2241-2242. McMillan, pp 1824-1826. Rudolph, pp 1735-1739.)* The findings described point to posterior urethral valves; the radiograph shows an area of obstruction and proximal dilatation of the bladder. The clinical picture of posterior valves ranges from that described in the question to severe renal obstruction with renal failure and pulmonary hypoplasia. Urinary tract infections are common complications in older children, and sepsis occasionally can be the presenting sign in afflicted newborns. Despite early recognition and correction of the obstruction, the prognosis in these children for normal renal function is guarded. Prenatal diagnosis is often accomplished because of widespread use of ultrasound.

Ureteropelvic junction obstruction, a common urinary obstruction in children that results in isolated hydronephrosis, can be found either on a prenatal ultrasound or after birth when the child is noted to have a mass, pain, or infection. Serial ultrasounds of the kidney assist in following the associated hydronephrosis. Prune belly syndrome occurs almost exclusively in males; it is diagnosed in a child with absent abdominal muscular tone, undescended testes, and urinary tract anomalies including hydronephrosis and dilated ureters and bladder. Duplication of the collecting system is often asymptomatic, but can present with symptoms of obstruction and reflux. Horseshoe kidney is often an asymptomatic condition, and results when both kidneys are joined at the lower pole by a fibrous band of tissue or by renal parenchyma; symptoms may arise resulting from obstruction and/or reflux.

287. The answer is a. *(Kliegman et al, pp 2223-2227. McMillan et al, p 1839. Rudolph et al, p 1669.)* The patient in the question has acute lobar nephronia, which is in the middle of the spectrum between pyelonephritis and renal abscess. Patients have prolonged fever curves despite appropriate antibiotics. A CT scan is most useful in diagnosing nephronia, but a renal ultrasound can identify the process as well. Treatment is prolonged IV and then PO antibiotics. Shorter courses like the typical treatment for pyelonephritis can lead to recurrence and renal abscess. Surgery and biopsy are not necessary, and a DMSA scan, while identifying alterations in flow consistent with pyelonephritis, would not add to the patient's care. (Note that there is an error in the McMillan text referenced above, referring to labor [sic] nephronia in both the figure accompanying the text as well as the index.)

288. The answer is b. *(Hay, pp 698-700. Kliegman, pp 1989-1995. McMillan, pp 1532-1536. Rudolph, pp 1877-1885.)* Blood pressures in children must be interpreted in relation to the child's age and height. Nomograms are available to assist in all general texts and on governmental websites. Routine BP measurement is performed on children of age 3 and beyond and for subgroups of children at younger ages, including children who were premature, had frequent urinary tract infection, had umbilical artery catheters, and so on. Hypertension is usually asymptomatic, but with marked hypertension (that which is demonstrated by this 4-year-old) children can develop headache, dizziness, visual disturbances, irritability, and nocturnal wakening. Hypertensive encepha-lopathy can be preceded or accompanied by vomiting, hyperreflexia, ataxia, and focal or generalized seizures. Isolated facial nerve palsy can be the sole manifestation of severe hypertension. Isolated left ventricular hypertrophy, decreased urine output, and abdominal bruits are possible. When marked fundoscopic changes are present or when there are signs of vascular compromise, emergency treatment of the accompanying hypertension is warranted. Such hypertensive persons require immediate hospitalization for diagnosis and therapy.

289. The answer is c. *(Hay et al, pp 967-968. Kliegman et al, pp 2260-2261. McMillan et al, pp 1831-1832. Rudolph et al, pp 1740-1742.)* The child in the photograph has an undescended testis, or cryptorchidism. By 6 months of life, 0.8% of boys born at term still have cryptorchidism. In adults with cryptorchidism, the risk of testicular malignancy is much higher than in unaffected men. Orchiopexy does not eliminate this risk, but repositioning the testes makes them accessible for periodic examinations. Whether the testes are brought into the scrotum or not, the sperm count can be reduced. The failure of the testes to develop, and their subsequent atrophy, can be detected by 6 months of age. Torsion of the testis is a potential risk because of the excessive mobility of the undescended testis. Orchiopexy helps to eliminate this problem. The incidence of UTI and epididymitis are not affected by the position of the testes.

290. The answer is d. (*Hay et al, pp 705-706. Kliegman et al, pp 2225-2226. McMillan et al, pp 438-439. Rudolph et al, p 1668.*) The mechanism by which urine is collected is paramount in determining the interpretation of cultures. No bacteria should grow in a properly obtained urine sample from a suprapubic tap unless infection is present. For children who undergo bladder catheterization, colony counts of 10^3 to 10^4 are considered significant. Ileal-loop bags are usually contaminated and are not useful. Bag specimens in smaller children (obtained by placing an adhesive, sealed, sterile collection system onto the perineum) can be helpful if the culture is negative. Contamination is common, especially in girls and in uncircumcised boys; positive cultures in this latter group of children, especially if they contain more than one organism, are suspect. In properly obtained midstream clean-catch urines, colony counts greater than 10^5 in the asymptomatic child and colony counts of 10^4 in the symptomatic child may be significant. Clean-catch urine samples in an uncircumcised male who cannot retract the foreskin are also suspect.

291. The answer is b. (*Hay et al, pp 689-690. Kliegman et al, pp 2173-2175. McMillan et al, pp 1856-1858. Rudolph et al, pp 1677-1681.*) Acute poststreptococcal glomerulonephritis follows a skin or throat infection with certain nephritogenic strains of group A β-hemolytic streptococci; the photograph demonstrates impetigo. Hematuria often colors the urine dark, and decreased urinary output can result in circulatory congestion from volume overload with pulmonary edema, periorbital edema, tachycardia, and hepatomegaly; these complications are avoided by fluid restriction. Acute hypertension is common and can be associated with headache, vomiting, and encephalopathy with seizures. Pyelonephritis and sexually transmitted diseases can cause bloody urine, but rarely present with impetigo. IgA nephropathy is rare in black children and rarely presents with hypertension. Idiopathic hypercalciuria presents with blood and renal stones, but the other findings are distinctly unusual. It should be noted that while "rheumatogenic" strains of group A streptococci are only associated with pharyngitis, "nephritogenic" strains can be associated with either pharyngeal or skin infections.

292. The answer is e. *(Hay et al, pp 694-695. Kliegman et al, pp 2181-2182. McMillan et al, pp 2600-2602. Rudolph et al, pp 1696-1698.)* Hemolytic-uremic syndrome is most common in children younger than 4 years of age and is characterized by an acute microangiopathic hemolytic anemia, thrombocytopenia from increased platelet utilization, and renal insufficiency from vascular endothelial injury and local fibrin deposition. Ischemic changes result in renal cortical necrosis and damage to other organs such as colon, liver, heart, brain, and adrenal. Laboratory findings associated with hemolytic-uremic syndrome include low hemoglobin level, decreased platelet count, hypoalbuminemia, and evidence of hemolysis on peripheral smear (burr cells, helmet cells, schistocytes). Urinalysis reveals hematuria and proteinuria. A marked reduction of renal function leads to oliguria and rising levels of blood urea nitrogen (BUN) and creatinine. Gastrointestinal bleeding and obstruction, ascites, and central nervous system findings such as somnolence, convulsions, and coma can occur. In the past decade, infection by the verotoxin-producing *E coli* 0157:H7 has been implicated as a cause of hemolytic-uremic syndrome. This organism is epizootic in cattle. Outbreaks associated with undercooked contaminated hamburgers have been reported in several states. Roast beef, cow's milk, and fresh apple cider have been implicated as well. The Coombs test is not positive in this type of hemolytic anemia.

Henoch-Schönlein purpura is a vasculitis that presents with petechial-like rash on the lower extremities (but the platelet count is normal); it is not usually associated with fever, but microscopic blood in the stool or urine are possible as is colicly abdominal pain. IgA nephropathy can cause hematuria, but none of the other findings in the question typically are noted. Intussusception is seen in children of this age, but the lack of episodic colicky abdominal pain or emesis makes this diagnosis unlikely. Meckel diverticulum causes painless bloody stool without fever or other associated symptoms; it does not cause anuria.

293. The answer is d. *(Hay et al, pp 685-687. Kliegman et al, pp 2168-2171. Rudolph et al, pp 1659-1660.)* A number of pH-dependent substances can impart a red color to urine. Use of phenolphthalein, a cathartic agent, or phenindione, an anticoagulant, can cause red urine; ingestion of blackberries, red Kool-Aid, or beets also can lead to red coloration ("beeturia"). None of these choices, however, would cause the heme test to be positive. Myoglobin, on the other hand, is the only choice listed that can test positive for heme. Myoglobinuria occurs in rhabdomyolysis with skeletal muscle damage and increased serum creatine kinase. Another possible cause of heme positive urine with no red cells is hemoglobinuria resulting from hemolysis. "Hematuria," therefore, should be confirmed by dipstick testing as well as by microscopic examination of urinary sediment.

294. The answer is a. (*Hay, pp 625-627, 689-690. Kliegman, pp 1015-1019, 2173-2175. McMillan, pp 1856-1858, 2543-2546. Rudolph, pp 847-850, 1687-1688.*) The figure accompanying the question depicts a red blood cell cast characteristically found in the urine of patients with glomerular disease. The fever, malaise, and weight loss as well as the arthritis involving mainly small joints are common findings of systemic lupus erythematosus (SLE). Raynaud phenomenon resulting in digital ulceration and gangrene in a few patients may also be seen. Not described in this patient is the oft-seen malar rash in a butterfly distribution across the bridge of the nose and the cheeks.

Simultaneous urine and serum electrolytes for bicarbonate determination hint at renal tubular acidosis that often presents with failure to thrive and unexplained acidosis, sometimes with repeated episodes of dehydration and anorexia. Poststreptococcal glomerulonephritis can present with red cell casts, but the symptoms usually develop 8 to 14 days after the acute throat infection. Urinary tract infections, especially of the upper system, can result in casts, but they would be expected to consist of white rather than red cells.

Elevation of the erythrocyte sedimentation rate may be found in SLE, but this is a nonspecific finding noted in many other chronic and acute inflammatory conditions; its diagnostic usefulness in this situation is limited.

295. The answer is a. (*Kliegman et al, p 2262. McMillan et al, p 1832. Rudolph et al, pp 1740-1741.*) The majority of all cases of acute scrotal pain and swelling in boys 12 years of age and older are caused by testicular torsion. If surgical exploration occurs within 4 to 6 hours, the testes can be saved 90% of the time. Too often, delay caused by scheduling imaging and laboratory tests, such as those outlined in the question, results in an unsalvageable gonad.

One of the more important diagnoses in the differential is epididymitis. It is often gradual in onset, and the physical examination usually will reveal the testicle to be in its normal vertical position and to be of equal size to its counterpart. Epididymitis usually presents with redness, warmth, and scrotal swelling (but normal cremasteric reflex); the pain is posterior (over the epididymis). Pain relief upon elevation of the testicle (Prehn sign) may be helpful to diagnose epididymitis although it is not specific.

296. The answer is c. (*Hay et al, pp 142-143. Kliegman et al, pp 2274-2278.*) The symptoms listed are those of vulvovaginitis, with nonspecific (or chemical) vulvovaginitis accounting for 70% of all pediatric vulvovaginitis cases. The discharge in nonspecific vulvovaginitis is usually brown or green and with a fetid odor. The burning with urination occurs because of contact between raw skin and urine. Further history in this case might reveal use of tight-fitting clothing (including swimsuits or dance outfits), nylon undergarments, prolonged bubble baths with contamination of the vagina with soap products, use of perfumed lotions in the vaginal area, or improper toilet habits (wiping of fecal material toward rather than away from vagina). Attention to these causative conditions usually results in resolution of the symptoms. The finding of a normal hymen, the history of a single caretaker, and the absence of behavioral changes all point away from, but do not completely exclude, sexual abuse. A vaginal examination under general anesthesia is usually required when a vaginal foreign body is suspected. Pinworms can infest the vagina, but symptoms usually include significant itching of the rectum and vagina. Estrogen cream, as well as antibiotic creams, are sometimes helpful in reducing the discomfort of vaginitis. In a sexually active adolescent (or in a sexually abused younger child), a variety of infectious agents, such as candida, *Chlamydia trachomatis, Trichomonas vaginalis, Gardnerella vaginalis,* and *Neisseria gonorrhoeae,* would be higher on the differential.

297. The answer is b. (*Hay et al, pp 690, 871. Kliegman et al, pp 1043-1045. McMillan et al, pp 2559-2562. Rudolph et al, pp 842-844, 1688-1689.*) Henoch-Schönlein purpura (HSP), or anaphylactoid purpura, is a systemic IgA-mediated vasculitis. The rash of anaphylactoid purpura most often involves extensor surfaces of the extremities; the face, soles, palms, and trunk are less often affected. Other significant symptoms include edema, arthralgia or arthritis, colicky abdominal pain with GI bleeding, acute scrotal pain, and renal abnormalities ranging from microscopic hematuria to acute renal failure. As HSP is a systemic vasculitis, any organ system can be affected.

The prognosis, however, is excellent, with only a small percentage of children going on to end-stage renal failure. Seizures are an uncommon complication of CNS involvement; more commonly, patients will complain of headache and will have behavioral changes. Unilateral lymphadenopathy and non-purulent conjunctivitis are not typical of HSP (but are criteria for Kawasaki disease, another pediatric vasculitis).

298. The answer is e. *(Kliegman et al, pp 2263, 2264 (photo). McMillan et al, pp 1832-1833. Rudolph et al, p 1742.)* Varicocele, a common condition seen after 10 years of age, occurs in about 15% of adult males. It results from the dilatation of the pampiniform venous plexus (usually on the left side) due to valvular incompetence of the spermatic vein. Reduced sperm counts are possible with this condition; surgery may ultimately be indicated for infertility problems. Typically, this condition is not painful but can become tender with strenuous exercise. Its typical "bag of worms" appearance on palpation makes its diagnosis apparent in most cases. For a 13-year-old boy, reassurance and education seem appropriate.

A Doppler flow study of testes or a radionuclide scan might be indicated if the area were painful and the diagnosis of a torsion were being entertained. The child does not have evidence of a urinary tract infection (dysuria or fever) so a urinalysis and culture are unlikely to be helpful. If this sexually active child had painful testes and the diagnosis of epididymitis were being entertained, then ceftriaxone intramuscularly and doxycycline orally might be considered.

299. The answer is d. *(Hay et al, p 618. Kliegman et al, p 2264. McMillan et al, p 1832. Rudolph et al, p 1742.)* The description is that of a hydrocele, an accumulation of fluid in the tunica vaginalis. Small hydroceles usually resolve spontaneously in the first year of life. Larger ones or those that have a variable fluid level with time will likely need surgical repair. This is a common condition affecting 2% of males; thus, chromosomes are not indicated. Incision and drainage and antibiotics are not indicated for this developmental condition.

300. The answer is a. *(Hay et al, p 691. Kliegman et al, pp 2172-2173. McMillan et al, pp 1875-1878. Rudolph et al, pp 1699-1700.)* The most common type of hereditary nephritis is Alport syndrome. Clinically, patients present with asymptomatic microscopic hematuria, but gross hematuria is also possible, especially after an upper respiratory infection. Hearing loss, eventually leading to deafness, is associated with Alport syndrome in 30% to 75% of cases. End-stage renal disease, as hinted in the question (the father was at a dialysis center), is common by the second or third decades of life. This syndrome is mostly commonly an X-linked dominant disorder, which explains the more severe course in males. Other findings include ocular abnormalities (30% to 40%) and, rarely, leiomyomatosis of the esophagus or respiratory tree.

Berger nephropathy (IgA nephropathy) results from IgA deposits within the mesangium of the glomerulus in the absence of systemic disease; it can be associated with microscopic or gross hematuria, but is not associated with a heredity condition resulting in deafness and end-stage renal disease. Idiopathic hypercalciuria, which may be autosomal dominant, causes recurrent gross hematuria, persistent microscopic hematuria, and complaints of dysuria or abdominal pain without stone formation. Membranous glomerulopathy is an unusual cause of hematuria in children occurring in the second decade of life when seen; it is the most common cause of nephritic syndrome in adults. It usually presents with signs and symptoms of nephrotic syndrome. Goodpasture syndrome results in pulmonary hemorrhages in addition to the signs and symptoms of glomerulonephritis; it is a rare disease in children.

301. The answer is c. (*Hay et al, pp 204-206. Kliegman et al, pp 2249-2250. McMillan et al, pp 670-672. Rudolph et al, pp 1742-1743.*) Nocturnal enuresis is involuntary voiding at night at an age when control of micturition is expected. Nocturnal enuresis can be split into two categories: primary nocturnal enuresis, when the child has never been dry at night; and secondary nocturnal enuresis, when the child has had a few months of dry nights before developing enuresis. By 5 years of age, most children (90%-95%) are completely dry during the day, and 80% to 85% are dry during the night. Over the years, the incidence of nocturnal enuresis decreases, dropping to 7% at 7 to 8 years of age, and down to 1% at 14. A careful history and physical examination will usually identify any potential organic causes. In most cases, no etiology is found. A family history is common. Minimal laboratory testing beyond screening urinalysis is indicated. The condition is more common in boys than in girls. Therapy is aimed at reassurance to the parents that the condition is self-limited, avoidance of punitive measures, and consideration of purchasing a bed-wetting alarm. Spontaneous cure rates are high regardless of therapy. Short courses of desmopressin (a synthetic analog of antidiuretic hormone) lead to control in 60% to 75% of cases while the patient takes the medication, and would be appropriate to consider in this boy and in other situations in which patients need episodic control of their enuresis. However, desmopressin is not a cure, and episodes frequently return when the medication is stopped.

302. The answer is b. *(Hay et al, p 1044. Kliegman et al, p 2221. McMillan et al, pp 405-406, 1850-1851. Rudolph et al, p 1639.)* Oligohydramnios can cause a number of serious problems in the infant, including constraint deformities (such as clubfoot) and pulmonary hypoplasia. These infants have usually experienced intrauterine growth retardation and frequently have an associated serious renal abnormality. Ultrasound of the kidneys is important to rule out renal involvement as a cause of the oligohydramnios. None of the other testing would be expected to identify an etiology for the oligohydramnios and pulmonary hypoplasia, although this child's ultimate clinical course might necessitate additional testing. The finding of bilateral renal agenesis is termed Potter sequence.

303-306. The answers are 303-f, 304-d, 305-a, 306-c. *(Hay et al, pp 689-693, 703, 871. Kliegman et al, pp 1043-1045, 2173-2175, 2178-2179, 2184, 2190-2195, 2201-2202. McMillan et al, pp 1854-1856, 1858-1859, 1864-1874, 1904-1906, 1912, 2559-2562. Rudolph et al, pp 1677-1686, 1710-1713.)* Idiopathic hypercalciuria causes recurrent gross hematuria, persistent microscopic hematuria, and complaints of dysuria or abdominal pain without initial stone formation. Over time, however, stones may form in 15% of cases.

With acute glomerulonephritis, oliguria (often presenting with dark, cola-colored urine) frequently occurs as a direct consequence of the disease process itself; on occasion, it can be profound, with virtual anuria for several days. During this period of time, it is vital to monitor and restrict fluid intake lest massive edema, hypervolemia, and even pulmonary edema and death occur.

Elevated levels of cholesterol and triglycerides are common in nephrotic syndrome because of increased generalized protein synthesis in the liver (including lipoproteins) and because of a decrease in lipid metabolism due to reduced plasma lipoprotein lipase levels. In the nephrotic syndrome, albumin is lost in the urine and, despite increased hepatic synthesis, serum levels drop. The upper limit of protein excretion in healthy children is 0.15 g/24 h; in nephrotic syndrome, proteinuria can exceed 2.0 g/24 h. When the serum protein level drops low enough, the oncotic pressure of the plasma becomes too low to balance the hydrostatic pressure. Plasma volume, therefore, decreases as edema occurs. Periorbital edema in the morning and scrotal edema in boys during the day is commonly reported. Endocrine and renal mechanisms then partially compensate by retaining water and salt. Overzealous monitoring and restriction of water and salt intake are usually not required.

Hypertension commonly accompanies glomerulonephritis, but only occasionally accompanies nephrotic syndrome. Diuretics are sometimes used in both nephrotic syndrome and glomerulonephritis with temporary effect, but are not curative. A combination of albumin infusions followed by a diuretic also has been used to temporarily decrease the edema in patients with nephrotic syndrome. Because both illnesses are usually self-limited, temporary measures are important. In all cases, blood pressure must be evaluated for the age of the child (eg, the 6-year-old girl with a blood pressure of 120/80 mm Hg is significantly hypertensive).

Bartter syndrome (also known as juxtaglomerular hyperplasia) is an autosomal recessive condition that causes hypokalemia, hypercalciuria, alkalosis, hyperaldosteronism, and hyperreninemia; blood pressure is usually normal. Clinical presentations occurring frequently between 6 and 12 months of age include failure to thrive with constipation, weakness, vomiting, polyuria, and polydipsia. Treatment is aimed at preventing dehydration, providing nutritional support, and returning the potassium level to normal.

Henoch-Schönlein purpura nephritis presents with a purpuric rash, arthritis, and abdominal pain, and has an associated glomerulonephritis that can cause gross or microscopic hematuria. IgA (Berger) nephropathy is the most common chronic glomerulonephritis. Initially thought to be benign, it is now known to progress over decades to chronic renal failure in many afflicted patients. IgA is found in the mesangium, but this occurs with other disease processes as well. The most common clinical finding is hematuria; episodic gross hematuria is frequently associated with a febrile illness.

The Neuromuscular System

Questions

307. A 6-year-old child has had repeated episodes of otitis media. She undergoes an uneventful surgical placement of pressure-equalization (PE) tubes. In the recovery room she develops a fever of 40°C (104°F), rigidity of her muscles, and metabolic and respiratory acidosis. Which of the following is the most likely explanation for her condition?

a. Otitis media
b. Septicemia
c. Malignant hyperthermia
d. Dehydration
e. Febrile seizure

308. The 7-year-old boy now in your office was last seen 2 weeks ago with a mild viral upper respiratory tract infection. Today, however, he presents with fever, ataxia, weakness, headache, and emesis. In the office he has a 3 minute left-sided tonic-clonic seizure. You send him to the hospital and order a magnetic resonance imaging (MRI) of the brain, the results of which show disseminated multifocal white matter lesions that enhance with contrast. This boy's likely diagnosis is which of the following?

a. Multiple sclerosis
b. Acute disseminated encephalomyelitis
c. Malignant astrocytoma
d. Bacterial meningitis
e. Neurocysticercosis

309. The examination of a child's back is shown below. Evaluation with ultrasound of this lesion may demonstrate which of the following?

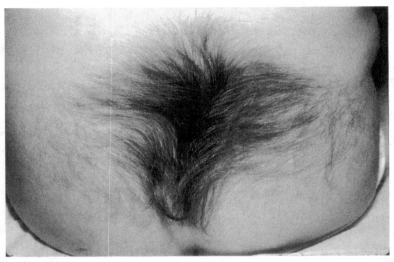

(Courtesy of Adelaide Hebert, MD.)

a. Epstein pearl
b. Mongolian spot
c. Cephalohematoma
d. Omphalocele
e. Occult spina bifida

310. A 6-month-old child was noted to be normal at birth, but over the ensuing months you have been somewhat concerned about his slowish weight gain and his mild delay in achieving developmental milestones. The family calls you urgently at 7:00 AM noting that their child seems unable to move the right side of his body. Which of the following conditions might explain this child's condition?

a. Phenylketonuria
b. Homocystinuria
c. Cystathioninuria
d. Maple syrup urine disease
e. Histidinemia

311. On a newborn boy's first examination, you note a prominent occiput, a broad forehead, and an absent anterior fontanelle. The baby's head is long and narrow. The remainder of the physical examination, including a careful neurological evaluation, is normal. You note that the baby was born via cesarean section for cephalopelvic disproportion. When you enter the mother's room, the first question she asks is about her baby's head shape. Which of the following is the most appropriate statement to the mother about this infant's condition?

a. The condition is usually associated with other genetic defects.
b. The condition is usually associated with hydrocephalus.
c. Patients with this condition usually develop seizures.
d. The condition is associated with pituitary abnormalities.
e. The condition requires referral to a surgeon.

312. A 4-year-old child is observed to hold his eyelids open with his fingers and to close one eye periodically, especially in the evening. He has some trouble swallowing his food. He usually appears sad, although he laughs often enough. He can throw a ball, and he runs well. Which of the following is most likely to aid in the diagnosis?

a. Muscle biopsy
b. Creatine phosphokinase (CPK)
c. Effect of a test dose of edrophonium
d. Chest x-ray
e. Antinuclear antibodies (ANAs)

313. A 14-year-old girl with a history of seizures is admitted to the hospital with the diagnosis of status epilepticus. Her valproic acid level is in the therapeutic range. You arrange a 24-hour video electroencephalogram (EEG). During the EEG, she has several episodes of tonic and clonic movements with moaning and crying, with no loss of bowel or bladder control. The neurologist tells you that during the events the EEG had excessive muscle artifact but no epileptiform discharges. Which of the following treatments is the most appropriate for this condition?

a. Add a scheduled benzodiazepine for her muscular symptoms
b. Add carbamazepine to her current seizure medication
c. Increase her dose of valproic acid
d. Withdraw all seizure medications
e. Request a psychiatric evaluation

314. A previously healthy 7-year-old child suddenly complains of a headache and falls to the floor. When examined in the emergency room (ER), he is lethargic and has a left central facial weakness and left hemiparesis with conjugate ocular deviation to the right. Which of the following is the most likely diagnosis?

a. Hemiplegic migraine
b. Supratentorial tumor
c. Todd paralysis
d. Acute subdural hematoma
e. Acute infantile hemiplegia

315. A 5-month-old child was normal at birth, but the family reports that the child does not seem to look at them any longer. They also report the child seems to "startle" more easily than he had before. Testing of his white blood cells (WBCs) identifies the absence of β-hexosaminidase A activity, confirming the diagnosis of which of the following?

a. Niemann-Pick disease, type A
b. Infantile Gaucher disease
c. Tay-Sachs disease
d. Krabbe disease
e. Fabry disease

316. The family of a 4-year-old boy has just moved into your area. The child was recently brought to the emergency department (ED) for an evaluation of abdominal pain. Although appendicitis was ruled out in the ED and the child's abdominal pain has resolved, the ED physician requested that the family follow up in your office to evaluate an incidental finding of an elevated creatine kinase. The family notes that he was a late walker (began walking independently at about 18 months of age), that he is more clumsy than their daughter was at the same age (especially when trying to hold onto small objects), and that he seems to be somewhat sluggish when he runs, climbs stairs, rises from the ground after he sits, and rides his tricycle. A thorough history and physical examination are likely to reveal which of the following?

a. Hirsutism
b. Past seizure activity
c. Proximal muscle atrophy
d. Cataracts
e. Enlarged gonads

317. A 9-year-old girl is brought by her sister to her pediatrician with the complaint of severe, intermittent headaches for the past several months, one of which resulted in her going to the ER. The physical examination today, including a careful neurologic examination, is normal. The headache is diffuse, throbbing, lasts several hours, and is not associated with vomiting or other symptoms. The child cannot feel the headaches coming on; they appear on all days of the week; and usually the headaches are gone when she awakens from a nap. The child reports that she is doing well in school, plays clarinet in the school band, and has "lots of friends." The sister is not sure, but she thinks their father, who lives in another state, may have headaches. The most likely explanation for this girl's headache is which of the following?

a. Migraine
b. Tension headache
c. Brain tumor
d. Sinusitis
e. Fungal meningitis

318. Examination of the cerebrospinal fluid (CSF) of an 8-year-old, mildly febrile child with nuchal rigidity and intermittent stupor shows the following: WBCs 85/μL (all lymphocytes), negative Gram stain, protein 150 mg/dL, and glucose 15 mg/dL. A computed tomographic (CT) scan with contrast shows enhancement of the basal cisterns by the contrast material. Which of the following is the most likely diagnosis?

a. Tuberous sclerosis
b. Tuberculous meningitis
c. Stroke
d. Acute bacterial meningitis
e. Pseudotumor cerebri

319. An irritable 6-year-old child has a somewhat unsteady but nonspecific gait. Physical examination reveals a very mild left facial weakness, brisk stretch reflexes in all four extremities, bilateral extensor plantar responses (Babinski reflex), and mild hypertonicity of the left upper and lower extremities; there is no muscular weakness. Which of the following is the most likely diagnosis?

a. Pontine glioma
b. Cerebellar astrocytoma
c. Tumor of the right cerebral hemisphere
d. Subacute sclerosing panencephalitis
e. Progressive multifocal leukoencephalopathy

320. A 2-year-old boy has been doing well despite his diagnosis of tetralogy of Fallot. He presented to an outside ER a few days ago with a complaint of an acute febrile illness for which he was started on a "pink antibiotic." His mother reports that for the past 12 hours or so he has had a headache and is more lethargic than normal. On your examination he seems to have a severe headache, nystagmus, and ataxia. Which of the following would be the most appropriate first test to order?

a. Urine drug screen
b. Blood culture
c. Lumbar puncture
d. CT or MRI of the brain
e. Stat echocardiogram

321. A 6-year-old child is hospitalized for observation because of a short period of unconsciousness after a fall from a playground swing. He has developed unilateral pupillary dilatation, focal seizures, recurrence of depressed consciousness, and hemiplegia. Which of the following is the most appropriate management at this time?

a. Spinal tap
b. CT scan
c. Rapid fluid hydration
d. Naloxone
e. Gastric decontamination with charcoal

322. A 6-year-old boy is seen in the office for evaluation of polyuria. Further questioning reveals several months of headache with occasional emesis. Your physical examination reveals a child who is less than 5% for weight. He has mild papilledema. His glucose is normal, and his first urine void specific gravity after a night without liquids is 1.005 g/mL. Which of the following might also be expected to be seen in this patient?

a. Sixth nerve palsy
b. Unilateral cerebellar ataxia
c. Unilateral pupillary dilatation
d. Unilateral anosmia
e. Bitemporal hemianopsia

323. A 6-year-old boy had been in his normal state of good health until a few hours prior to presentation to the ER room. His mother reports that he began to have difficulty walking, and she noticed that he was falling and unable to maintain his balance. Which of the following is the most likely cause for his condition?

a. Drug intoxication
b. Agenesis of the corpus callosum
c. Ataxia telangiectasia
d. Muscular dystrophy
e. Friedreich ataxia

324. A 9-year-old child has developed headaches that are more frequent in the morning and are followed by vomiting. Over the previous few months, his family has noted a change in his behavior (generally more irritable than usual) and his school performance has begun to drop. Imaging of this child is most likely to reveal a lesion in which of the following regions?

a. Subtentorial
b. Supratentorial
c. Intraventricular
d. Spinal canal
e. Peripheral nervous system

325. A young infant is noted to have developed constipation over the past week, and then facial diplegia and difficulty sucking and swallowing. The child has been colicky, and the maternal grandmother has been treating the child with a mixture of weak tea, rice water, and honey. Which of the following disorders is the most likely culprit in this child?

a. Infantile spinal muscular atrophy
b. Myasthenia gravis
c. Congenital myotonic dystrophy
d. Duchenne muscular dystrophy
e. Botulism

326. At birth, an infant is noted to have an abnormal neurologic examination. Over the next few weeks he develops severe progressive central nervous system (CNS) degeneration, an enlarged liver and spleen, macroglossia, coarse facial features, and a cherry-red spot in the eye. Which of the following laboratory findings most likely explains this child's problem?

a. Reduced serum hexosaminidase A activity
b. Deficient activity of acid β-galactosidase
c. Defective gene on the X chromosome
d. Complete lack of acid β-galactosidase activity
e. Deficient activity of galactosyl-3-sulfate-ceramide sulfatase (cerebroside sulfatase)

327. The parents of a 2-year-old bring her to the emergency center after she had a seizure. Although the parents report she was in a good state of health, the vital signs in the emergency center reveal a temperature of 39°C (102.2°F). She is now running around the room. Which part of the story would suggest the best outcome in this condition?

a. A CSF white count of 100/μL.
b. Otitis media on examination.
c. The seizure lasted 30 minutes.
d. The child was born prematurely with an intraventricular hemorrhage.
e. The family reports the child to have had right-sided tonic-clonic activity only.

328. About 12 days after a mild upper respiratory infection, a 12-year-old boy complains of weakness in his lower extremities. Over several days, the weakness progresses to include his trunk. On physical examination, he has the weakness described and no lower extremity deep tendon reflexes, muscle atrophy, or pain. Spinal fluid studies are notable for elevated protein only. Which of the following is the most likely diagnosis in this patient?

a. Bell palsy
b. Muscular dystrophy
c. Guillain-Barré syndrome
d. Charcot-Marie-Tooth disease
e. Werdnig-Hoffmann disease

329. The developmentally delayed 6-month-old child in the picture below had intrauterine growth retardation (including microcephaly), hepatospleno-megaly, prolonged neonatal jaundice, and purpura at birth. The calcific densities in the skull x-ray shown are likely the result of which of the following?

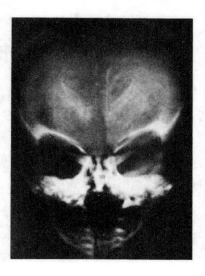

a. Congenital cytomegalovirus (CMV) infection
b. Congenital toxoplasmosis infection
c. Congenital syphilis infection
d. Tuberculous meningitis
e. Craniopharyngioma

330. The infant pictured below develops infantile spasms. Which of the following disorders is most likely to be affecting this infant?

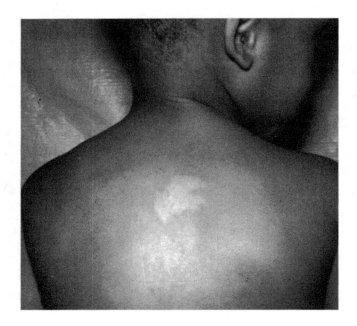

a. Neurofibromatosis
b. Tuberous sclerosis
c. Incontinentia pigmenti
d. Pityriasis rosea
e. Psoriasis

331. A newborn infant has respiratory distress and trouble feeding in the nursery. The mother has no significant medical history, but the pregnancy was complicated by decreased fetal movement. On physical examination, you note that aside from shallow respirations and some twitching of the fingers and toes, the infant is not moving, and is very hypotonic. In the mouth there is pooled saliva and you note tongue fasciculations. Deep tendon reflexes are absent. Spinal fluid is normal. Appropriate statements about this condition include which of the following statements?

a. The condition is caused by the absence of the muscle cytoskeletal protein dystrophin.
b. The condition is caused by the degeneration of anterior horn cells in the spinal cord.
c. The condition is caused by the antibodies that bind the acetylcholine receptor at the postsynaptic muscle membrane.
d. The condition is caused by progressive autoimmune demyelination.
e. The condition is caused by birth trauma.

332. A 3-year-old boy's parents complain that their child has difficulty walking. The child rolled, sat, and first stood at essentially normal ages and first walked at 13 months of age. Over the past several months, however, the family has noticed an increased inward curvature of the lower spine as he walks and that his gait has become more "waddling" in nature. On examination, you confirm these findings and also notice that he has enlargement of his calves. Which of the following is the most likely diagnosis?

a. Occult spina bifida
b. Muscular dystrophy
c. Brain tumor
d. Guillain-Barré syndrome
e. Botulism

333. Your 6-year-old son awakens at 1:00 AM screaming. You note that he is hyperventilating, is tachycardic, and has dilated pupils. He cannot be consoled, does not respond, and is unaware of his environment. After a few minutes, he returns to normal sleep. He recalls nothing the following morning. Which of the following is the most likely diagnosis?

a. Seizure disorder
b. Night terrors
c. Drug ingestion
d. Psychiatric disorder
e. Migraine headache

334. A previously healthy 16-year-old girl presents to the emergency center with the complaint of "falling out." She was with her friends at a local fast food restaurant when she felt faint and, according to her friends, lost consciousness for about a minute. There was no seizure activity noted, but the friends did notice her arms twitching irregularly. She is now acting normally. She denies chest pain or palpitations, and her electrocardiogram (ECG) is normal. Further management of this patient should include which of the following?

a. Obtain an EEG
b. Refer to a child psychiatrist
c. Begin β-blocker therapy
d. Encourage adequate fluid and salt intake
e. Obtain serum and urine drug screens

Questions 335 to 337

Headache in children can often be a concerning symptom to parents, but usually can be explained with a careful history and physical examination. Choose the headache associated with the clinical presentation listed below. Each lettered option may be used once, more than once, or not at all.

a. Tension headache
b. Factitious headache
c. Vascular headache (migraine)
d. Increased intracranial pressure
e. Hemiplegic migraine

335. A 15-year-old girl has an acute, recurrent, pulsatile headache localized behind the eyes that tends to occur more frequently around menses. She has no symptoms that occur prior to the headache; her neurologic examination is normal.

336. A 7-year-old boy has chronic, worsening headache without preceding symptoms. He complains of emesis in the morning before breakfast for the last 2 weeks.

337. A 12-year-old boy has chronic headache that worsens during the school day. These headaches are not associated with nausea or emesis, and he does not have any symptoms prior to the headache.

Questions 338 to 340

For each description, select the most likely diagnosis. Each lettered option may be used once, more than once, or not at all.

a. Transient tic disorder of childhood
b. Tourette syndrome
c. Sydenham chorea
d. Dystonia
e. Cerebral palsy

338. Eye blinking or throat-clearing noises in an otherwise healthy 8-year-old boy.

339. A 6-year-old boy with eye twitching and echolalia.

340. An 8-year-old hospitalized boy with unusual "spasms" of his neck and arms shortly after receiving Phenergan for nausea caused by his chemotherapy.

Questions 341 to 343

For each diagnosis listed, select the most common clinical sign or symptom. Each lettered option may be used once, more than once, or not at all.

a. A 6-month-old with blindness on the same side as a large facial lesion
b. An infant with infantile spasms, a hypsarrhythmic EEG pattern, and ash-leaf depigmentation on her back
c. An 18-year-old with a history of fractures and optic gliomas, who now has developed a malignant schwannoma
d. A 2-year-old with multiple episodes of skin infection and failure to thrive
e. A 14-year-old girl with a history of precocious puberty who now develops a large goiter

341. Neurofibromatosis type 1

342. PHACE syndrome

343. Tuberous sclerosis

The Neuromuscular System

Answers

307. The answer is c. (*Hay et al, pp 331-332. Kliegman et al, p 2552. McMillan et al, p 2326. Rudolph et al, p 2296.*) In addition to the findings listed in the question, patients experiencing malignant hyperthermia (MH) also have clinical findings of tachycardia, arrhythmia, tachypnea, and cyanosis, as well as laboratory findings of myoglobinuria, elevated serum creatine kinase levels, and evidence of acute renal failure. This myopathy is usually inherited as an autosomal dominant trait; the gene is on chromosome 19 and codes for the ryanodine receptor, a calcium release channel. A family history of similarly affected relatives would suggest the need to evaluate all family members for this condition; prevention (or treatment) is with dantrolene sodium. The test of choice to identify a patient at risk for this condition is the caffeine contracture test, in which a muscle biopsy tissue specimen is attached to a strain gauge and then exposed to caffeine. Patients at risk for malignant hyperthermia have a diagnostic muscle spasm.

Otitis media would have been diagnosed during the surgical procedure. An uneventful, minor surgical procedure such as PE tube placement is not likely to result in septicemia, nor would it be anticipated to be noted so quickly. Dehydration, especially in a newborn, can cause mild elevation of temperature, but this child is too old for this to be seen. Febrile seizures are rare beyond 5 years of age.

308. The answer is b. (*Kliegman et al, pp 2506-2507. McMillan et al, p 2263. Rudolph et al, p 2314.*) Acute disseminated encephalomyelitis (ADEM) is an autoimmune-demyelinating disease seen in children less than 10 years of age. It may follow many different types of infections, including upper respiratory tract infections, varicella, mycoplasma, herpes simplex virus, rubella, rubeola, and mumps; it may also follow immunizations. The history and physical examination is similar to multiple sclerosis; differences include age of onset (ADEM is usually seen in < 10-year olds), the presence of systemic findings like fever and emesis, and the lack of progression in the lesions once identified. Mortality is high, with 10% to 30% of affected patients dying. Treatment is high-dose corticosteroids. Meningitis is not usually diagnosed with MRI, but rather a lumbar puncture. Malignancies and neurocysticercosis (CNS infection by the tapeworm *Taenia solium*) do not present with the MRI findings described.

309. The answer is e. *(Kliegman et al, pp 2443-2444. McMillan et al, p 266. Rudolph et al, p 2185.)* The child in the photograph has a hairy nevus over the spine; virtually any abnormality (except Mongolian spots) over the lower spine points to the possibility of occult spinal dysraphism. This designation includes a number of spinal cord and vertebral anomalies that frequently produce severe loss of neurologic function, particularly in the region of the back, the lower extremities, and the urinary system. Examples of these abnormalities are subcutaneous lipomeningomyelocele, diastematomyelia, hamartoma, lipoma, tight filum terminale, tethered cord, dermal and epidermal cysts, dermal sinuses, neurenteric canals, and angiomas. Occasionally, the loss of neurologic function from such anomalies is mild and, as a result, easily overlooked. Prompt evaluation of these lesions via CT, MRI, or ultrasound is indicated. Epstein pearls are benign, small, white lesions noted on a newborn's hard palate. Mongolian spots are flat, hyperpigmented lesions on the lower back, buttocks, and occasionally elsewhere; they are more common on blacks, Hispanic, and Asian children and are not pathologic (although they are sometimes confused for bruising by the inexperienced observer). A cephalohematoma is a subperiosteal collection of blood that does not cross the suture line found on a newborn's scalp. Omphalocele, extravasations of intestinal contents into an abdominal wall sac, would be noted on the ventral surface.

310. The answer is b. *(Hay et al, p 998. Kliegman et al, pp 536-539. McMillan et al, pp 2158-2160. Rudolph et al, p 614.)* Homocystinuria is an autosomal recessive metabolic disease caused by deficiencies of cystathionine β-synthase, methylenetetrahydrofolate reductase, or the coenzyme for N^5-methyltetrahydrofolate methyltransferase. Manifestations include poor growth, arachnodactyly, osteoporosis, dislocated lenses, and mental retardation. In addition, thromboembolic phenomena may be seen in the pulmonary and systemic arteries and particularly in the cerebral vasculature; vascular occlusive disease is, in turn, one of the many causes of acute infantile hemiplegia. None of the other disorders listed in the question is associated with acute hemiplegia.

Phenylketonuria causes retardation and, on occasion, seizures; maple syrup urine disease, an abnormality of the metabolism of leucine, leads to seizures and rapid deterioration of the CNS in newborn infants; and histidinemia and cystathioninuria are most likely a benign aminoaciduria with no effect on the CNS. Many states now include these diseases in their newborn screening programs.

311. The answer is e. *(Hay et al, pp 745, 1037. Kliegman et al, pp 2455-2456. McMillan et al, pp 472-477. Rudolph et al, pp 11-12.)* The infant in the question, who is completely healthy otherwise, appears to have simple, primary craniosynostosis (simple = only one suture; primary = not because of failure of brain growth). This condition is usually sporadic (occurring in 1 in 2000 births) and more commonly affects the sagittal suture, which results in scaphocephaly (a long and narrow skull). In general, premature fusion of a single suture does not cause increased intracranial pressure or hydrocephalus; these features are more common with premature fusion of two or more sutures. The therapy for this condition is controversial, but usually involves surgery; consultation with a neurosurgeon would be indicated.

Craniosynostosis is associated with genetic defects in 10% to 20% of cases. A child whose examination or history is not normal (developmental delay, polydactyly or syndactyly, unusually shaped digits or eyes, etc) is more likely to have a genetic defect as the cause of the craniosynostosis. In these patients, chromosome evaluation for conditions such as Chotzen, Pfeiffer, Crouzon, Carpenter, or Apert syndromes is appropriate.

312. The answer is c. *(Hay et al, pp 777-779. Kliegman et al, pp 2554-2557. McMillan et al, pp 2317-2319. Rudolph et al, pp 2285-2287.)* Myasthenia gravis is an autoimmune disorder in which circulating acetylcholine receptor-binding antibodies result in neuromuscular blockade. The earliest signs of myasthenia gravis are ptosis and weakness of the extraocular muscles, followed by dysphagia and facial muscle weakness. The distinguishing hallmark of this disease is rapid fatiguing of the involved muscles. The conduction velocity of the motor nerve is normal in this condition. When the involved muscle is repetitively stimulated for diagnostic purposes, the electromyogram (EMG) shows a decremental response, which can be reversed by the administration of cholinesterase inhibitors. In older children this test is accomplished with edrophonium chloride, but it should be avoided in young infants, as cardiac arrhythmias may result (neostigmine would be used instead). Cholinesterase inhibitors are the primary therapeutic agents. Other therapeutic modalities for myasthenia gravis include immunosuppression, plasmapheresis, thymectomy (an enlarged thymus is frequently seen on chest x-ray), and treatment of hypothyroidism. CPK should be normal.

313. The answer is e. *(Hay et al, p 728. Kliegman et al, p 2478.)* Seizure-like activity with no epileptiform activity on EEG is consistent with pseudoseizure. These episodes may be very convincing for seizures and may include unusual posturing and sounds, but typically do not involve loss of bowel or bladder control. In addition, the patient usually will not cause self-injury, and pupillary response to light is normal. These episodes can be deliberate or part of a conversion disorder, and do not require treatment with antiepileptic medications. However, many patients with pseudoseizures also have true epileptic seizures, so withdrawal of antiepileptic medication would be inappropriate at this point. Psychiatric or psychologic evaluation is the best way to start managing pseudoseizures.

314. The answer is e. *(Hay et al, pp 741-743. Kliegman et al, pp 2508-2512. McMillan et al, pp 2270-2280. Rudolph et al, pp 2257-2258.)* The abrupt onset of a hemisyndrome, especially with the eyes looking away from the paralyzed side, strongly indicates a diagnosis of acute infantile hemiplegia. Most frequently, this represents a thromboembolic occlusion of the middle cerebral artery or one of its major branches. The diagnosis has also been used to describe an acute syndrome of fever and partial seizure with resulting hemiparesis. Childhood stroke can result from trauma, infection, a hypercoagulable state, arteritis, and congenital structural or metabolic disorders.

Hemiplegic migraine commonly occurs in children with a history of migraine and during a headache episode. Todd paralysis follows after a focal or Jacksonian seizure and generally does not last more than 24 to 48 hours. The clinical onset of supratentorial brain tumor is subacute, with repeated headaches and gradually developing weakness. A history of trauma usually precedes the signs of an acute subdural hematoma. Clinical signs of other diseases can appear fairly rapidly, but not often with the abruptness of occlusive vascular disease.

315. The answer is c. *(Hay et al, p 754. Kliegman et al, pp 594-595. McMillan et al, p 2207. Rudolph et al, pp 2324-2325.)* Children who have Tay-Sachs disease are characterized by progressive developmental deterioration;

physical signs include macular cherry-red spots and exquisite and characteristic sensitivity to noise. Diagnosis of this disorder can be confirmed biochemically by the absence of β-hexosaminidase A activity in WBCs. The other GM_2 gangliosidosis, Sandhoff disease, results from a deficiency of both β-hexosaminidase A and B. Tay-Sachs disease is inherited as an autosomal recessive trait; frequently, affected children are of Eastern European Jewish ancestry.

The other disorders listed in the question are associated with enzyme deficiencies as follows: Niemann-Pick disease (type A) sphingomyelinase, which results in a normal-appearing child at birth who then develops hepatosplenomegaly, lymphadenopathy, and psychomotor retardation in the first 6 months, followed by regression after that; infantile Gaucher disease, β-glucosidase, which presents in infancy with increased tone, strabismus, organomegaly, failure to thrive, strider, and several years of psychomotor regression before death; Krabbe disease (globoid cell leukodystrophy), galactocerebroside β-galactosidase, which presents early in infancy with irritability, seizures, hypertonia, and optic atrophy, with severe delay and death usually occurring in the first 3 years of life; and Fabry disease, β-galactosidase, which presents in childhood with angiokeratomas in the "bathing trunk area," ultimately resulting in severe pain episodes.

316. The answer is d. (*Hay et al, pp 772-776, 1040. Kliegman et al, pp 2544-2547. McMillan et al, p 2325. Rudolph et al, pp 2293-2294, 2406.*) The child in the question appears to have myotonic muscular dystrophy. An elevated creatine kinase (especially in the preclinical phase) often is found, and psychomotor retardation can be the presenting complaint (but may be identified only in retrospect). Ptosis, baldness, hypogonadism, facial immobility with distal muscle wasting (in older children), and neonatal respiratory distress (in the newborn period) are major features of this disorder. Cataracts are commonly seen, presenting either congenitally or at any point during childhood. The prominence of distal muscle weakness in this disease is in contrast to the proximal muscle weakness seen in most other forms of myopathies. The diagnosis is confirmed by identifying typical findings on muscle biopsy. Seizures are not a feature of myotonic dystrophy. Enlarged gonads are associated with fragile X syndrome, and hirsutism is found (among other things) in children with congenital adrenal hyperplasia.

317. The answer is a. (*Hay et al, 737-739. Kliegman et al, pp 2479-2482. McMillan et al, pp 2389-2392. Rudolph et al, pp 2274-2276.*) In contrast to adults, children with migraine most often have "common" migraine: bifrontal headache without an aura or diffuse throbbing headache of only a few hours' duration. As with adults, the headaches can be terminated with vomiting or sleep. Family history is frequently positive. Tension headaches are possible, but the severity of this child's headache and the throbbing nature suggests migraine. One always considers the possibility of brain tumor in children with headaches, but the duration of this headache, lack of findings on clinical examination, and lack of changes in behavior or school performance suggest this is not likely. Sinusitis is likely to give symptoms related to the upper airway, and fungal meningitis is unlikely to be this indolent.

318. The answer is b. (*Hay et al, pp 1197-1200. Kliegman et al, pp 1248-1249. McMillan et al, p 1149. Rudolph, pp 900-904, 953.*) Included among those processes that can cause the clinical picture are viral meningitis, tuberculous meningitis, meningeal leukemia, and medulloblastoma, all of which can cause pleocytosis as well as elevated protein and lowered glucose concentrations in CSF. Of the four diseases (and the likely diagosis of this patient), tuberculous meningitis is associated with the lowest glucose levels in CSF. The CT scan with contrast can be an excellent clue for diagnosing tuberculous meningitis. Exudate in the basal cisterns that shows enhancement by contrast material is typical; tuberculomas, ringed lucencies, edema, and infarction can be apparent; and hydrocephalus can develop. Confirmation with culture is mandatory. The x-ray of the chest will be likely to show signs of pulmonary tuberculosis. A high index of suspicion is necessary to diagnose tuberculous meningitis early.

In pseudotumor cerebri, the constituents of CSF are generally normal except for low-protein content in some instances and high opening pressure. Acute bacterial disease must be considered for this patient, but typically causes polymorphonuclear cells and positive Gram stains. Neither tuberous sclerosis nor stroke typically cause these findings on CSF examination.

319. The answer is a. (*Hay et al, pp 893-896. Kliegman et al, pp 2128-2137. McMillan et al, pp 1771-1775. Rudolph et al, pp 47, 2219-2221.*) A child who has a subacute disorder of the CNS that produces cranial nerve abnormalities (especially of cranial nerve VII and the lower bulbar nerves), long-tract signs, unsteady gait secondary to spasticity, and some behavioral changes is most likely to have a pontine glioma. These diffuse tumors are difficult to treat. Tumors of the cerebellar hemispheres can, in later stages, produce upper motor neuron signs, but the gait disturbance would be ataxia.

Dysmetria and nystagmus also would be present. Supratentorial tumors are quite common in 6-year-old children; headache and vomiting likely would be the presenting symptoms and papilledema a finding on physical examination. Subacute sclerosing panencephalitis (SSPE) is a rare disorder seen in children having experienced an episode of measles; extremely rare cases of SSPE can be associated with the vaccine. The patients have insidious behavior changes, deterioration in schoolwork, and finally dementia. No other findings are usually seen. Progressive multifocal leukoencephalopathy, caused by a chronic polyomavirus infection, is usually found in patients with immune deficiencies; although still rare, it has become more common as the incidence of AIDS increased.

320. The answer is d. (*Hay et al, pp 765-766. Kliegman et al, pp 2524-2525. McMillan et al, pp 1040-1043. Rudolph et al, pp 2319-2321.*) The patient in the question has a brain abscess, a condition more commonly seen in patients with cardiac defects that have right-to-left shunts associated with them. The antibiotics that he received from the ER kept the condition somewhat under control, but was unlikely to cure the condition, which ultimately progressed. The diagnostic tool of choice is imaging, and either CT or MRI is indicated. Lumbar puncture would be contraindicated in this patient until after imaging (the patient is at risk for brain herniation) and the CSF (and blood) cultures are usually negative. The patient is not experiencing new cardiac problems, so an echocardiogram is not indicated. If the patient has negative imaging of the brain, then a urine drug screen might be indicated, but not as a test of first choice.

321. The answer is b. (*Kliegman et al, pp 433-434. McMillan et al, pp 743-745. Rudolph et al, pp 2246-2248.*) Compression of cranial nerve III and distortion of the brainstem, resulting in unilateral pupillary dilatation, hemiplegia, focal seizures, and depressed consciousness, suggest a progressively enlarging mass, most likely an epidural hematoma. Such a hematoma displaces the temporal lobe into the tentorial notch and presses on the ipsilateral cranial nerve III. Brainstem compression by this additional tissue mass leads to progressive deterioration in consciousness. Rising blood pressure, irregular respiration, and falling pulse rate ("Cushing's triad") are characteristic of increasing intracranial pressure. The most urgent test to diagnose this condition is a CT scan.

Spinal taps in a patient with evidence of an expanding intracranial mass are contraindicated and may result in herniation and death; this patient has no evidence of intravascular fluid depletion, and rapid fluid hydration may exacerbate the increased intracranial process. Naloxone is indicated for an opiate ingestion, but such an ingestion would be expected to produce bilateral pinpoint pupils. Gastric decontamination with charcoal rarely is used, but would be indicated for some suspected ingestions.

322. The answer is e. (*Hay et al, p 945. Kliegman et al, p 2135. McMillan et al, p 2089. Rudolph et al, pp 2226-2227.*) The findings of poor growth, diabetes insipidus, and papilledema could be explained by a craniopharyngioma. This tumor is one of the most common supratentorial tumors in children, often causing growth failure through disruption of pituitary excretions such as growth hormone. Upward growth of a craniopharyngioma results in compression of the optic chiasm. Particularly affected are the fibers derived from the nasal portions of both retinas (ie, from those parts of the eyes receiving stimulation from the temporal visual field). Early in the growth of a craniopharyngioma, a unilateral superior quadrantanopsic defect can develop, and an irregularly growing tumor can impinge upon the optic chiasm and cause homonymous hemianopia. Treatment is surgical excision and may include radiation therapy for large lesions. However, significant morbidity is associated with these tumors and their removal, including vision loss, growth failure, and panhypopituitarism.

323. The answer is a. (*Hay et al, pp 752-760. Kliegman et al, pp 340-341. McMillan et al, p 749. Rudolph et al, pp 2314-2315.*) Cerebellar ataxia in childhood can occur in association with infection, metabolic abnormalities, ingestion of toxins, hydrocephalus, cerebellar lesions, multiple sclerosis, labyrinthitis, polyradiculopathy, and neuroblastoma. Although the other listed diagnoses (except agenesis of the corpus callosum) can cause ataxia, symptoms would be more chronic in nature than the acute episode described. Ingestion (intentional or accidental) of barbiturates, phenytoin, alcohol, and other drugs also must be considered. Agenesis of the corpus callosum is usually diagnosed by imaging studies; however, it does not cause acute ataxia.

324. The answer is a. (*Hay et al, pp 893-896. Kliegman et al, pp 2128-2137. McMillan et al, pp 1771-1775. Rudolph et al, pp 2207-2210.*) Brain tumors are the most common solid tumor in childhood, and account for 25% to 30% of all pediatric malignancies. While supratentorial tumors predominate in the first year of life (including choroid plexus tumors and teratomas), brain tumors in children 1 to 10 years old are more frequently infratentorial (posterior fossa) and include cerebellar and brainstem tumors such as medulloblastoma or cerebellar astrocytoma. After 10 years of age, supratentorial tumors (eg, diffuse astrocytoma) are again more common.

325. The answer is e. (*Hay et al, pp 1172-1173. Kliegman et al, pp 1224-1227. McMillan et al, pp 1034-1036, 2319-2320. Rudolph et al, pp 2287-2288.*) Although the other possibilities listed in the question may be the etiology, it seems most likely that botulism is the culprit for this child's problem. Botulism clearly has been associated with the ingestion of raw honey, and in young children often presents with constipation before the development of the other symptoms listed; constipation is an unusual presenting feature in the other disorders.

Constipation in a young infant is a common complaint of parents, and potentially is unrelated to this child's problem. Some of the other diagnostic considerations listed in the question are possibilities if the constipation is a red herring. Spinal muscular atrophy in a neonate is associated with hypotonia and feeding difficulties; a muscle biopsy can confirm this diagnosis. Neonatal myasthenia gravis, although uncommon, must be considered in a newborn infant who has the symptoms described in the question. The symptoms presented (excepting prominent constipation) also could represent myotonic dystrophy; this diagnosis is confirmed by examination of both parents for percussion and grip myotonia, and by EMG depiction of myotonic discharges. Duchenne (pseudohypertrophic) muscular dystrophy clinically appears in children who are about 2 or 3 years of age.

326. The answer is b. (*Hay et al, pp 754-757. Kliegman et al, pp 593-595. McMillan et al, pp 2205-2211. Rudolph et al, pp 668, 2205, 2323-2324.*) The cherry-red spot represents the center of a normal retinal macula that is surrounded by ganglion cells in which an abnormal accumulation of lipid has occurred, thus altering the surrounding retinal color so that it is yellowish or grayish white; it is seen more often in such disorders as GM_1 generalized gangliosidosis type 1, Sandhoff disease, and Niemann-Pick disease type A, in which there is lipid material deposited in the ganglion cells. Generalized gangliosidosis type 1 (type 1 GM_1 gangliosidosis) presents as noted in the question, with symptoms often present at birth; these infants have a complete lack of acid β-galactosidase activity. Other findings with generalized gangliosidosis type 1 (and not listed in the question) include gingival hyperplasia, hernias, joint stiffness, dorsal kyphosis, and edema of the extremities. β-Hexosaminidase A deficiency (GM$_2$ gangliosidosis, type 1, or Tay-Sachs disease) presents as psychomotor retardation and hypotonia beginning at about 6 to 12 months of age; the children are usually normal at birth. A pronounced startle reflex and severe hyperacusis, seizures, loss of vision (with cherry-red macular spots), and macrocephaly are seen. Reduced activity of α-galactosidase (Fabry disease) presents in older children as acroparesthesia (numbness or tingling in one or more extremities), intermittent painful crises of the extremities or the abdomen, frequently low-grade fevers, and sometimes cataracts. Patients with Rett syndrome (the etiology of which has been traced to a defective gene called MECP2 on the X chromosome) present as normal children at birth, but then have a rapid decline in motor and cognitive functions beginning between 6 and 18 months of age. Affected girls demonstrate loss in the use of their hands and loss in their ability to communicate and socialize.

Metachromatic leukodystrophy (deficient activity of galactosyl-3-sulfate-ceramide sulfatase) has its onset between 1 and 2 years of age and is notable for progressive ataxia, weakness, and peripheral neuropathy. In this disorder, gray macular lesions can be seen that look somewhat similar to cherry-red spots.

327. The answer is b. *(Hay et al, pp 720, 726. Kliegman et al, pp 2457-2458. McMillan et al, pp 2297-2299. Rudolph et al, pp 2270-2271.)* The child in the question likely had a febrile seizure. Febrile seizures usually occur in children between the ages of 9 months and 5 years, generally in association with upper respiratory illness, roseola, shigellosis, or gastroenteritis. The generalized seizures are mostly brief (2-5 minutes), and the CSF is normal. Since other more serious processes cause seizure and fever, each child must be carefully evaluated. Children younger than 12 to 18 months do not have a reliable neck examination for meningismus, so they will probably need a lumbar puncture to rule out CNS infection as a cause. In a simple febrile seizure, EEG and CNS imaging are not usually necessary. Infants who have seizures that are prolonged (longer than 15 minutes), focal, or lateralized, or who had neurologic problems before the febrile seizure (including intraventricular hemorrhage), are at a higher risk of developing an afebrile seizure disorder during the subsequent 5 to 7 years. CSF is usually normal after a seizure, so a pleocytosis requires evaluation for meningitis or encephalitis.

328. The answer is c. *(Hay et al, pp 767-771. Kliegman et al, pp 2565-2566. McMillan et al, pp 2311-2312. Rudolph et al, pp 2281-2283.)* The paralysis of Guillain-Barré often occurs about 10 days after a nonspecific viral illness. Weakness is gradual over days or weeks, beginning in the lower extremities and progressing toward the trunk. Later, the upper limbs and the bulbar muscles can become involved. Involvement of the respiratory muscles is life-threatening. The syndrome seems to be caused by a demyelination in the motor nerves and, occasionally, the sensory nerves. Measurement of spinal fluid protein is helpful in the diagnosis; protein levels are increased to more than twice normal, while glucose and cell counts are normal. Hospitalization for observation is indicated. Treatment can consist of observation alone, intravenous immunoglobulin, steroids, or plasmapheresis. Recovery is not always complete. Bell palsy usually follows a mild upper respiratory infection, resulting in the rapid development of weakness of the entire side of the face. Muscular dystrophy encompasses a number of entities that include weakness over months. Charcot-Marie-Tooth disease has a clinical onset including peroneal and intrinsic foot muscle atrophy, later extending to the intrinsic hand muscles and proximal legs. Werdnig-Hoffmann disease is an anterior horn disorder that presents either *in utero* (in about one-third of cases) or by the first 6 months of life with hypotonia, weakness, and delayed developmental motor milestones.

329. The answer is a. (*Hay et al, pp 1120-1123. Kliegman et al, pp 1377-1379, McMillan et al, pp 511-515. Rudolph et al, pp 1031-1035.*) Periventricular calcifications are a characteristic finding in infants who have congenital CMV infection. The encephalitic process especially affects the subependymal tissue around the lateral ventricles and thus results in the periventricular deposition of calcium. Calcified tuberculomas, if visible radiographically, are not particularly periventricular; congenital tuberculosis presenting such as the patient described would be extraordinarily unusual. Granulomatous encephalitis caused by congenital toxoplasmosis is associated with scattered and soft-appearing intracranial calcification, and suprasellar calcifications are typical of craniopharyngiomas. Congenital syphilis does not produce intracranial calcifications. The unscientific, but sometimes useful, way of keeping intracranial calcifications caused by CMV differentiated from those caused by toxoplasmosis is to remember that "CMV" has a *V* in it, as does "periventricular"; "toxoplasmosis" has an *X* in it, and the lesions associated with it are scattered throughout the "cortex," which also has an *X* in it.

330. The answer is b. (*Hay et al, pp 750-751. Kliegman et al, pp 2485-2487. McMillan et al, pp 2385-2386. Rudolph et al, pp 770-772.*) In infants, achromic skin patches, especially in association with infantile spasms, are characteristic of tuberous sclerosis, an autosomal dominantly acquired condition. Other dermal abnormalities (adenoma sebaceum and subungual fibromata) associated with this disorder appear later in childhood. Children with this condition may present with infantile spasms, and a Wood lamp evaluation of their skin may assist in the identification of the hypopigmented, "ash-leaf" lesions. CT scan of the brain may demonstrate calcified tubers, but these may not be evident until 3 to 4 years of age.

Although children who have neurofibromatosis may have a few achromic patches, the identifying dermal lesions are café au lait spots. Incontinentia pigmenti also is associated with seizures; the skin lesions typical of this disorder begin as bullous eruptions that later become hyperpigmented lesions. Pityriasis rosea and psoriasis are not associated with infantile spasms.

331. The answer is b. *(Hay et al, pp 783, 1038-1039. Kliegman et al, pp 2557-2559. McMillan et al, pp 2307-2309. Rudolph et al, pp 2001-2002.)* The infant described has spinal muscular atrophy (SMA) type I, also referred to as Werdnig-Hoffman disease, or infantile progressive spinal muscular atrophy. The defect is found in the survivor motor neuron (SMN) gene that stops apoptosis of motor neuroblasts. During development, an excess of motor neuroblasts is noted, and through apoptosis only about half survive in the normal newborn; the SMN gene regulates this natural destruction. A defect in the SMN gene results in a continuation of apoptosis, resulting in progressive destruction of motor neurons in the brain stem and spinal cord. The only currently available treatment is supportive care, and infants with SMA I usually die of respiratory complications by the second or third year of life. Three other types of SMA have been described: SMA 0, a rare severe form that is fatal in the perinatal period; SMA II, in which infants may suck normally and despite progressive weakness may survive into the school-aged years; and SMA III, which usually presents later and with a better prognosis. Intelligence is normal, and the heart is not affected.

Absence of dystrophin is seen in muscular dystrophy. Antibodies binding to the acetylcholine (ACh) receptor at the postsynaptic membrane are the underlying cause of myasthenia gravis. Progressive postinfectious autoimmune demyelination is the underlying problem in Guillain-Barré syndrome. Birth trauma may cause CNS bleeding which would be expected to result in seizures, but not generalized weakness. It should be noted that congenital Guillain-Barré syndrome rarely has been described, but in those cases CSF protein is elevated. In addition, congenital myasthenia gravis has been described in patients born to mothers with myasthenia.

332. The answer is b. *(Hay et al, pp 772-773, 1039. Kliegman et al, pp 2540-2550. McMillan et al, pp 2322-2329. Rudolph et al, pp 2289-2294.)* The most common form of muscular dystrophy is Duchenne muscular dystrophy. It is inherited as an X-linked recessive trait. Male infants are rarely diagnosed at birth or early infancy since they often reach gross milestones at the expected age. Soon after beginning to walk, however, the features of this disease become more evident. While these children walk at the appropriate age, the hip girdle weakness is seen by the age of 2 years. Increased lordosis, while standing, is evidence of gluteal weakness. Gower sign (use of the hands to "climb up" the legs in order to assume the upright position) is seen by 3 to 5 years of age, as is the hip waddle gait. Ambulation ability remains through about 7 to 12 years of age, after which use of a wheelchair is common. Associated features include mental impairment and cardiomyopathy. Death caused by respiratory failure, heart failure, pneumonia, or aspiration is common by early adulthood.

333. The answer is b. *(Hay et al, p 89. Kliegman et al, p 2476. Rudolph et al, p 418.)* Night terrors are most common in children between the ages of 5 and 7 years. Children awaken suddenly, appear frightened and unaware of their surroundings, and have the clinical signs outlined in the question. The child cannot be consoled by the parents. After a few minutes, sleep returns, and the patient cannot recall the event in the morning. Sleepwalking is common in these children. Exploring the family dynamics for emotional disorders may be helpful; usually pharmacologic therapy is not required, and family reassurance is indicated.

334. The answer is d. *(Hay et al, pp 736-737. Kliegman et al, pp 2477-2478. McMillan et al, pp 2722-2733. Rudolph et al, pp 1892-1894.)* Simple syncope occurs following an alteration in brain blood flow, possible as a result of hypotension. The majority of syncopal episodes are vasovagal. Other considerations include cardiac causes (such as prolonged QTc, arrhythmia or outflow obstruction), migraine, seizure, hypoglycemia, hyperventilation, and vertigo. Ischemia of the higher cortical levels results in neuronal discharges from the reticular formation (which is no longer influenced by the cortical level) producing brief tonic contractions of muscles of the upper extremities, trunk, and face. The sequence of events described in the question probably resulted from vasovagal stimulation, often precipitated by pain, fear, excitement, or standing for long periods. This condition is common in adolescent girls. After a careful history and physical examination, an organic cause of this fainting episode is unlikely to be identified; reassurance is usually all that is required. Counseling on proper diet and fluid intake is appropriate; patients should also increase their salt intake. Occasionally patients with recurrent vasovagal syncope may be managed using β-blockers or fludrocortisone.

335 to 337. The answers are 335-c, 336-d, 337-a. *(Hay et al, pp 737-739. Kliegman et al, pp 2479-2483. McMillan et al, pp 2388-2395. Rudolph et al, pp 424-425, 2274-2276.)* Headaches can be a concerning symptom in the pediatric population, especially to parents; it is a common pediatric complaint. Vascular headaches can occur in all ages, and patients usually have a family history of migraine. While the typical scotomata discussed in adult migraine is not normally associated in children with migraine, pediatric migraines may have a nonspecific prodrome consisting of a change in mood, temperament, or appetite. Worsening headaches with nausea and emesis (particularly early morning emesis) are concerning for increased intracranial pressure from a mass lesion. Other associated findings may be decreased school performance, behavioral changes, or focal neurologic deficits. Papilledema may be present. Imaging would be necessary with this presentation.

Tension headaches are common in the older child and adolescent. They will worsen during the day, and may worsen with stressful situations like tests. They are typically described as squeezing, but are not usually pulsatile. Nausea and vomiting are not typical.

Factitious headache, as with any factitious diagnosis, should be one of exclusion. Hemiplegic migraine is descriptive of a typical aura that involves unilateral sensory or motor signs with a migraine headache. Patients can have unilateral weakness, numbness, and aphasia. These signs may resolve quickly or may last for days. This particular type of migraine is more common in children than in adults.

338 to 340. The answers are 338-a, 339-b, 340-d. *(Hay et al, pp 760-763, 784-786. Kliegman et al, pp 2490-2495. McMillan et al, pp 2368-2375. Rudolph et al, pp 462, 2166, 2197-2202.)* Tics are commonly seen in a pediatric practice. All have in common the nonrhythmic, spasmodic, involuntary, stereotypical behaviors that involve any muscle group. Transient tic disorder is the most common and is seen more often in boys; a family history is often noted. In this condition, the patient has eye blinking, facial movements, or throat clearing lasting for weeks to about a year. No medications are needed. Chronic motor tics persist throughout life and can incorporate motor movements involving up to three muscle groups.

Gilles de la Tourette syndrome is a lifelong condition that is characterized by motor and vocal tics, obsessive-compulsive behavior, and a high incidence of attention deficit disorder with hyperactivity (ADDH). Therapy for the ADDH is helpful, as is medication to control the motor or vocal tics. Multiple psychosocial problems exist with these children; a multidisciplinary approach is helpful.

Dystonic reactions are sometimes seen in patients receiving phenothiazine medications. They have unusual neck, arm, or leg muscle twitches that are sometimes confused with seizure activity. Diphenhydramine, infused intravenously, usually rapidly reverses this relatively common idiosyncratic drug reaction.

Cerebral palsy is a static condition of movement and posture disorders frequently associated with epilepsy and abnormalities of vision, speech, and intellect. A defect in the developing brain is felt to be the cause. No significant change in the incidence of cerebral palsy has been noted in the past few decades despite drastically improved obstetric and neonatal care. No treatment for cerebral palsy is available; a multidisciplinary approach to manage the many medical problems associated with the condition is helpful.

The term chorea describes involuntary uncoordinated jerks of the arms and legs. Sydenham chorea is the most common acquired chorea of childhood, is seen after infections with group A β-hemolytic streptococci, and is associated with rheumatic heart disease and arthritis. In addition to the motor symptoms, patients may be hypotonic, emotionally labile and have a "milkmaid" grip with sequential grip tightening and relaxing. Other findings include a darting tongue and "spooning" of an extended hand (flexion at the wrist and extension of the fingers).

341 to 343. The answers are 341-c, 342-a, 343-b. *(Hay et al, pp 748-751. Kliegman et al, pp 2483-2488. McMillan et al, pp 2379-2388. Rudolph et al, pp 769-773, 2344-2348.)* Neurofibromatosis type 1 (NF1) is a progressive neurocutaneous syndrome that results from a defect in neural crest differentiation and migration during the early stages of development. It has an autosomal dominant pattern of inheritance; the gene locus has been identified on chromosome 17. Any organ or system can be affected, neurologic complications are frequent, and patients are at high risk of developing malignant neoplasms of various types. The presence of any two of the following findings confirms the diagnosis of NF1: (1) Five or more café au lait spots over 5 mm in diameter in prepubertal patients; six or more over 15 mm in diameter in postpubertal patients; (2) axillary freckling; (3) two or more Lisch nodules (hamartomas of the iris); (4) two or more neurofibromas, typically involving the skin and appearing during adolescence or pregnancy, or one plexiform neuroma involving a nerve track present at birth; (5) bony lesions leading to pathologic fracture and kyphoscoliosis; (6) optic glioma; (7) NF1 in a first-degree relative.

The child with a unilateral facial lesion and blindness suggests either Sturge-Webber or PHACE syndrome (posterior fossa malformations, hemangiomas, arterial anomalies, coarctation of the aorta or other cardiac defects, and eye abnormalities). These patients can have seizures, hemiparesis, intracranial calcifications, and mental retardation.

Tuberous sclerosis, an autosomal dominant condition, can result in severe mental retardation and seizures. Infantile spasms, a hypsarrhythmic EEG pattern, hypopigmented lesions (ash-leaf spots), cardiac tumors, sebaceous adenomas, a shagreen patch (a roughened, raised lesion over the sacrum), and calcifications on the CT scan are all features of this condition. No specific treatment is available.

McCune-Albright syndrome (the 14-year-old child with precocious puberty and goiter) and NF1 share many of the same clinical findings: skin, bones, and endocrine glands can be involved in both. The characteristic features of McCune-Albright syndrome include large, irregular, usually unilateral café au lait spots and fibrous dysplasia of bones in association with precocious puberty in girls.

Infectious Diseases and Immunology

Questions

344. A 10-year-old patient (pictured below) calls his parents from summer camp to state that he has had fever, muscular pain (especially in the neck), headache, and malaise. He describes the area from the back of his mandible toward the mastoid space as being full and tender and that his earlobe on the affected side appears to be sticking upward and outward. Drinking sour liquids causes much pain in the affected area. When his father calls your office, you remind him that he had refused immunizations for his child on religious grounds. Which of the following preventable diseases has this child acquired?

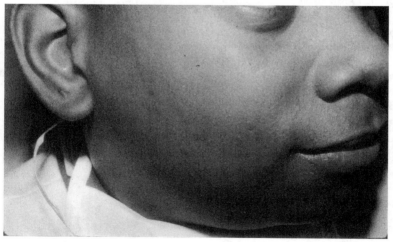

(Courtesy of Adelaide Hebert, MD.)

a. Mumps
b. Varicella
c. Rubella
d. Measles
e. Diphtheria

345. A 2-month-old child of an HIV-positive mother is followed in your pediatric practice. Which of the following therapies should be considered for this child?

a. Monthly evaluation for Kaposi sarcoma
b. Prophylaxis against *Pneumocystis jiroveci* pneumonia (*Pneumocystis carinii*)
c. Vitamin C supplementation
d. Oral polio virus vaccine
e. Bone marrow transplantation

346. A 10-month-old infant on long-term aspirin therapy for Kawasaki disease develops sudden onset of high fever, chills, diarrhea, and irritability. A rapid swab in your office identifies influenza A, adding her to the long list of influenza patients you have seen this December. Over the next few days, she slowly improves and becomes afebrile. However, 5 days after your last encounter you hear from the hospital that she has presented to the emergency center obtunded and posturing with evidence of liver dysfunction. Which of the following statements about her current condition is correct?

a. With proper supportive care, the overall mortality rate is low.
b. With her progressive liver dysfunction, increased total serum bilirubin is anticipated.
c. Administration of *N*-acetylcysteine is first-line therapy.
d. Seizures are uncommon with this condition.
e. Death is usually associated with increased intracranial pressures and herniation.

347. An 18-month-old child presents to the emergency center having had a brief, generalized tonic-clonic seizure. He is now postictal and has a temperature of 40°C (104°F). During the lumbar puncture (which ultimately proves to be normal), he has a large, watery stool that has both blood and mucus in it. Which of the following is the most likely diagnosis in this patient?

a. *Salmonella*
b. Enterovirus
c. Rotavirus
d. *Campylobacter*
e. *Shigella*

348. A 2-year-old child is admitted to your hospital team. The child's primary care doctor has been following the child for several days and has noted her to have had high fever, peeling skin, abdominal pain, and a bright red throat. You are concerned because two common pediatric problems that could explain this child's condition have overlapping presenting signs and symptoms. Which of the following statements comparing these two diseases in your differential is true?

a. Neither has cardiac complications.
b. Serologic tests are helpful in diagnosing both.
c. Only one of the diseases has mucocutaneous and lymph node involvement.
d. Pharyngeal culture aids in the diagnosis of one of the conditions.
e. A specific antibiotic therapy is recommended for one of the conditions, but only supportive care is recommended for the other.

349. A patient with hair loss is shown below. The lesion does not fluoresce with a Wood lamp and has not responded well to a variety of topical agents. The lesion is boggy, is spreading, and has tiny pinpoint black dots throughout. Which of the following is the most likely diagnosis?

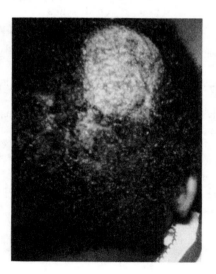

a. Traction alopecia from tight hair braids
b. Infection with *Trichophyton tonsurans*
c. Alopecia areata
d. Biotinidase deficiency
e. Hypothyroidism

350. An 8-year-old sickle-cell patient arrives at the emergency room (ER) in respiratory distress. Over the previous several days, the child has become progressively tired and pale. The child's hemoglobin concentration in the ER is 3.1 mg/dL. Which of the following viruses commonly causes such a clinical picture?

a. Roseola
b. Parvovirus B19
c. Coxsackie A16
d. Echovirus 11
e. Cytomegalovirus

351. A 10-year-old boy was healthy until about 10 days ago when he developed 7 days of fever, chills, severe muscle pain, pharyngitis, headache, scleral injection, photophobia, and cervical adenopathy. After 7 days of symptoms he seemed to get better, but yesterday he developed fever, nausea, emesis, headache and mild nuchal rigidity. Cerebrospinal fluid (CSF) shows 200 white blood cells (WBC) per microliter (all monocytes) and an elevated protein. Correct statements about this infection include which of the following?

a. The condition is obtained from arthropod vectors
b. CNS involvement is uncommon
c. Most cases are mild or subclinical
d. Appropriate treatment includes intravenous (IV) immune globulin (IVIG) and aspirin
e. Hepatic and renal involvement occurs in the majority of cases

352. A previously healthy 8-year-old boy has a 3-week history of low-grade fever of unknown source, fatigue, weight loss, myalgia, and headaches. On repeated examinations during this time, he is found to have developed a heart murmur, petechiae, and mild splenomegaly. Which of the following is the most likely diagnosis?

a. Rheumatic fever
b. Kawasaki disease
c. Scarlet fever
d. Endocarditis
e. Tuberculosis

353. A 15-month-old boy is brought to the ER because of fever and a rash. Six hours earlier he was fine, except for tugging on his ears; another physician diagnosed otitis media and prescribed amoxicillin. During the interim period, the child has developed an erythematous rash on his face, trunk, and extremities. Some of the lesions, which are of variable size, do not blanch on pressure. The child is now very irritable, and he does not interact well with the examiner. Temperature is 39.5°C (103.1°F). He continues to have injected, immobile tympanic membranes, but you are concerned about his change in mental status. Which of the following is the most appropriate next step in the management of this infant?

a. Begin administration of IV ampicillin
b. Begin diphenhydramine
c. Discontinue administration of ampicillin and begin trimethoprim with sulfamethoxazole
d. Perform bilateral myringotomies
e. Perform a lumbar puncture

354. The 3-year-old sister of a newborn baby develops a cough diagnosed as pertussis by nasopharyngeal culture. The mother gives a history of having been immunized as a child. Which of the following is a correct statement regarding this clinical situation?

a. The mother has no risk of acquiring the disease because she was immunized.
b. Hyperimmune globulin is effective in protecting the infant.
c. The risk to the infant depends on the immune status of the mother.
d. Erythromycin should be administered to the infant.
e. The 3-year-old sister should be immediately immunized with an additional dose of pertussis vaccine.

355. A 14-year-old boy is seen in the ER because of a 3-week history of fever between 38.3°C and 38.9°C (101°F and 102°F), lethargy, and a 2.7-kg (6-lb) weight loss. Physical examination reveals marked cervical and inguinal adenopathy, enlarged tonsils with exudate, small hemorrhages on the soft palate, a WBC differential that has 50% lymphocytes (10% atypical), and a palpable spleen 2 cm below the left costal margin. Which of the following therapies should be initiated?

a. Initiation of zidovudine
b. IV acyclovir
c. IV infusion of immunoglobulins and high-dose aspirin
d. Intramuscular penicillin
e. Avoidance of contact sports

356. A 2-year-old child is seen in the emergency center with a 10-day complaint of fever and a limp. The child has an elevated erythrocyte sedimentation rate (ESR) and the radiograph shown below. Which of the following statements about this child's condition is correct?

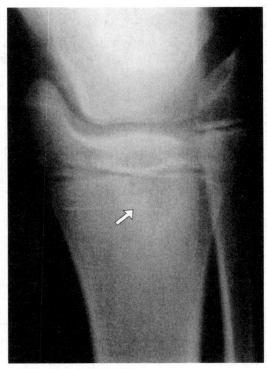

(Courtesy of Susan John, MD.)

a. It is most commonly caused by *Streptococcus pyogenes*.
b. It can arise following development of deep cellulitis.
c. It usually results in tenderness in the region of infection that is diffuse, not localized.
d. It causes diagnostic radiographic changes on plain films within 48 hours of the beginning of symptoms.
e. It requires antibiotic therapy usually for 10 to 14 days.

357. A 16-day-old infant presents with fever, irritability, poor feeding, and a bulging fontanelle. Spinal fluid demonstrates gram-positive cocci. Which of the following is the most likely diagnosis?

a. *Listeria monocytogenes*
b. Group A streptococci
c. Group B streptococci
d. *Streptococcus pneumoniae*
e. *Staphylococcus aureus*

358. A 16-year-old boy presents to the emergency center with a 2-day history of an abscess with spreading cellulitis. While in the emergency center, he develops a high fever, hypotension, and vomiting with diarrhea. On examination you note a diffuse erythematous macular rash, injected conjunctiva and oral mucosa, and a strawberry tongue. He is not as alert as when he first arrived. This rapidly progressive symptom constellation is likely caused by which of the following disease processes?

a. Kawasaki disease
b. TSST-1–secreting *S aureus*
c. Shiga toxin–secreting *Escherichia coli*
d. α-Toxin–secreting *Clostridium perfringens*
e. Neurotoxin-secreting *Clostridium tetani*

359. A 14-month-old infant suddenly develops a fever of 40.2°C (104.4°F). Physical examination shows an alert, active infant who drinks milk eagerly. No physical abnormalities are noted. The WBC count is 22,000/μL with 78% polymorphonuclear leukocytes, 18% of which are band forms. Which of the following is the most likely diagnosis?

a. Pneumococcal bacteremia
b. Roseola
c. Streptococcosis
d. Typhoid fever
e. Diphtheria

360. A 21-year-old woman has just delivered a term infant. She has had only one visit to her obstetrician, and that was at about 6 weeks of pregnancy. She provides her laboratory results from that visit. The delivered infant is microcephalic, has cataracts, a heart murmur, and hepatosplenomegaly. Your further evaluation of the child demonstrates thrombocytopenia, mild hemolytic anemia, and, on the echocardiogram, patent ductus arteriosus and peripheral pulmonary artery stenosis. Which of the following maternal laboratory tests done at 6 weeks gestation is likely to explain the findings in this child?

a. Positive hepatitis B surface antibody
b. Positive rapid plasma reagin (RPR) with negative Microhemagglutination-Treponema pallidum test (MHATP)
c. Negative rubella titer
d. Negative triple screen
e. Positive varicella titer

361. The parents of a 7-day-old infant bring her to your office for a swollen eye. Her temperature has been normal, but for the last 2 days she has had progressive erythema and swelling over the medial aspect of the right lower lid near the punctum. Her sclera and conjunctiva are clear. Gentle pressure extrudes a whitish material from the punctum. Which of the following ophthalmic conditions is the correct diagnosis?

a. Chalazion
b. Dacryocystitis
c. Preseptal cellulitis
d. Hyphema
e. Congenital Sjögren syndrome

362. The parents of a 3-year-old patient followed in your clinic recently took their child on quickly planned 5-day trip to Africa to visit an ill grandparent. Everyone did well on the trip, but since their return about 10 days ago the boy has been having intermittent, spiking fevers associated with headache, sweating, and nausea. The parents had not been too concerned since he was relatively well, except for being tired, between the fevers. Today, however, they feel that he looks a bit pale and his eyes appear "yellow." Which of the following is likely to reveal the source of his problem?

a. Hepatitis A IgG and IgM titers
b. Complete blood count (CBC) with smear
c. Hemoglobin electrophoresis
d. Tuberculosis skin test
e. Hepatitis B IgG and IgM titers

363. The child shown below presents with a 3-day history of malaise, fever to 41.1°C (106°F), cough, coryza, and conjunctivitis. He then develops the erythematous, maculopapular rash pictured. He is noted to have white pinpoint lesions on a bright red buccal mucosa in the area opposite his lower molars. Which of the following is the most likely diagnosis?

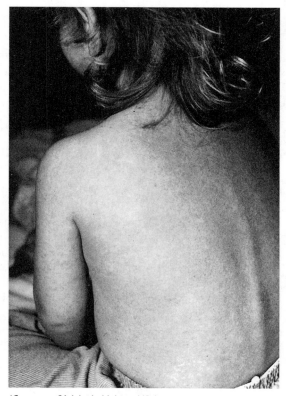

(Courtesy of Adelaide Hebert, MD.)

a. Parvovirus
b. Rubella
c. Herpes
d. Rubeola
e. Varicella

364. A 14-year-old girl awakens with a mild sore throat, low-grade fever, and a diffuse maculopapular rash. During the next 24 hours, she develops tender swelling of her wrists and redness of her eyes. In addition, her physician notes mild tenderness and marked swelling of her posterior cervical and occipital lymph nodes. Four days after the onset of her illness, the rash has vanished. Which of the following is the most likely diagnosis?

a. Rubella
b. Rubeola
c. Roseola
d. Erythema infectiosum
e. Erythema multiforme

365. A 4-year-old child presents in the clinic with an illness notable for swelling in front of and in back of the ear on the affected side, as well as altered taste sensation. Correct statements about this condition include which of the following?

a. Arthritis is a common presenting complaint in children.
b. The disease could have been prevented by prior immunization with killed whole-cell vaccine.
c. Involvement of the central nervous system (CNS) may occur 10 days after the resolution of the swelling.
d. Orchitis can occur and is almost exclusively seen in prepubertal males.
e. Subendocardial fibroelastosis is a common complication in a child of this age.

366. A bat is found in the bedroom of a 4-year-old patient while the boy is sleeping. The family and the patient deny close contact with or bites from the bat. Which of the following is a correct statement regarding this situation?

a. Therapy is only required if the patient shows signs of rabies infection.
b. Bats are not a natural reservoir for rabies virus; no therapy is required.
c. The patient should be started on the rabies vaccine series.
d. The patient needs immediate treatment with acyclovir.
e. The patient needs immediate treatment with ribavirin.

367. An 8-year-old Cub Scout who returned from an outing 9 days ago is brought to the clinic with the rapid onset of fever, headache, muscle pain, and rash. The maculopapular rash began on the flexor surfaces of the wrist and has become petechial as it spread inward to his trunk. Which of the following is the most likely diagnosis?

a. Lyme disease
b. Tularemia
c. Measles
d. Toxic shock syndrome
e. Rocky Mountain spotted fever

368. The parents of a 7-month-old boy arrive in your office with the child and a stack of medical records for a second opinion. The boy first started having problems after his circumcision in the nursery when he had prolonged bleeding. Studies were sent at the time for hemophilia, but factor VIII and IX activity were normal. At 2 months he developed bloody diarrhea, which his doctor assumed was a milk protein allergy and changed him to soy; his parents note he still has occasional bloody diarrhea. He has seen a dermatologist several times for eczema, and he has been admitted to the hospital twice for pneumococcal bacteremia. During both admissions, the parents were told that the infant's platelet count was low, but they have yet to attend the hematology appointment arranged for them. The child's WBC count and differential were normal. Which of the following is the most likely diagnosis in this child?

a. Idiopathic thrombocytopenic purpura
b. Wiskott-Aldrich syndrome
c. Acute lymphocytic leukemia
d. Adenosine deaminase deficiency
e. Partial thymic hypoplasia

369. A 10-year-old boy from the Connecticut coast is seen because of discomfort in his right knee. He had a large, annular, erythematous lesion on his back that disappeared 4 weeks prior to the present visit. His mother recalls pulling a small tick off his back. Which of the following is a correct statement about this child's likely illness?

a. The tick was probably a *Dermacentor andersoni*.
b. The disease is caused by a rickettsial agent that is transmitted by the bite of a tick.
c. In addition to skin and joint involvement, CNS and cardiac abnormalities may be present.
d. Therapy with antibiotics has little effect on the resolution of symptoms.
e. The pathognomonic skin lesion is required for diagnosis.

370. Two weeks ago, a 5-year-old boy developed diarrhea, which has persisted to the present time despite dietary management. His stools have been watery, pale, and frothy. He has been afebrile. Microscopic examination of his stools is likely to show which of the following?

a. *Salmonella sonnei*
b. *Enterobius vermicularis*
c. *Sporothrix schenckii*
d. *Toxoplasma gondii*
e. *Cryptosporidium*

371. The rash and mucous membrane lesions shown in the photograph below develop in an infant 5 days into the course of an upper respiratory infection with otitis media; the child is being treated with amoxicillin. The child's condition is likely which of the following?

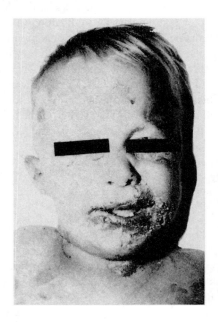

a. Urticaria
b. Rubeola
c. Stevens-Johnson syndrome
d. Kawasaki disease
e. Scarlet fever

372. An 8-year-old immigrant from rural Central America presents with complaints of weakness, facial swelling, muscle pain, and fever. A CBC reveals marked eosinophilia. Which of the following parasites is most likely to be responsible?

a. *Cryptosporidium parvum*
b. *Sporothrix schenckii*
c. *Giardia lambila*
d. *Enterobius vermicularis*
e. *Trichinella spiralis*

373. A patient presents to the emergency center with a 6-hour history of fever to 38.9°C (102°F). Her mother reports that the patient appeared to be feeling poorly, that she had been eating less than normal, and that she vomited once. About 2 hours prior to arrival at the ER, the mother states that she noted a few purple spots scattered about the body on the patient, especially on the buttocks and legs. On the 30-minute ride to the ER, the purple areas spread rapidly and became coalesced in areas, and the patient is now obtunded. Which of the following is the most likely diagnosis?

a. Henoch-Schönlein purpura
b. Toxic shock syndrome caused by *S aureus*
c. Measles
d. Rocky Mountain spotted fever
e. Meningococcemia

374. A 2-month-old infant comes to the emergency center with fever for 2 days, emesis, a petechial rash, and increasing lethargy. In the ambulance he had a 3-minute generalized tonic/clonic seizure that was aborted with lorazepam. He does not respond when blood is drawn or when an IV is placed, but he continues to ooze blood from the skin puncture sites. On examination, his anterior fontanelle is open and bulging. His CBC shows a WBC of 30,000 cells/µL with 20% band forms. Which of the infant's problems listed below is a contraindication to lumbar puncture?

a. Uncorrected bleeding diathesis
b. Bulging fontanelle
c. Dehydration
d. History of recent seizure
e. Significantly elevated WBC count consistent with bacteremia

375. The mother of one of your regular patients calls your office. She reports that her daughter has a 3-day history of subjective fever, hoarseness, and a bad barking cough. You arrange for her to be seen in your office that morning. Upon seeing this child, you would expect to find which of the following?

a. A temperature greater than 38.9°C (102°F)
b. Expiratory stridor
c. Infection with parainfluenza virus
d. Hyperinflation on chest x-ray
e. A child between 6 and 8 years of age

Questions 376 to 379

For each set of immunologic abnormalities listed in the table below, select the most likely clinical presentation. Each lettered option may be used once, more than once, or not at all.

a. A 5-year-old boy who, after 3 months of age, developed recurrent otitis media, pneumonia, diarrhea, and sinusitis, often with simultaneous infections at two or more disparate sites
b. A distinctive-appearing 8-month-old boy with an interrupted aortic arch, hypocalcemia, and cleft palate
c. A 1-year-old boy with severe eczema, recurrent middle-ear infections, lymphopenia, and thrombocytopenia
d. A 9-year-old with an eczema-like rash and recurrent severe staphylococcal infections
e. A 4-month-old who has had failure to thrive, chronic diarrhea, a variety of rashes, and recurrent serious bacterial, fungal, and viral infections

	Serum IgG	Serum IgA	Serum IgM	T-Cell Function	Parathyroid Function
376.	Normal	Normal	Normal	Decreased	Decreased
377.	Low	Low	Low	Normal	Normal
378.	Low	Low	Low	Decreased	Normal
379.	Normal	High	Low	Decreased	Normal

Questions 380 to 385

Match the disease with the associated organism. Each lettered option may be used once, more than once, or not at all.

a. *Bartonella henselae*
b. *Pseudomonas*
c. Rubivirus
d. Human herpesvirus 6
e. *Escherichia coli*
f. *Helicobacter pylori*
g. Group B streptococci
h. *Listeria monocytogenes*
i. Epstein-Barr virus
j. *Toxocara cati*
k. *Campylobacter jejuni*

380. An 18-year-old college girl with an extremely sore throat and high fever who develops a rash upon administration of ampicillin

381. Foot puncture wound through a tennis shoe of an adolescent exploring a construction site

382. Warm, red, tender axillary lymph nodes in a 5-year-old girl; she has a few red papules on her hand at the site of a feline scratch

383. The appearance of an evanescent, erythematous, maculopapular rash following the rapid defervescence of several days of high fever in a 9-month-old boy

384. A 3-week-old uncircumcised boy with fever and urinary tract infection

385. Several weeks' history of epigastric and periumbilical pain that worsens with fasting and is relieved by eating, in a 9-year-old with guaiac-positive stools

Questions 386 to 388

Match the diagnostic test with the associated disease state. Each lettered option may be used once, more than once, or not at all.

a. A 15-year-old sexually active girl with a single non-tender lesion on her labia and regional nontender lymphadenopathy
b. An otherwise healthy 9-year-old boy with pinpoint black dots in the center of an itchy 3-cm boggy patch of hair loss on his scalp
c. An infant born at home 2 days ago who has profuse purulent drainage from both eyes, lid edema, and chemosis
d. A toddler with bloody diarrhea, anemia, and acute renal failure
e. Recurring fever and anemia in an immigrant from central Africa

386. Culture on sorbitol MacConkey medium

387. Culture on modified Thayer-Martin medium

388. Dark field microscopy

Questions 389 to 392

Match each clinical state with the most likely form of pneumonia. Each lettered option may be used once, more than once, or not at all.

a. Mycoplasmal pneumonia
b. Pneumococcal pneumonia
c. Chlamydial pneumonia
d. Viral pneumonia
e. Tuberculous pneumonia
f. Fungal pneumonia
g. Staphylococcal pneumonia

389. A 6-week-old infant with tachypnea and history of eye discharge at 2 weeks of age.

390. A 14-year-old girl with low-grade fever, cough of 3 weeks' duration, and interstitial infiltrate.

391. A 2-month-old boy with a 3-day history of upper respiratory infection who suddenly develops high fever, cough, and respiratory distress; within 48 hours, the patient has developed a pneumatocele and a left-sided pneumothorax.

392. An 8-year-old girl with fever, tachypnea, and lobar infiltrate. She has failed outpatient therapy of amoxicillin, has developed empyema, and has had to have chest tubes placed.

Infectious Diseases and Immunology

Answers

344. The answer is a. *(Hay et al, pp 1134-1135. Kliegman et al, pp 1341-1344. McMillan et al, pp 1279-1281. Rudolph et al, pp 1056-1058.)* In addition to the findings described, mumps typically swells to the opposite side in a day or so after symptoms appear on the first side. Other findings include redness and swelling at the opening of Stensen's duct, edema and swelling in the pharynx, and displacement of the uvula on the affected side. A rash would not be expected. It is important to note that while mumps has largely been eliminated with vaccination, other organisms still may cause parotitis. Measles presents in a child with a several days' history of malaise, fever, cough, coryza, and conjunctivitis followed by the typical, widespread, erythematous, maculopapular rash. Koplik spots, white pinpoint lesions on a bright red buccal mucosa often in the area opposite his lower molars, appear transiently and are pathognomonic. Symptoms of rubella, usually a mild disease, include a diffuse maculopapular rash that lasts for 3 days, marked enlargement of the posterior cervical and occipital lymph nodes, low-grade fever, mild sore throat, and, occasionally, conjunctivitis, arthralgia, or arthritis. Signs and symptoms of varicella include a prodrome of fever, anorexia, headache, and mild abdominal pain, followed 24 to 48 hours later by the typical clear, fluid-filled vesicles (dewdrop on a rose petal). The rash of varicella typically starts on the scalp, face, or trunk. The lesions are pruritic and appear in crops over the next several days, with old lesions crusting over as new lesions develop.

Diphtheria (caused by *Corynebacterium diphtheria*) starts with a mild sore throat and malaise (only 50% have fever), but quickly progresses with an adherent membrane that covers the tonsils and can extend to cover the uvula, palate, posterior oropharynx, hypopharynx, and glottic area. Lymphadenopathy and soft tissue swelling lead to a "bull neck" appearance and potential airway compromise.

345. The answer is b. *(Hay et al, pp 1249-1252. Kliegman et al, pp 1325-1327. McMillan et al, pp 947-948, 1404-1407. Rudolph et al, pp 1045-1053,*

1144-1145.) In certain situations, such as in an infant born to an HIV-positive mother, prophylaxis against *P jiroveci* (formerly known as *P carinii*) infection is instituted. While awaiting final determination of this infant's HIV status, which can take several months, prophylaxis with trimethoprim-sulfamethoxazole starting at 6 weeks is usually appropriate.

Severe anemia can be associated with AIDS and can require blood transfusion, especially if there is evidence of respiratory compromise. Bone marrow transplants in AIDS patients have been unsuccessful thus far because of the persistence of virus in macrophages throughout the body. HIV-positive and AIDS patients should receive primary and booster immunization with diphtheria-pertussis-tetanus (DPT) vaccine, measles-mumps-rubella (MMR) vaccine (unless severely immunocompromised), hepatitis B vaccine, and *Haemophilus influenzae* type B conjugated vaccine (HibCV). Inactivated polio vaccine (IPV) is recommended in place of oral polio vaccine (OPV) for all patients now (not just immunosuppressed patients) because of the theoretical risk of paralytic polio. If children with HIV are exposed to measles, they should receive a protective dose of measles immunoglobulin regardless of their immunization history. Pneumovax at age 2 and influenza vaccine are recommended annually. Eventually, all patients infected with HIV will lose weight and fail to grow. The factors responsible include reduced caloric intake because of poor appetite, intestinal malabsorption, and increased resting energy expenditure associated with chronic infection. Maintaining adequate nutrition in AIDS patients is very difficult, but vitamin C supplementation, by itself, has no special benefits. Kaposi sarcoma is rare in children.

346. The answer is e. (*Hay et al, pp 663-664. Kliegman et al, pp 1697-1998. McMillan et al, pp 2019-2020. Rudolph et al, p 1490.*) Reye syndrome is an acquired mitochondrial hepatopathy that results from the interaction of an influenza (or varicella) infection and aspirin use. While prevalence has decreased over the last few decades, mortality remains the same at more than 40% of cases. Liver enzymes and ammonia are elevated, but total bilirubin is not. Patients initially present toward the end of a viral infection with sleepiness, emesis, and abnormal liver functions. As the disease progresses, the patient may develop seizures, coma, hyperventilation, and decorticate posturing. Ultimately they may develop respiratory arrest, loss of deep tendon reflexes (DTRs), and fixed and dilated pupils. Death is usually from cerebral edema and subsequent herniation. While aspirin is no longer routinely used in children as an antipyretic or pain reliever, the increase in the use of aspirin in adults with heart disease requires specific counseling for parents of children with influenza and varicella to avoid aspirin use. In addition, both of these infections are preventable with proper immunization. *N*-acetylcysteine is protective of hepatocytes in acetaminophen overdose.

347. The answer is e. (*Hay et al, pp 1185-1186. Kliegman et al, pp 1191-1193. McMillan et al, pp 1116-1120. Rudolph et al, pp 985-987.*) Clinical manifestations of shigellosis range from watery stools for several days to severe infection with high fever, abdominal pain, and generalized seizures. In addition, there is a rare and fatal "toxic encephalopathy" seen with *Shigella* infection known as Ekiri syndrome. In general, about 50% of infected children have emesis, greater than two-thirds have fever, 10% to 35% have seizures, and 40% have blood in their stool. Often, the seizure precedes diarrhea and is the complaint that brings the family to the physician. Fever usually lasts about 72 hours, and the diarrhea resolves within 1 to 2 weeks. Presumptive diagnosis can be made on the clinical history; confirmation is through stool culture. Supportive care, including adequate fluid and electrolyte support, is the mainstay of therapy. Antibiotic treatment is problematic; resistance to trimethoprim-sulfamethoxazole and ampicillin is common, necessitating therapy with third-generation cephalosporins in many cases. As always, knowledge of the susceptibility patterns of the bacteria in your area is the key to using the right antibiotic.

348. The answer is d. (*Hay et al, pp 582-583, 1152-1156. Kliegman et al, pp 1036-1041, 1135-1140. McMillan et al, pp 1015-1020, 1125-1130. Rudolph et al, pp 844-845, 993-999.*) The two conditions in consideration are Kawasaki disease and scarlet fever caused by a group A β-hemolytic streptococci. Kawasaki disease is an acute febrile illness of unknown etiology and shares many of its clinical manifestations with scarlet fever. Scarlatiniform rash, desquamation, erythema of the mucous membranes that produces an injected pharynx and strawberry tongue, and cervical lymphadenopathy are prominent findings in both. The most serious complication of Kawasaki disease and scarlet fever is cardiac involvement. Erythrogenic toxin-producing group A β-hemolytic streptococci is the agent responsible for scarlet fever. Isolation of the organism from the nasopharynx and a rise in antistreptolysin titers will confirm the diagnosis. Serologic tests for a variety of infectious agents, both viral and bacterial, have been negative in Kawasaki disease. Rheumatic heart disease is a serious sequela of streptococcal pharyngitis, which can be prevented by appropriate treatment with penicillin. Coronary artery aneurysm and thrombosis are the most serious complications of Kawasaki disease.

The current approach to treatment of Kawasaki disease, which includes specific therapy with aspirin and IV γ-globulin administered within a week of the onset of fever, appears to lower the prevalence of coronary artery dilatation and aneurysm and to shorten the acute phase of the illness.

349. The answer is b. *(Hay et al, p 410. Kliegman et al, pp 2746-2748. McMillan et al, pp 870-873. Rudolph et al, pp 1226-1230.)* Trichophyton tonsurans is a major cause of tinea capitis. It produces an infection within the hair follicle that is unresponsive to topical treatment alone and requires long-term oral therapy with griseofulvin or another antifungal for eradication. Fluorescence is absent on examination by Wood lamp. Diagnosis is made by microscopic examination of KOH preparation of infected hairs and by culture on appropriate media. A severe form of tinea capitis known as *kerion* is shown in the photograph. Enlarged occipital lymph nodes are a common finding. A diagnosis of tinea capitis, and not seborrhea, should be considered in any child between the ages of 6 months and puberty who presents with scaliness and hair loss, even if mild. Seborrhea rarely occurs in that age group. *Microsporum canis* is an occasional cause of tinea capitis, and it does fluoresce under a Wood lamp.

Traction alopecia typically is seen in children who have their hair tied tightly in bows or braids; the hair loss is linear following the area of traction, and is often associated with regional adenopathy. Alopecia areata can appear similar to fungal infections, but the hairs near the active lesion often can be extracted with gentle traction resulting in an attenuated or catagen bulb at the termination of the hair shaft (exclamation hair); it does not produce a kerion as shown in the photograph. Children with biotinidase deficiency and those with hypothyroidism would be unlikely to have only isolated hair loss as the presenting symptom; rather, symptoms might include a variety of neurologic, dermatologic, and ocular complaints.

350. The answer is b. *(Hay et al, pp 1129-1130. Kliegman et al, pp 1357-1360. McMillan et al, pp 1230-1232. Rudolph et al, pp 1058-1059.)* Fifth disease (erythema infectiosum), long recognized as a benign mild exanthem of school-age children, is now known to be caused by human parvovirus B19. Replication of the virus occurs in the erythroid progenitor cells resulting in a decrease in red cell production for about a week in infected patients. While this transient drop in reticulocytes is not noticeable in normal children, patients with hemolytic conditions (such as sickle-cell anemia) thus develop a transient aplastic crisis. A poorly functioning bone marrow (for a week or more) in a patient with a reduced red-cell life span (about 30 days) can result in profound anemia. Other problems can result in patients infected with parvovirus B19. In patients with immunodeficiency, the B19 infection can be persistent and lead to life-threatening chronic anemia. Infection in a pregnant woman can result in severe anemia in the infected fetus, with secondary hydrops fetalis and death. Roseola is now thought to be caused most often by the human herpesvirus 6. Coxsackie A16 virus causes hand-foot-and-mouth disease. Echo-11 virus frequently causes viral meningitis, and cytomegalovirus causes a congenital infection.

351. The answer is c. *(Hay et al, pp 1209-1210. Kliegman et al, pp 1271-1272. McMillan et al, pp 1076-1078. Rudolph et al, pp 944-945.)* Leptospirosis is the most common zoonotic infection worldwide, and is often a mild or subacute illness, frequently escaping detection. Usually a history of exposure to dogs, cats, livestock, rats, or other wild animals is obtained. Two distinct courses of infection are described: "anicteric" leptospirosis and "icteric" leptospirosis (also called Weil syndrome). Both courses start with similar symptoms, as described in the case vignette, termed the "septicemic" phase. The majority of cases are anicteric, and after a few days of symptom resolution, patients go on to the "immune" phase in which meningitic symptoms return and can last up to a month. Between 50% to 90% of cases have meningeal involvement. Less than 10% of leptospirosis cases are "icteric," but these patients go on to have more severe symptoms involving liver and kidney dysfunction. Penicillin and tetracycline (in children 10 years and older) are appropriate treatments, and seem to shorten the duration of the illness if started in the first week of symptoms. Some recommend prophylaxis with weekly doxycycline in endemic areas of the world. IVIG and aspirin are appropriate treatments for Kawasaki disease, but not leptospirosis.

352. The answer is d. *(Hay et al, p 588. Kliegman et al, pp 1953-1960. McMillan et al, pp 1648-1661. Rudolph et al, pp 909-913.)* The presentation of infective endocarditis can be quite variable, ranging from prolonged fever with few other symptoms to an acute and severe course with early toxicity. A high index of suspicion is necessary to make the diagnosis quickly. Identification of the causative organism (frequently *Streptococcus* sp. or *Staphylococcus* sp.) through multiple blood cultures is imperative for appropriate treatment. Echocardiography may identify valvular vegetations and can be predictive of impending embolic events, but a negative echocardiogram does not rule out endocarditis. Treatment usually consists of 4 to 6 weeks of appropriate antimicrobial therapy. Bed rest should be instituted only for heart failure. Antimicrobial prophylaxis prior to and after dental cleaning is indicated. The child is older than typical for Kawasaki disease (80% will present under the age of 5 years), and the history is not consistent with the diagnosis. Scarlet fever is typically self-limited and would not be consistent with the 3-week time course. Tuberculosis can cause prolonged low-grade fever, but cardiac involvement is unusual, consisting of pericarditis; thus a friction rub would be the typical examination finding.

353. The answer is e. *(Hay et al, pp 708-711, 764-765. Kliegman et al, pp 2440-2441, 2513-2521. McMillan et al, pp 924-933, 2679-2680. Rudolph et al, pp 900-904, 2169.)* Unsuspected bacteremia caused by H influenzae type B (now rare), *Neisseria meningitidis*, or S pneumoniae (decreasing in frequency secondary to vaccination) should be considered before prescribing treatment for otitis media in a young, febrile, toxic-appearing infant. In this situation, blood culture should be performed before antibiotic therapy is initiated, and examination of the CSF is indicated if meningitis is suspected.

The classic signs of meningitis are found with increasing reliability in children older than 6 months. Nevertheless, a febrile, irritable, inconsolable infant with an altered state of alertness deserves a lumbar puncture even in the absence of meningeal signs. A petechial rash, characteristically associated with meningococcal infection, has been known to occur with other bacterial infections as well. Organisms may be identified on smear of these lesions.

A fever accompanied by inability to flex rather than rotate the neck immediately suggests meningitis (a sign more reliable in children older than 12 to 18 months of age). An indolent clinical course does not rule out bacterial meningitis. A lumbar puncture is of prime diagnostic importance in determining the presence of bacterial meningitis, which requires immediate antibiotic therapy. A delay in treatment can lead to complications such as cerebrovascular thrombosis, obstructive hydrocephalus, cerebritis with seizures or acute increased intracranial pressure, coma, or death. A missed diagnosis of meningitis is one of the most common reasons for civil litigation involving a pediatrician. In the described patient, lumbar puncture is warranted because of the change in his clinical status.

354. The answer is d. *(Hay et al, pp 1194-1196. Kliegman et al, pp 1178-1182. McMillan et al, pp 1094-1097. Rudolph et al, pp 973-975.)* Newborn infants exposed to pertussis are at considerable risk of being infected regardless of the immune status of the mother. In contrast to other childhood infectious diseases, pertussis is not entirely prevented by transplacentally acquired antibody. Hyperimmune globulin is ineffective and not recommended. Natural immunity conferred by infection is lifelong. Because immunity acquired by immunization declines with age, however, many adults who were immunized in infancy are susceptible to pertussis. The Tdap vaccine has been introduced specifically to address this waning immunity; now, instead of merely receiving a scheduled tetanus (and diphtheria) booster with Td, adults may receive the Tdap which includes a pertussis booster. Erythromycin achieves high concentrations in respiratory secretions and is effective in eliminating organisms from the respiratory tract of patients. In exposed, susceptible persons, erythromycin may be effective in preventing or lessening severity of the disease if administered during the preparoxysmal stage. Immunization against pertussis is unnecessary if the patient has had culture-proven pertussis.

355. The answer is e. *(Hay et al, pp 1123-1124. Kliegman et al, pp 1372-1376. McMillan et al, pp 1241-1246. Rudolph et al, pp 1035-1039.)* To prove a diagnosis of infectious mononucleosis caused by Epstein-Barr virus (EBV), a triad of findings should be present. First, physical findings can include diffuse adenopathy, tonsillar enlargement, an enlarged spleen, small hemorrhages on the soft palate, and periorbital swelling. Second, the hematologic changes should reveal a predominance of lymphocytes with at least 10% of these cells being atypical. Third, the characteristic antibody response should be present. Traditionally, heterophil antibodies can be detected when confirming a diagnosis of infectious mononucleosis. These antibodies may not be present, however, particularly in young children. Alternatively, specific antibodies against viral antigens on the EBV can be measured. Antibodies to viral capsid antigen (VCA) and to anti-D early antigen are elevated prior to the appearance of Epstein-Barr nuclear antigen (EBNA) and are therefore markers for acute infection. IgG VCA and EBNA persist for life, whereas anti-D disappears after 6 months. Adolescents with this condition, because of the enlarged spleen, should avoid contact sports until the splenomegaly has resolved.

While some features of the other conditions can overlap with EBV infection, the totality of the presentation in the case strongly suggests EBV as the causative agent. Initiation of zidovudine would be indicated if the child were proven to have HIV disease. IV acyclovir might be indicated for varicella infection. IV infusion of immunoglobulins and high dose aspirin suggest a diagnosis of Kawasaki disease, which is usually not seen at this age. Intramuscular penicillin might be helpful in streptococcal pharyngitis, but atypical lymphocytes are not usually seen with this condition.

356. The answer is b. *(Hay et al, pp 797-799. Kliegman et al, pp 2841-2845. McMillan et al, pp 2497-2499. Rudolph et al, pp 835, 904-907.)* Acute osteomyelitis tends to begin abruptly, with fever and marked, localized bone tenderness that usually occurs at the metaphysis. Redness and swelling frequently follow. Although usually the result of hematogenous bacterial spread, particularly of *S aureus*, acute osteomyelitis can follow an episode of deep cellulitis or septic joint and should be suspected whenever these occur. Diagnosis often must be based on clinical grounds because early soft tissue changes on plain radiograph often take 3 days to develop, and diagnostic bone changes may not be visible on plain films for up to 12 days after onset of the disease; the radiograph shown demonstrates lytic lesions in the proximal tibia. Bone scans with radionuclides, however, can be useful in the diagnosis of osteomyelitis within 24 to 48 hours of symptoms and in its differentiation from cellulitis and septic arthritis. Magnetic resonance imagining (MRI) has become more widely used for the diagnosis of osteomyelitis, as it is very sensitive and specific.

Caution must be exercised, however, when interpreting a normal bone scan in a patient suspected of having osteomyelitis; falsely normal bone scans do occur in patients with active bone infection. Antibiotic treatment must be initiated immediately to avoid further extension of infection into bone, where adequate drug levels are difficult to achieve. Treatment is usually continued for at least 3 weeks.

357. The answer is c. *(Hay et al, pp 764-765, 1089-1090. Kliegman et al, pp 1145-1149, 2513-2521. McMillan et al, pp 924-933. Rudolph et al, pp 900-904, 999-1001.)* Many organisms can cause meningitis in the neonate, including *E coli, L monocytogenes, H influenzae,* gram-negative rods, group B and D streptococci, and coagulase-positive and coagulase-negative staphylococci; statistically, the most likely cause in this case is late-onset group B streptococci (GBS). Early onset GBS is seen in the first 7 days of life and is associated with maternal complications such as prolonged rupture and chorioamnionitis; late onset GBS occurs after 7 days of life and is not related to maternal issues but rather environmental exposures. As expected, the incidence of early onset GBS has been steadily dropping with maternal prophylaxis; the incidence of late onset GBS has remained unchanged during the same time period. Clinical manifestations of meningitis in neonates include lethargy, bulging fontanelle, seizures, and nuchal rigidity. The diagnosis is made with examination and culture of the CSF. Treatment is begun while awaiting the results of the spinal fluid analysis. Appropriate initial antibiotic coverage must include activity against gram-positive and gram-negative organisms (ampicillin and gentamicin or ampicillin and cefotaxime).

358. The answer is b. *(Hay et al, p 1164. Kliegman et al, pp 1128-1129. McMillan et al, pp 1124-1125. Rudolph et al, p 992.)* Toxic shock syndrome (TSS) is usually caused by *S aureus*, but a similar syndrome (sometimes called toxic shock-like syndrome [TSLS]) may be caused by *Streptococcus* sp. The strains of *S aureus* responsible secrete toxic shock syndrome toxin 1 (TSST-1), and can cause "menstrual" TSS (associated with intravaginal devices like tampons, diaphragms, and contraceptive sponges) or "nonmenstrual" TSS associated with pneumonia, skin infection (as in this patient), bacteremia, or osteomyelitis. The diagnosis is made clinically, and the case description is typical. Treatment includes blood cultures followed by aggressive fluid resuscitation and antibiotics targeting *S aureus*. Kawasaki is not typically seen in adolescents, and is not as rapidly progressive. Shiga toxin–producing strains of *E coli* and *Shigella* are usually associated with hemolytic-uremic syndrome. *Clostridium perfringens* can secrete several toxins; one is an α-toxin that causes hemolysis, platelet lysis, increased vascular permeability, and hepatotoxicity. The neurotoxin secreted by *C tetani* causes tetanus.

359. The answer is a. *(Hay et al, pp 1160-1163. Kliegman et al, pp 1087-1089. McMillan et al, pp 908-911, 1103. Rudolph et al, pp 307-308.)* In an infant who appears otherwise normal, the sudden onset of high fever, together with a marked elevation and shift to the left of the WBC count, suggests pneumococcal bacteremia. The incidence of pneumococcal disease producing this picture may be decreasing with the widespread use of a pneumococcal vaccine. Viral infections such as roseola occasionally can present in a similar fashion but without such profound shifts in the blood leukocyte count. Streptococcosis refers to prolonged, low-grade, insidious nasopharyngitis that sometimes occurs in infants infected with group A β-hemolytic streptococci. Neither typhoid fever nor diphtheria produces markedly high WBC counts; both are characterized by headache, malaise, and other systemic signs. Other bacteria that should be considered in a child with this presentation include *H influenzae* type B (rare in the vaccinated child) and meningococcus.

360. The answer is c. *(Hay et al, pp 1132-1133. Kliegman et al, pp 1337-1341. McMillan et al, pp 1272-1275. Rudolph et al, pp 1075-1079, 2312-2313.)* When German measles (rubella) occurs during the first 2 months of pregnancy, it has a severe effect on the fetus, including cardiac defects, cataracts, and glaucoma. The most common cardiac defects are patent ductus arteriosus, which can be accompanied by peripheral pulmonary artery stenosis, and atrial and ventricular septal defects. A myriad of other complications vary in incidence with the timing of the infection during pregnancy, including thrombocytopenia, hepatosplenomegaly, hepatitis, hemolytic anemia, microcephaly, and a higher risk of developing insulin-dependent diabetes mellitus. The mother's negative rubella titer early in the pregnancy indicates she is susceptible to the infection and its sequelae; her titer undoubtedly now is positive.

A positive hepatitis B surface antibody indicates successful vaccination or old, resolved infection. The positive RPR (a screening test for syphilis) with negative MHATP (the confirmatory test for syphilis) points away from this TORCH infection, but can be associated with a variety of conditions, such as systemic lupus erythematosus or other collagen vascular diseases. The triple screen, usually done at 16 to 18 weeks' gestation, identifies infants at risk for conditions such as Down syndrome or neural tube defects. The positive varicella titer indicates either previous natural infection or successful vaccination.

361. The answer is b. (*Hay et al, pp 430-432. Kliegman et al, p 2587. McMillan et al, pp 809-810. Rudolph et al, p 2367.*) Dacryocystitis is an infection of the nasolacrimal sac. In newborns it is associated with congenital nasolacrimal duct obstruction, which is seen in 6% of normal infants. Nasolacrimal duct obstruction is thought to be caused by the failure of epithelial cells forming the duct to canalize. Treatment of this benign, usually self-limited condition involves nasolacrimal massage and cleaning the area with warm washcloths; failure to open the duct by 6 months usually results in a referral to ophthalmology for surgical opening. When the lacrimal sac is infected, as in dacryocystitis, the patient requires a course of antibiotics to clear the infection.

Chalazion is a firm, nontender nodule that results from a chronic granulomatous inflammation of the meibomian gland. Preseptal (periorbital) and orbital cellulitis may be distinguished by clinical examination. Blood in the anterior chamber of the eye is called a hyphema. Congenital Sjögren syndrome doesn't exist as an entity; however, mothers with Sjögren syndrome may have infants with congenital lupus.

362. The answer is b. (*Hay et al, pp 1214-1222. Kliegman et al, pp 1477-1484. McMillan et al, pp 1341-1350. Rudolph et al, pp 1136-1142.*) The child in the question likely has malaria; a Giemsa-stained smear of peripheral blood will assist in the identification of the malaria species. Blood smears over several days may be required to identify the organism; a single negative "malaria prep" does not eliminate the diagnosis from the differential. Depending on the species of malaria causing the infection, a patient classically presents with paroxysms of fever with intervening periods of relative wellness (except for fatigue). Other symptoms commonly reported include sweating, rigors, headache; abdominal, back, and muscle pain; nausea and vomiting; and, as in this case, pallor and jaundice. Children can present with anorexia, hepatosplenomegaly, thrombocytopenia, and low WBC count.

The family in the question had a hastily arranged trip and did not get prophylaxis prior to departure. Therapy for this condition is complicated by a variety of resistance problems, depending on the location of the travel. Visiting the Centers for Disease Control and Prevention's Web site (www.cdc.gov) provides up-to-date data on recommended prophylaxis prior to travel, as well as therapy for the infected patient.

Of the other answers, hepatitis A is a possibility, but the pattern of high, spiking fevers after visiting an endemic area and without prophylaxis makes malaria a more likely choice. Sickle-cell anemia is a possibility, but this child had no previous history of this condition. Tuberculosis is unlikely to present so quickly after a trip, and the skin test would not be expected to become positive for 2 to 12 weeks after exposure. Hepatitis B is unlikely in this time course.

363. The answer is d. *(Hay et al, pp 1130-1131. Kliegman et al, pp 1331-1337. McMillan et al, pp 1275-1279. Rudolph et al, pp 1053-1056.)* The picture and clinical history presented are most common for the diagnosis of measles (rubeola). This is an uncommon disease in areas where immunization rates are high, but sporadic outbreaks do occur. The rash typically lasts 6 days. Complications are common, including pneumonia, laryngitis, myocarditis, and encephalitis.

Parvovirus B19 causes erythema infectiosum (fifth disease), which presents with low-grade fever, headache, and mild upper respiratory infection (URI) symptoms; the rash is "slapped cheek" in appearance. Rubella in this age of child would present with mild URI symptoms, retroauricular, posterior cervical and postoccipital lymphadenopathy, and then a diffuse erythematous macular-papular rash that clears in about 72 hours. Herpes, depending on where it presents, usually is found to have thin-walled vesicles on an erythematous bases. Varicella presents with fever, malaise, headache, moderate fever 37.8°C to 38.9°C (100°F to 102°F), and then crops of intensely pruritic red macules that evolve into fluid-filled vesicles.

364. The answer is a. (*Hay et al, pp 1132-1133. Kliegman et al, pp 1337-1341. McMillan et al, pp 1272-1275. Rudolph et al, pp 1075-1079.*) Symptoms of rubella (German measles), usually a mild disease, include a diffuse maculopapular rash that lasts for 3 days, marked enlargement of the posterior cervical and occipital lymph nodes, low-grade fever, mild sore throat, and, occasionally, conjunctivitis, arthralgia, or arthritis; it has become a rare disease in the United States. Persons with rubeola (measles) develop a severe cough, coryza, photophobia, conjunctivitis, and a high fever that reaches its peak at the height of the generalized macular rash, which typically lasts for 5 days. Koplik spots on the buccal mucosa are diagnostic; it, too, is a rare disease in the United States. Roseola is a viral exanthem of infants in which the high fever abruptly abates as a rash appears. Erythema infectiosum (fifth disease) begins with bright erythema on the cheeks ("slapped cheek" sign), followed by a red maculopapular rash on the trunk and extremities, which fades centrally at first. Erythema multiforme is a poorly understood syndrome consisting of skin lesions and involvement of mucous membranes. A number of infectious agents and drugs have been associated with this syndrome.

365. The answer is c. (*Kliegman et al, pp 1035-1036. McMillan et al, pp 1141-1142. Rudolph et al, pp 1056-1058.*) The child in this question likely has mumps. Although mumps is usually thought of as a parotitis (presenting as swelling as described in the question), it is a generalized infection and, as such, can have widespread effects and a variety of clinical presentations. Many infections with the mumps virus are unrecognized because of the substantial rate of subclinical attacks. Meningitis, pancreatitis, and renal involvement can occur as part of the disease. Many patients with mumps have some WBCs in their spinal fluid. The meningitis that occurs with mumps can occur at the same time as the parotitis, or following the parotitis by about 10 days. Orchitis, seen most frequently in postpubertal males, has been reported in young children as well. All of these problems can be prevented by prior immunization with live attenuated virus vaccine; widespread use of this vaccine has reduced the number of cases in the United States to less than 500 per year. Arthritis is rare in children. Subendocardial fibroelastosis in a newborn was once thought to be associated with prenatal infection with mumps, but this does not appear to be true.

366. The answer is c. (*Hay et al, pp 277-278, 1135-1136. Kliegman et al, pp 1423-1426. McMillan et al, p 710. Rudolph et al, pp 1062-1064.*) Rabies infection is rare in the United States, but about 50,000 cases occur annually worldwide. While dogs are the most frequent vector of the infection in most parts of the world, immunization of pets in the United States has minimized this reservoir. The most common animal to be infected with rabies in the United States is the raccoon; other potential vectors include skunks, bats, foxes, and coyotes. Small rodents such as mice, squirrels, and rabbits rarely carry the disease. Bats have been associated with the majority of the rabies cases in the United States, with most victims not having an obvious bite. Therefore, the CDC recommends that postexposure prophylaxis (PEP) be considered for any close encounter with a bat, even without an obvious bite, such as the one described above. PEP consists of wound cleansing (if there is a wound), rabies immune globulin (RIG) and the five injection rabies vaccine series. Modifications may be made for patients who have received PEP in the past. Rabies is almost uniformly fatal; many different medications have been attempted, including ribavirin and α-interferon, without success. Of the six reported cases of survival from rabies infection, five had some of the recommended PEP.

367. The answer is e. *(Hay et al, p 1138. Kliegman et al, pp 1289-1293. McMillan et al, pp 987-991. Rudolph et al, pp 1013-1015.)* The incubation period for Rocky Mountain spotted fever (RMSF) has a range of 1 to 14 days. A brief prodromal period consisting of headache and malaise is typically followed by the abrupt onset of fever and chills. A maculopapular rash starts on the second to fourth day of illness on the flexor surfaces of the wrists and ankles before moving in a central direction. Typically, the palms and soles are involved. The rash can become hemorrhagic within 1 or 2 days. Hyponatremia and thrombocytopenia may be seen. Doxycycline is the appropriate treatment, and it must be started early in the course to be effective.

Tularemia has a variable presentation including abrupt onset of fever, chills, malaise, weakness, and headache, and also a variety of skin rashes. Children often have fever, pharyngitis, hepatosplenomegaly, and nonspecific constitutional symptoms.

In the differential diagnosis of RMSF are a number of other diseases. A morbilliform eruption can precede a petechial rash caused by *N meningitidis*. Viral infections, particularly by the enteroviruses, can cause a severe illness that resembles RMSF. Atypical measles is seen primarily in persons who received the killed measles vaccine before 1968. After exposure to wild-type measles, such a person can develop a prodrome consisting of fever, cough, headache, and myalgia. This is usually followed by the development of pneumonia and an urticarial rash beginning on the extremities. TSS is a disease characterized by sudden onset of fever, diarrhea, shock, inflammation of mucous membranes, and a diffuse macular rash resulting in desquamation of the hands and feet.

Lyme disease is seen with an early period of localized disease including erythema migrans, possibly with flu-like symptoms, followed by a distinctive period of erythema migrans, arthralgia, arthritis, meningitis, neuritis, and carditis.

368. The answer is b. *(Hay et al, pp 927-928. Kliegman et al, pp 890-891. McMillan et al, pp 2467-2468. Rudolph et al, p 799.)* The patient described has Wiskott-Aldrich syndrome, an X-linked recessive combined immunodeficiency characterized by thrombocytopenia, eczema, and increased susceptibility to infection. Problems occur early, and frequently prolonged bleeding from the circumcision site is the first clue. The thrombocytopenia also manifests as bloody diarrhea and easy bruising. Patients have impaired humoral immunity with a low serum IgM and a normal or slightly low IgG; they also have cellular immunity problems, with decreased T cells and depressed lymphocyte response. Few live past their teens, frequently succumbing to malignancy caused by EBV infection.

Idiopathic thrombocytopenic purpura (ITP) is an isolated and usually transient thrombocytopenia thought to be secondary to a viral infection. These children do not have increased susceptibility to infection. Acute lymphocytic leukemia (ALL) usually presents with abnormalities in all three cell lines, and does not have a prolonged course as in the described patient. Adenosine deaminase (ADA) deficiency is a type of severe combined immunodeficiency (SCID) but patients always have lymphopenia from birth; platelets are not affected. Partial thymic hypoplasia (partial DiGeorge) patients usually do not have problems early on and can grow up normally, and they do not have thrombocytopenia.

369. The answer is c. *(Hay et al, pp 1211-1213. Kliegman et al, pp 1274-1278. McMillan et al, pp 1046-1049. Rudolph et al, pp 946-948.)* Lyme disease, caused by the spirochete *Borrelia burgdorferi* and transmitted mostly by ticks of the Ioxodes family, is characterized by a unique skin lesion, recurrent attacks of arthritis, and occasional involvement of the heart and CNS. Illness usually appears in late summer or early fall, 2 to 30 days after a bite by an infecting tick. Erythema chronicum migrans begins as a red macule, usually on the trunk at the site of tick attachment, which enlarges in a circular fashion with central clearing. Nonspecific systemic signs include headache, fever, and malaise. Joint involvement generally occurs days to years after onset of the rash. Cardiac disease consists primarily of disturbances of rhythm. Involvement of the CNS is evidenced by headache and stiff neck. The diagnosis should be suspected when any of the signs and symptoms occur, because the disease can present in an atypical manner. The characteristic lesion of erythema chronicum migrans, as well as the history of tick bite, have frequently not been noted by the patient. It is not until late joint, heart, or neurologic manifestations occur, and Lyme disease is suspected, that serologic evidence confirms the etiology. Serologic evidence is sought when the patient has spent time in summer months in endemic areas or there is a risk of tick bite. Treatment with penicillin or tetracycline results in a faster resolution of symptoms and prevention of later complications, especially if given early in the course of the disease. The *Dermacentor* family of ticks is typically associated with RMSF, while the *Ixodes* family is associated with Lyme disease. *Borrelia* is a spirochete, not a *Rickettsia*.

370. The answer is e. (*Hay et al, p 1229. Kliegman et al, p 1465. McMillan et al, pp 1327-1329. Rudolph et al, pp 1126-1128.*) *Cryptosporidium* has become an important cause of diarrhea in immunocompromised patients, particularly those with AIDS. It can also affect patients who are immunocompetent, and has been recognized as an agent responsible for epidemics of diarrhea in day-care centers. Although the disease is self-limited in immunocompetent individuals, treatment with the antiparasitic nitazoxanide can improve symptoms quickly. Persistent, nonsuppurative diarrhea as described in the question can be caused by such organisms as amebas, whipworms (trichuriasis), *Cryptosporidium*, or *Giardia lamblia*. *Salmonella sonnei* can be grown in culture, but microscopy is not helpful other than finding fecal leukocytes. *Enterobius vermicularis* is pinworms, which causes rectal itching and not diarrhea. Sporotrichosis is a fungal infection of the cutaneous and subcutaneous tissue that typically does not cause diarrhea. Acquired *Toxoplasma gondii* can infest any body tissue. Infection can result in fever, myalgia, lymphadenopathy, maculopapular rash, hepatomegaly, pneumonia, encephalitis, chorioretinitis, or myocarditis. This intracellular parasite does not ordinarily cause diarrhea and is not found in stools.

371. The answer is c. (*Hay et al, p 418. Kliegman et al, p 2687. McMillan et al, pp 848-849. Rudolph et al, pp 1195-1197.*) The combination of erythema multiforme and vesicular, ulcerated lesions of the mucous membranes of the eyes, mouth, anus, and urethra defines the Stevens-Johnson syndrome (erythema multiforme major). Fever is common, and even pulmonary involvement occasionally is noted; the mortality rate can approach 10%. Common complications include corneal ulceration; dehydration due to severe stomatitis, and, subsequently, poor fluid intake; and urinary retention caused by dysuria. Among the known causes of the Stevens-Johnson syndrome are allergy to various drugs (including phenytoin, barbiturates, sulfonamides, and penicillin) and infection with a variety of organisms including *Mycoplasma pneumoniae* or herpes type 1. Erythema multiforme is sometimes confused with urticaria early in the course because both can have a target-like lesion. The former has a target center that contains a papule or vesicle, which progresses to blister and necrosis. In contrast, urticaria can have a bluish center, but the lesions are transient (often lasting less than 24 hours) and are pruritic. Kawasaki disease is an acute febrile illness of unknown etiology, sharing many of its clinical manifestations with scarlet fever. Scarlatiniform rash, desquamation, erythema of the mucous membranes that produces an injected pharynx and strawberry tongue (but not sloughing, as in the case presentation), and cervical lymphadenopathy are prominent findings in both. Persons with rubeola develop a severe cough, coryza, photophobia, conjunctivitis, and a high fever that reaches its peak at the height of the generalized macular rash, which typically lasts for 5 days. The oral changes include Koplik spots (transient white pinpoint lesions on a bright red buccal mucosa often in the area opposite the lower molars) but not sloughing.

DRESS (drug rash, eosinophilia, and systemic symptoms) is another consideration in this patient. The condition is usually associated with anticonvulsants, but has been associated with other medications such as antibiotics. The skin findings are the same as erythema multiforme (EM), but patients may also have lymphadenopathy; eosinophilia; leukocytosis; fever; and liver, kidney, and lung involvement.

372. The answer is e. *(Hay et al, pp 1234-1235. Kliegman et al, p 1508. McMillan et al, pp 1368-1369. Rudolph at al, pp 1111-1112.)* One to seven days following the ingestion of pork or other improperly cooked meat infected with *T spiralis*, symptoms develop, including abdominal pain, nausea, vomiting, and malaise. During the second week, muscle invasion occurs, which causes edema of eyelids, myalgia, weakness, fever, and eosinophilia. The muscle organisms can become encysted and remain viable for years.

Enterobius vermicularis (pinworm) causes a localized infestation resulting in perianal pruritus and does not have a tissue phase that would cause eosinophilia. Sporotrichosis is a chronic fungal infection that typically is limited to cutaneous and subcutaneous tissues. *Giardia* and *Cryptosporidium* rarely penetrate the gut wall, instead causing gas, diarrhea, and bloating as common findings, but not fever and eosinophilia.

373. The answer is e. *(Hay et al, pp 1167-1169. Kliegman et al, pp 1164-1168. McMillan et al, pp 1082-1087. Rudolph et al, pp 970-972.)* The patient in the question likely has meningococcemia, but RMFS is also a consideration. RMFS and meningococcemia can present in a similar fashion, although a rapid course as outlined in the question is more common of meningococcemia. Meningococcemia can be complicated by a variety of disorders, including meningitis, purulent pericarditis, endocarditis, pneumonia, otitis media, and arthritis. (Arthritis associated with meningococcemia may be mediated by an immune mechanism rather than by bacterial invasion of the joint.) The potent endotoxin of the causative organism, *N meningitidis*, can induce shock, disseminated intravascular coagulation with associated hemorrhaging, and acute adrenal failure caused by localized intra-adrenal bleeding; these reactions can be collectively referred to as the Waterhouse-Friderichsen syndrome. Vaccines against *N meningitidis* groups A, C, Y, and W135 are now available, and the CDC's Advisory Committee on Immunization Practices now recommends meningococcal immunization of all adolescents (11-18 years old). Prophylaxis with sulfadiazine for sensitive organisms or with rifampin for those in close contact with affected persons is recommended.

In contrast, RMFS is often a more indolent infection, with rash developing days after the onset of the fever and other symptoms. This course is not invariable, however, and antibiotic therapy for the patient for whom RMFS and meningococcemia cannot be differentiated should not be delayed.

Measles presents in a child with a several days' history of malaise, fever, cough, coryza, and conjunctivitis followed by the typical, widespread, erythematous, maculopapular rash. Koplik spots, white pinpoint lesions on a bright red buccal mucosa often in the area opposite his lower molars, appear transiently and are pathognomonic. Henoch-Schönlein purpura can have a distribution of rash that appears purpuric (actually a vasculitis) over the lower extremities, but its rapid progression and shocklike state as presented in the question would be distinctly unusual.

374. The answer is a. *(Hay et al, pp 708-709. Kliegman et al, pp 2440-2441. McMillan et al, pp 2679-2680. Rudolph et al, p 2169.)* The importance and urgency of the lumbar puncture in cases of suspected meningitis outweigh the usual niceties in the performance of procedures. Infants and children require adequate restraints, preferably local anesthesia, and sometimes sedation.

Contraindications are few and include increased intracranial pressure in the patient without an open fontanelle that can result in herniation; severe cardiorespiratory distress; skin infection at the puncture site; and severe thrombocytopenia or other coagulation disorder, suggested by the oozing IV and venipuncture sites.

375. The answer is c. (*Hay et al, pp 500-502. Kliegman et al, pp 1763-1766. McMillan et al, pp 694-695. Rudolph et al, pp 1275-1277.*) The description is that of croup. This infection involves the larynx and trachea; it usually is caused by parainfluenza or respiratory syncytial viruses. The usual age range for presentation is 6 months to 6 years. Symptoms include low-grade fever, barking cough, and hoarse, inspiratory stridor without wheezing. The pharynx can be normal or slightly red, and the lungs are usually clear. In children in severe respiratory distress, prolonged dyspnea can progress to physical exhaustion and fatal respiratory failure. Expiratory stridor is usually associated with a fixed obstruction, such as a tumor or vascular ring. Because agitation can be a sign of hypoxia, sedation should not be ordered. Hyperinflation on chest x-ray is seen in asthma, not croup. One condition in the differential in this child is epiglottitis, a now rare disease owing to widespread use of the *H influenza* b vaccine. Its presentation is more abrupt, with higher fever in rather toxic-appearing patients.

376 to 379. The answers are 376-b, 377-a, 378-e, 379-c. (*Hay et al, pp 922, 925-928. Kliegman et al, pp 879-880, 884-891. McMillan et al, pp 2445-2446, 2462-2464, 2467-2468. Rudolph et al, pp 793-800.*) Many primary immunologic deficiencies can be classified as defects of T-lymphocyte function (containment of fungi, protozoa, acid-fast bacteria, and certain viruses) and B-lymphocyte function (synthesis and secretion of immunoglobulins). Among the T-cell diseases is DiGeorge anomaly, in which defective embryologic development of the third and fourth pharyngeal pouches results in hypoplasia of both thymus and parathyroid glands. Associated findings with DiGeorge anomaly include CATCH: *C* for cardiac, *A* for abnormal faces, *T* for thymic hypoplasia, *C* for cleft palate, and *H* for hypocalcemia.

Primary B-cell diseases include X-linked agammaglobulinemia (XLA, or Bruton disease), a deficiency of all three major classes of immunoglobulins, as well as other selective deficiencies of the immunoglobulins or their subgroups. This condition usually presents after 3 months of age (after maternal antibodies wane) with recurrent and often simultaneous bouts of otitis media, pneumonia, diarrhea, and sinusitis, but usually without fungal and viral infections. Combined T- and B-cell diseases include the X-linked recessive Wiskott-Aldrich syndrome of mild T-cell dysfunction, diminished serum IgM, marked elevation of IgA and IgE, eczema, recurrent middle-ear infections, lymphopenia, and thrombocytopenia. Patients with the catastrophic combined T- and B-cell disease, known as severe combined immunodeficiency disease (Swiss-type lymphopenic agammaglobulinemia or SCID), have deficient T and B cells. Consequently, they have both, lymphopenia and agammaglobulinemia, as well as thymic hypoplasia. Chronic diarrhea; rashes; recurrent, serious bacterial, fungal, or viral infections; wasting; and early death are characteristic. Other T- and B-cell deficiencies include ataxia telangiectasia and chronic mucocutaneous candidiasis.

Job-Buckley syndrome is a disorder of phagocytic chemotaxis associated with hypergammaglobulin E, eczema-like rash, and recurrent severe staphylococcal infections.

380 to 385. The answers are 380-i, 381-b, 382-a, 383-d, 384-e, 385-f.

(Hay et al, pp 608-609, 1119-1120, 1123-1124, 1132-1133, 1156-1158, 1178-1182, 1196-1197, 1204-1205. Kliegman et al, pp 1145-1149, 1157-1159, 1193-1196, 1208-1210, 1219-1222, 1337-1341, 1372-1376, 1572-1573. McMillan et al, pp 438, 482-483, 1053-1058, 1079-1081, 1106-1110, 1241-1246, 1260-1261, 1272-1275. Rudolph et al, pp 923-928, 945-946, 987-990, 999-1001, 1035-1040, 1110-1111, 1430-1431.) EBV can produce a number of clinically important syndromes, one of which is mononucleosis as described in the college-age patient with fever and sore throat. Other symptoms might include headache, profound fatigue, abdominal pain, and myalgia. Splenic enlargement is common, and contact sports are to be avoided. The rash ("ampicillin rash") is poorly understood but occurs so commonly as to be diagnostic when seen; it is self-resolving.

Pseudomonas is a ubiquitous organism. Most infections with the organism are opportunistic, involving several organs. Skin infections related to burns, trauma (such as in a puncture wound through a tennis shoe), and use of swimming pools are not uncommon. Injuries through a tennis shoe are prone to pseudomonal infections because of the warm, moist nature of the shoe's environment. In contrast, a wound through a bare foot would be associated with cutaneous flora such as *Staphylococcus*.

Bartonella henselae is the major etiologic agent for cat-scratch disease (the 5-year-old with a feline scratch). History of a scratch or a bite from a kitten is often positive, and fleas are often a factor in transmission. Diagnosis is usually by history and presenting signs and symptoms, as described in the question. Another form of the disease, Parinaud oculoglandular syndrome, occurs when the primary site of inoculation occurs in or near the conjunctivae, resulting in a moderately severe conjunctivitis and preauricular lymph adenopathy.

Roseola (exanthema subitum) is a common acute illness of young children (such as the 9-month-old child with fever and transient rash), characterized by several days of high fever followed by a rapid defervescence and the appearance of an evanescent, erythematous, maculopapular rash. Human herpesvirus 6 (HHV-6) has been identified as its main cause.

Urinary tract infections are the most common cause of bacterial infections in the young child. The incidence is slightly higher in the uncircumcised as compared to the circumcised male. *E coli* is a leading cause.

Infection with *H pylori* is associated with antral gastritis and primary duodenal ulcer disease, with the symptoms described in the question of the 9-year-old with abdominal pain and blood in the stool. Culture for *H pylori* requires endoscopy and gastric biopsy. The biopsied tissue can be tested for urease activity and examined histologically after special staining. Alternatively, noninvasive tests involving detection of metabolic products of *H pylori* (urease activity) or antibodies against *H pylori* can be demonstrated.

386 to 388.   The answers are 386-d, 387-c, 388-a. *(Hay et al, pp 1171, 1179, 1206. Kliegman et al, pp 1171, 1196, 1266. McMillan et al, pp 1066, 1088-1090, 1139-1140. Rudolph et al, pp 969, 987, 1003.)* Certain pathogens do not grow on routine culture media. A routine stool culture will not make the diagnosis of enterohemorrhagic *E coli*, since some *E coli* strains are normal intestinal flora. To differentiate the pathogenic organism in the case of the patient with hemolytic uremic syndrome, stool culture on sorbitol MacConkey will help diagnose *E coli* O157:H7. While there are rapid gonorrhea assays available now, the gold standard is still culture. Regular chocolate agar can be used for specimens from usually sterile areas (blood, spinal fluid); a selective culture medium (such as modified Thayer-Martin media, which includes several antimicrobial compounds) is needed for cultures of sites normally colonized with other organisms (cervix, rectum). Syphilis is not usually cultured. It is identified by direct visualization of treponemes with dark field microscopy, or with the use of serological tests such as the nontreponemal rapid plasma reagin (RPR) test, or the treponemal-specific fluorescent treponemal antibody absorption (FTA-ABS) test.

389 to 392.   The answers are 389-c, 390-a, 391-g, 392-b.   *(Hay et al, pp 51, 518-525, 1160-1167, 1239-1252. Kliegman et al, pp 1125, 1245-1247, 1278-1280, 1286-1287, 1795-1799. McMillan et al, pp 537-540, 1102-1106, 1146-1147, 1395-1400, 1404-1410. Rudolph et al, pp 929-931, 949-959, 965-967, 1980-1986.)* Approximately 10% to 20% of infants born to mothers with *Chlamydia trachomatis* infection develop pneumonia. The presentation of this pneumonia usually occurs between 1 and 3 months of age, with cough, tachypnea, and lack of fever. Examination reveals rales but not wheezing. Laboratory data suggestive of *C trachomatis* infection include an increase in eosinophils in the peripheral blood. The chest radiograph shows hyperinflation with interstitial infiltrates.

Mycoplasma pneumoniae is a common cause of pneumonia in the school-age child or young adult. Usual presentation includes the gradual onset of headache, malaise, fever, and lower respiratory symptoms. Typically, the cough (often nonproductive) worsens for the first 2 weeks of the illness, and then slowly resolves over the ensuing 3 to 4 weeks. Early in the disease, the physical examination is remarkable for a paucity of signs; the patient usually has a few fine rales. Later, the dyspnea and fever become worse. Radiographic findings include an interstitial or bronchial pattern, especially in the lower lobes, and commonly on only one side. The diagnosis is usually made on clinical grounds.

Staphylococcal pneumonia is caused by *S aureus*. It is a rapidly progressive and life-threatening form of pneumonia most commonly seen in children less than 1 year of age. Commonly, the child has an upper respiratory infection for several days, with the abrupt onset of fever and respiratory distress. Pleural effusion, empyema, and pyopneumothorax are common complications. Laboratory evidence of this disease can include a markedly elevated WBC count with left shift. Radiographic findings include nonspecific bronchopneumonia early in the disease, which later becomes more dense and homogeneous and involves an entire lobe or hemithorax.

Pneumococcal pneumonia often presents with sudden onset of fever, cough, and chest pain. This child may have failed outpatient therapy because of increased incidence of resistant organisms. Pleural effusions or empyema are commonly seen; chest tube evacuation of the fluid is often required. Depending on sensitivity patterns in a particular community, therapy with high-dose penicillin, cefuroxime, amoxicillin/clavulanate, or even vancomycin may be required.

A high index of suspicion is needed to diagnose tuberculosis. An exposure history is helpful but not always present. Many children who are infected have a positive purified protein derivative (PPD) as the only evidence. Children at higher risk of active disease include those who are very young, malnourished, immunodeficient or immunosuppressed, or diabetic. Most active disease is pulmonary, but can also be disseminated and involve the CNS, bone, skin, and abdomen. Pulmonary disease includes a parenchymal focus and regional lymphadenopathy. The pleura is frequently involved.

Fungal infections can resemble TB, and can be difficult to diagnose. In the United States, *Histoplasma* is found in the Ohio and Mississippi river valleys. Human-to-human transmission does not occur, so exposure to an endemic area is required. About half of histoplasmosis infection is asymptomatic and diagnosed based on scattered calcifications in the lungs. In immunocompetent individuals, the disease usually resolves in 2 weeks. Other clinically significant fungi that cause lung disease include *Coccidioides, Cryptococcus, Blastomyces,* and *Aspergillus. Pneumocystis jiroveci* (formerly *Pneumocystis carinii*) is technically a fungus, but responds to antiparasitic medications.

Hematologic and Neoplastic Diseases

Questions

393. Two weeks after a viral syndrome, a 2-year-old child develops bruising and generalized petechiae, more prominent over the legs. No hepatosplenomegaly or lymph node enlargement is noted. The examination is otherwise unremarkable. Laboratory testing shows the patient to have a normal hemoglobin, hematocrit, and white blood cell (WBC) count and differential. The platelet count is 15,000/μL. Which of the following is the most likely diagnosis?

a. Von Willebrand disease (vWD)
b. Acute leukemia
c. Idiopathic (immune) thrombocytopenic purpura (ITP)
d. Aplastic anemia
e. Thrombotic thrombocytopenic purpura

394. An 11-month-old African American boy has a hematocrit of 24% on a screening laboratory done at his well-child checkup. Further testing demonstrates: hemoglobin 7.8 g/dL; hematocrit 22.9%; leukocyte count 12,200/μL with 39% neutrophils, 6% bands, 55% lymphocytes; hypochromia on smear; free erythrocyte protoporphyrin (FEP) 114 μg/dL; lead level 6 μg/dL whole blood; platelet count 175,000/μL; reticulocyte count 0.2%; sickle-cell preparation negative; stool guaiac-negative; and mean corpuscular volume (MCV) 64 fL. Which of the following is the most appropriate recommendation?

a. Blood transfusion
b. Oral ferrous sulfate
c. Intramuscular iron dextran
d. An iron-fortified cereal
e. Calcium EDTA

395. The parents of a previously healthy 2-year-old child note her to be pale and bring her to your clinic for evaluation. She currently has no fever, nausea, emesis, bone pain, or other complaints. Her examination is significant for pallor, tachycardia, and a systolic ejection murmur, but she has no organomegaly. Her complete blood count (CBC) reveals a hemoglobin of 4 g/dL, normal indices for age, a WBC count of 6.5/μL, and a platelet count of 750,000/μL. Her reticulocyte count is 0%. Coombs test is negative. Her peripheral blood smear shows no blast forms and no fragments. Red blood cell (RBC) adenosine deaminase levels are normal. A bone marrow reveals markedly decreased erythroid precursors. Which of the following is this child's likely diagnosis?

a. Diamond-Blackfan anemia
b. Sickle-cell anemia
c. Pearson marrow-pancreas syndrome
d. Iron deficiency anemia
e. Transient erythroblastopenia of childhood

396. On a routine-screening CBC, a 1-year-old is noted to have a microcytic anemia. A follow-up hemoglobin electrophoresis demonstrates an increased concentration of hemoglobin A2. The child is most likely to have which of the following?

a. Iron deficiency
b. β-Thalassemia trait
c. Sickle-cell anemia
d. Chronic systemic illness
e. Lead poisoning

397. After being delivered following a benign gestation, a newborn infant is noted to have a platelet count of 35,000/μL, decreased fibrinogen, and elevated fibrin spilt products. On examination you note a large cutaneous hemangioma on the abdomen that is purple and firm. Which of the following anomalies might also be expected in this infant?

a. Kaposiform hemangioendothelioma
b. Nevus simplex
c. Nevus flammeus
d. PHACE(S) syndrome
e. Infantile fibrosarcoma

398. A 4-year-old previously well African American boy is brought to the office by his aunt. She reports that he developed pallor, dark urine, and jaundice over the past few days. He stays with her, has not traveled, and has not been exposed to a jaundiced person, but he is taking trimethoprim sulfamethoxazole for otitis media. The CBC in the office shows a low hemoglobin and hematocrit, while his "stat" serum electrolytes, blood urea nitrogen (BUN), and chemistries are remarkable only for an elevation of his bilirubin levels. His aunt seems to recall his 8-year-old brother having had an "allergic reaction" to aspirin, which also caused a short-lived period of anemia and jaundice. Which of the following is the most likely cause of this patient's symptoms?

a. Hepatitis B
b. Hepatitis A
c. Hemolytic-uremic syndrome
d. Gilbert syndrome
e. Glucose-6-phosphate dehydrogenase deficiency

399. Your sister who lives in another state sends via e-mail photographs of her 6-month-old infant. You note the child has a white reflection from one of his eyes. You hastily assist in arranging an urgent pediatric ophthalmologic evaluation. Your sister immediately accesses the Internet and begins to ask questions of you. Which of the following statements found by your sister is correct?

a. Most cases of retinoblastoma are unilateral and hereditary.
b. Cure rates for retinoblastoma treated in the United States exceed 90%.
c. Biopsy is usually performed to confirm the diagnosis.
d. Intraocular calcifications are an unusual finding and suggest worse prognosis.
e. Patients with the hereditary form of retinoblastoma are at significantly increased risk of leukemia in later years.

400. A 2950-g (6.5-lb) black baby boy is born at home at term. On arrival at the hospital, he appears pale, but the physical examination is otherwise normal. Laboratory studies reveal the following: mother's blood type A, Rh-positive; baby's blood type O, Rh-positive; hematocrit 38%; and reticulocyte count 5%. Which of the following is the most likely cause of the anemia?

a. Fetomaternal transfusion
b. ABO incompatibility
c. Physiologic anemia of the newborn
d. Sickle-cell anemia
e. Iron-deficiency anemia

401. A father brings his 3-year-old daughter to the emergency center after noting her to be pale and tired and with a subjective fever for several days. Her past history is significant for an upper respiratory infection 4 weeks prior, but she had been otherwise healthy. The father denies emesis or diarrhea, but does report his daughter has had leg pain over the previous week, waking her from sleep. He also reports that she has been bleeding from her gums after brushing her teeth. Examination reveals a listless pale child. She has diffuse lymphadenopathy with splenomegaly but no hepatomegaly. She has a few petechiae scattered across her face and abdomen and is mildly tender over her shins, but does not have associated erythema or joint swelling. A CBC reveals a leukocyte count of 8,000/μL with a hemoglobin of 4 g/dL and a platelet count of 7,000/μL. The automated differential reports an elevated number of atypical lymphocytes. Which of the following diagnostic studies is the most appropriate next step in the management of this child?

a. Epstein-Barr virus titers
b. Serum haptoglobin
c. Antiplatelet antibody assay
d. Reticulocyte count
e. Bone marrow biopsy

402. While bathing her newly-received 2-year-old son, a foster mother feels a mass in his abdomen. A thorough medical evaluation of the child reveals aniridia, hypospadias, horseshoe kidney, and hemihypertrophy. Which of the following is the most likely diagnosis for this child?

a. Neuroblastoma
b. Wilms tumor
c. Hepatoblastoma
d. Rhabdomyosarcoma
e. Testicular cancer

403. A healthy 1-year-old child comes to your office for a routine checkup and for immunizations. His parents have no complaints or concerns. The next day, the CBC you performed as customary screening for anemia returns with the percentage of eosinophils on the differential to be 30%. Which of the following is the most likely explanation?

a. Bacterial infections
b. Chronic allergic rhinitis
c. Fungal infections
d. Helminth infestation
e. Tuberculosis

404. A 2-year-old child in shock has multiple nonblanching purple lesions of various sizes scattered about on the trunk and extremities; petechiae are noted, and oozing from the venipuncture site has been observed. The child's peripheral blood smear is shown below. Clotting studies are likely to show which of the following?

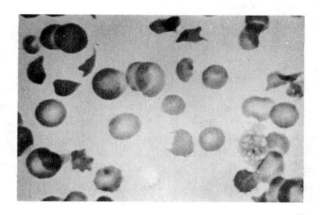

a. Increased levels of factor V and VIII
b. A decreased prothrombin level
c. An increased fibrinogen level
d. The presence of fibrin split products
e. Normal partial thromboplastin time (PTT)

405. A male infant was found to be jaundiced 12 hours after birth. At 36 hours of age, his serum bilirubin was 18 mg/dL, hemoglobin concentration was 12.5 g/dL, and reticulocyte count 9%. Many nucleated RBCs and some spherocytes were seen in the peripheral blood smear. The differential diagnosis should include which of the following?

a. Pyruvate kinase deficiency
b. Hereditary spherocytosis
c. Sickle-cell anemia
d. Rh incompatibility
e. Polycythemia

406. On a routine well-child examination, a 1-year-old boy is noted to be pale. He is in the 75th percentile for weight and the 25th percentile for length. Results of physical examination are otherwise normal. His hematocrit is 24%. The answer to which of the following questions is most likely to be helpful in making a diagnosis?

a. What is the child's usual daily diet?
b. Did the child receive phototherapy for neonatal jaundice?
c. Has anyone in the family received a blood transfusion?
d. Is the child on any medications?
e. What is the pattern and appearance of his bowel movements?

407. A 10-year-old boy is admitted to the hospital because of bleeding. Pertinent laboratory findings include a platelet count of 50,000/μL, prothrombin time (PT) of 15 seconds (control 11.5 seconds), activated partial thromboplastin time (aPTT) of 51 seconds (control 36 seconds), thrombin time (TT) of 13.7 seconds (control 10.5 seconds), and factor VIII level of 14% (normal 38%-178%). Which of the following is the most likely cause of his bleeding?

a. Immune thrombocytopenic purpura (ITP)
b. Vitamin K deficiency
c. Disseminated intravascular coagulation (DIC)
d. Hemophilia A
e. Hemophilia B

408. A 17-year-old adolescent comes to your office seeking help for "heavy" menses. Your review of systems also reveals weekly epistaxis. Her only significant past history includes a tonsillectomy at age 6 after which she required blood transfusion for excessive bleeding. Her family history includes several people who seem to bleed and bruise more easily than others. The patient's mother required a hysterectomy after child birth for excessive hemorrhage. You order a variety of laboratory tests. The patient has a hemoglobin of 6.5 mg/dL with an MCV of 60%; her platelet count is 350,000/μL. Her von Willebrand antigen and her von Willebrand factor (vWF) activity (ristocetin cofactor activity) are decreased. Her vWF is reported as normal but in decreased amounts. You have been unable to reach her to report the findings, but when she calls about 1 week later she reports she is having a mild to moderate nosebleed. You initiate therapy with which of the following?

a. Aminocaproic acid (Amicar)
b. vWF concentrate alone
c. vWF with factor VIII
d. Desmopressin (DDAVP)
e. Intravenous immunoglobulin (IVIG)

409. Over the previous 2 to 3 weeks, a very active 13-year-old white boy is noted by his family to have developed deep pains in his leg that awaken him from sleep. The family brings him to your office with a complaint of a swelling over his distal leg, which he attributes to his being kicked while playing soccer about 1 week ago. He has had no fever, headaches, weakness, bruising, or other symptoms. A radiograph of the leg is shown below. Which of the following is the most likely explanation for his pain?

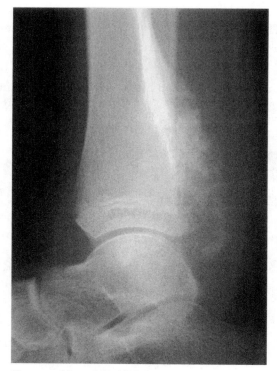

(Courtesy of Susan John, MD.)

a. Growing pains
b. Leukemia
c. Osteomyelitis
d. Bone fracture
e. Osteosarcoma

410. An otherwise healthy 17-year-old complains of swollen glands in his neck and groin for the past 6 months and an increasing cough over the previous 2 weeks. He also reports some fevers, especially at night, and possibly some weight loss. On examination, you notice that he has nontender cervical, supraclavicular, axillary, and inguinal nodes, no hepatosplenomegaly, and otherwise looks to be fairly healthy. Which of the following would be the appropriate next step?

a. Biopsy of a node
b. CBC and differential
c. Trial of antituberculosis drugs
d. Chest radiograph
e. Cat-scratch titers

411. An otherwise healthy child has on his 1-year-old routine CBC the polymorphonuclear neutrophil shown below. This child likely has which of the following?

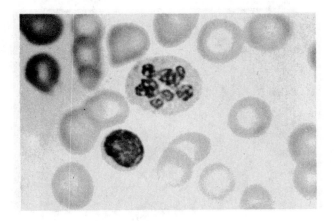

a. Malignancy
b. Iron deficiency
c. Folic acid deficiency
d. Döhle inclusion bodies
e. The Pelger-Huët nuclear anomaly

Questions 412 to 415

For each disorder listed below, select the peripheral blood smear with which it is most likely to be associated. Each lettered option may be used once, more than once, or not at all.

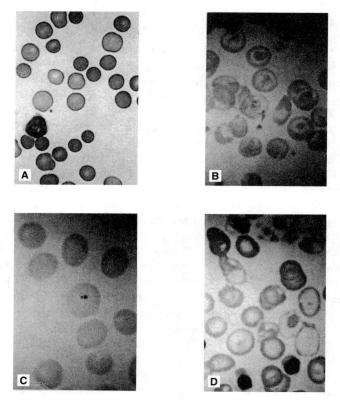

412. An 8-year-old patient with sickle-cell anemia

413. A 7-month-old boy with severe anemia requiring transfusions, heart failure, hepatosplenomegaly, and weakness

414. A 3-day-old newborn with anemia and pathologic hyperbilirubinemia requiring phototherapy

415. A completely asymptomatic, healthy 1-year-old whose routine CBC reveals an abnormality

Hematologic and Neoplastic Diseases

Answers

393. The answer is c. *(Hay et al, pp 860-862. Kliegman et al, pp 2082-2084. McMillan et al, pp 1731-1733. Rudolph et al, pp 1556-1557.)* In children, ITP is the most common form of thrombocytopenic purpura. In most cases, a preceding viral infection can be noted. No diagnostic test identifies this disease; exclusion of the other diseases listed in the question is necessary. In this disease, the platelet count is frequently less than 20,000/µL, but other laboratory tests yield essentially normal results, including the bone marrow aspiration (if done). Complications are uncommon; significant bleeding occurs in only 5% of cases and intracranial hemorrhage is even rarer. The treatment of childhood ITP is controversial. Patients with mild symptoms such as bruising and self-limited epistaxis may be observed, while patients with significant bleeding should be treated. IVIG and corticosteroids are effective in causing a rapid increase in platelet count, but controversy exists surrounding the use of prednisone before ruling out leukemia with a bone marrow aspirate. For Rh-positive patients with a working spleen, the use of anti-D immunoglobulin also results in an increase in platelet count. For patients with chronic (> 1 year) ITP, a splenectomy may be helpful.

Aplastic anemia is unlikely if the other cell lines are normal. Von Willebrand disease might be expected to present with bleeding and not just bruising. It is unlikely that acute leukemia would present with thrombocytopenia only. Thrombotic thrombocytopenic purpura is rare in children.

394. The answer is b. *(Hay et al, pp 837-838. Kliegman et al, pp 2014-2017. McMillan et al, pp 1692-1694. Rudolph et al, pp 1525-1528.)* Response to a therapeutic trial of iron is an appropriate and cost-effective method of diagnosing iron-deficiency anemia. A prompt reticulocytosis and rise in hemoglobin and hematocrit follow the administration of an oral preparation of ferrous sulfate. Intramuscular iron dextran should be reserved for situations in which compliance cannot be achieved, since this treatment is expensive, painful, and no more effective than oral iron. Dietary modifications, such as limiting the intake of cow's milk and including iron-fortified cereals along with a mixed diet, are appropriate long-term measures, but they will not make enough iron available to replenish iron stores. The gradual onset of iron-deficiency anemia enables a child to adapt to surprisingly low hemoglobin concentrations. Transfusion is rarely indicated unless a child becomes symptomatic or is further compromised by a superimposed infection.

When the iron available for production of hemoglobin is limited, free protoporphyrins accumulate in the blood. Levels of erythrocyte protoporphyrin (EP) are also elevated in lead poisoning. Iron-deficiency anemia can be differentiated from lead intoxication by measuring blood lead, which should be less than 10 μg/dL.

395. The answer is e. *(Hay et al, pp 836-837. Kliegman et al, pp 2006-2009. McMillan et al, pp 1707-1709 . Rudolph et al, pp 1566-1567.)* This child has transient erythroblastopenia of childhood (TEC), the most common acquired RBC aplasia in children. This condition is commonly diagnosed between the ages of 1 to 3 years and some affected children have a history of a recent viral infection; however, no specific virus has been implicated (parvovirus B19 is usually specifically excluded). Physical findings are minimal and include pallor and tachycardia. Laboratory studies reveal a profound anemia and reticulocytopenia with a marked reduction in erythrocyte precursors in the marrow. RBC adenosine deaminase (ADA) levels are normal. The condition lasts for several months, and may require 1 or 2 transfusions, but ultimately is self-limited. Steroids are not helpful.

Alternative diagnoses with this presentation include Diamond-Blackfan anemia (DBA), but this condition is congenital and usually presents in infancy; RBC ADA levels are usually elevated. In addition, about half of patients with DBA will have congenital anomalies including short stature, cranial abnormalities, and upper extremity abnormalities. Pearson marrow-pancreas is another form of congenital hypoplastic anemia, including poor growth, pancreatic fibrosis with insulin-dependant diabetes, and muscle and nerve involvement. Early death is typical. Sickle-cell patients usually have evidence of ongoing hemolysis on their smear, and iron deficiency causes a microscopic hypochromic anemia.

396. The answer is b. *(Hay et al, pp 844-845. Kliegman et al, pp 2033-2037. McMillan et al, pp 1699-1700. Rudolph et al, pp 1536-1538.)* The concentration of hemoglobin A2 is increased in β-thalassemia trait (also called β-thalassemia minor). Patients have a single abnormal gene for the β-globin component of hemoglobin; they do not typically have problems aside from a mild microcytic anemia. It is important to distinguish between β-thalassemia trait and the more common iron deficiency anemia, as iron is not useful to patients with β-thalassemia trait. In severe iron deficiency, hemoglobin A2 may be decreased. In mild to moderate iron deficiency, the level of hemoglobin A2 is normal. The level is also normal in sickle-cell anemia, chronic systemic illness, and lead poisoning.

397. The answer is a. *(Hay et al, p 863. Kliegman et al, pp 2156-2157, 2488. McMillan et al, pp 1813-1814. Rudolph et al, pp 1203-1208.)* The child in the question likely has Kasabach-Merritt phenomenon, which is seen with large vascular anomalies (ie, kaposiform hemangioendothelioma and tufted angioma). Platelet and RBC sequestration within the vascular tumor causes peripheral thrombocytopenia, coagulopathy, and microangiopathic hemolytic anemia. Treatment options include corticosteroids, α-interferon, and vincristine. Surgery frequently results in excessive bleeding.

Nevus simplex is a common minor vascular malformation seen on the glabella, eyelids, and nape of the neck in newborns; such lesions on the face are also called "angel kiss," while lesions on the back of the neck are called "stork bite." Nevus flammeus, or port wine stain, is a large sharply demarcated pink to purple vascular malformation that can occur anywhere. Port wine stain involving the V1 distribution of the trigeminal nerve should raise the suspicion of Sturge-Weber syndrome. PHACE(S) syndrome includes posterior fossa malformations, large facial hemangiomas, arterial abnormalities, coarctation of the aorta, eye abnormalities, and sternal defects. Infantile fibrosarcoma is a malignant congenital tumor that can be easily mistaken for an infantile hemangioma; a high index of suspicion is required to investigate further if a "hemangioma" is not resolving as expected.

398. The answer is e. *(Hay et al, pp 849-850. Kliegman et al, pp 2040-2042. McMillan et al, pp 2461-2462. Rudolph et al, pp 1542-1543.)* Synthesis of the RBC enzyme glucose-6-phosphate dehydrogenase (G6PD) is determined by genes on the X chromosome, and the pattern of inheritance is X-linked recessive. The enzyme found in most populations is termed G6PDB1. There are more than 380 deficient variants of the enzyme, affecting over 100 million people worldwide. Among them is variant G6PDA1, a mutant enzyme affecting about 13% of African American males and 2% of African American females. The disease occurs, though less commonly, in other ethnic groups, including Middle Eastern, African, and Asian groups. Deficiency of G6PD compromises the generation of reduced glutathione and upon exposure to oxidant agents such as sulfa drugs, antimalarials, nitrofurans, naphthalene mothballs, or infection, a hemolytic episode usually occurs. The degree of hemolysis depends on the nature of the oxidant and severity of the enzyme deficiency. In African Americans, the older, more G6PD-deficient cells are destroyed, but since young cells have sufficient enzyme to prevent further RBC destruction even if the inciting factor is still present, the hemolytic crisis is usually self-limited. Blood transfusion may be unnecessary. In African Americans, premature testing for the enzyme immediately after a hemolytic episode can lead to a false-negative result, since the newly produced RBCs in the circulation have a higher G6PD enzyme activity. The older RBCs containing Heinz bodies (insoluble precipitates resulting from oxidation), the "bite cells" (RBCs after the removal of the Heinz bodies), and cell fragments are removed from the circulation within 3 to 4 days. In the severe Mediterranean type, young as well as old RBCs are enzyme deficient. Recovery is signaled by the appearance of reticulocytes and a rise in hemoglobin.

Hepatitis A or B will often occur after an exposure, and usually does not cause anemia as a presenting sign. Gilbert syndrome presents with episodes of jaundice, but not anemia. Hemolytic-uremic syndrome must be considered in a clinical situation similar to that presented, but the absence of uremia makes the diagnosis less likely.

399. The answer is b. (*Hay et al, pp 908-909. Kliegman et al, pp 2151-2152. McMillan et al, pp 1786-1788. Rudolph et al, pp 2395-2396.*) Retinoblastoma is an uncommon malignancy in children, with a worldwide incidence of 1 case per 18 to 30,000 live births with an equal male to female incidence. Diagnosis is usually made in the first or second year of life, typically during a routine physical examination or by parents noting a white reflection in a flash photograph. With early detection, more than 90% of cases can be cured, but vision is frequently lost in the affected eye. The most common presentation is a spontaneous unilateral tumor, accounting for 60% of cases. Hereditary tumors are less common, with a bilateral hereditary presentation accounting for 25% of cases, and unilateral hereditary tumor accounting for 15%. Biopsy is not indicated; diagnosis is made by typical findings on ophthalmologic examination, including a white or pink mass protruding from the retina into the vitreous matter, and intraocular calcifications. The genetic defect involved in the hereditary form also puts the patient at significantly elevated risk of soft tissue tumors years later, most commonly osteosarcoma (40%) but also including soft tissue sarcomas and malignant melanoma.

400. The answer is a. (Hay et al, pp 59-60. Kliegman et al, pp 766-768. McMillan et al, pp 442-443. Rudolph et al, pp 197-199.) The absence of a major blood group incompatibility and the finding of a normal reticulocyte count argue strongly in favor of a recent fetomaternal transfusion, probably at the time of delivery. A Kleihauer-Betke stain for fetal hemoglobin-containing RBCs in the mother's blood would confirm the diagnosis. After birth, erythropoiesis ceases, and the progressive decline in hemoglobin values, reaching a nadir at 6 to 8 weeks of age, has been termed physiologic anemia of infancy. Iron-deficiency anemia can be seen in the term infant between 9 and 24 months of age when the iron stores derived from circulating hemoglobin have been exhausted and an exogenous dietary source of iron has not been provided. The manifestations of sickle-cell disease do not appear until 4 to 6 months of life, coincident with the replacement of fetal hemoglobin with sickle hemoglobin.

401. The answer is e. (Hay et al, pp 885-888. Kliegman et al, pp 2116-2120. McMillan et al, pp 1750-1758. Rudolph et al, pp 1594-1600.) Children who present with symptoms that suggest leukemia with bone marrow failure require a bone marrow biopsy as soon as possible to clarify the diagnosis. Leukemias are the most common childhood malignancy, accounting for about 40% of all malignancies in children less than 15 years of age. Two thousand children a year are diagnosed with acute lymphoblastic leukemia (ALL) in the United States. Most are between the ages of 2 and 6 years; a male predominance is noted. All of the symptoms in the vignette are typically found with leukemia: clinical and laboratory evidence of marrow failure with anemia and thrombocytopenia. The WBC count can be normal, high, or low. Automated systems initially may report blast forms as atypical lymphocytes. A reticulocyte count would reflect lack of marrow response, but is nonspecific. EBV can cause fever and listlessness with lymphadenopathy, but is usually not associated with significant anemia and thrombocytopenia as described here. Haptoglobin may help distinguish hemolytic from nonhemolytic anemia, and an antiplatelet antibody would not explain the anemia.

402. The answer is b. (Hay et al, pp 903-905. Kliegman et al, pp 2140-2143. McMillan et al, pp 1775-1777. Rudolph et al, pp 1614-1616.) An abdominal mass is palpated in 85% of patients with Wilms tumor; abdominal pain is present in 40%, hypertension in about 60%, and hematuria in 12% to 24%. Because of the association of hemihypertrophy and aniridia with Wilms tumor, children with these findings should be followed with periodic physical examinations and abdominal sonograms, especially during their first 5 years. Wilms tumor and aniridia are associated with abnormalities on chromosome 11.

Neuroblastoma should also be considered in the differential diagnosis of abdominal mass, especially if fever, irritability, bone pain, limp, and diarrhea are present; in the case presented, however, the other features such as aniridia and horseshoe kidney make this diagnosis less likely than Wilms tumor.

403. The answer is d. *(Hay et al, p 859. Kliegman et al, pp 902-903. McMillan et al, pp 1716-1717. Rudolph et al, p 1555.)* Some common causes of eosinophilia in the peripheral blood smear include asthma, recurrent urticaria, infantile eczema, drug reactions, angioneurotic edema, helminth infections, collagen vascular disease, and some neoplasms. Allergic rhinitis can cause eosinophilia in nasal secretions, but usually does not cause dramatic peripheral eosinophilia.

404. The answer is d. *(Hay et al, pp 868-869. Kliegman et al, pp 2080-2081. McMillan et al, pp 1745-1746. Rudolph et al, p 1575.)* The clinical history and blood smear findings (fragmented cells and few platelets) presented in the question are typical of disseminated intravascular coagulation. The disorder, which can be triggered by endotoxin shock, results ultimately in the initiation of the intrinsic clotting mechanism and the generation of thrombin (prolonged PT and PTT, decreased fibrinogen concentration, and an increase in fibrin split products). Fibrin deposited in the microcirculatory system can lead to tissue ischemia and necrosis, further capillary damage, release of thromboplastic substances, and increased thrombin generation. Simultaneous activation of the fibrinolytic system produces increased amounts of fibrin split products, which inhibit thrombin activity. Of utmost importance in the treatment of children who have disseminated intravascular coagulation is the management of the condition that precipitated the disorder.

405. The answer is b. *(Hay et al, pp 840-841. Kliegman et al, pp 2020-2023. McMillan et al, pp 1701-1703. Rudolph et al, pp 1539-1540.)* The patient in the question has a hemolytic anemia and spherocytes on the smear. An increased number of spherocytes on peripheral smear can be seen in such conditions as hyperthermia, hereditary spherocytosis, G6PD deficiency, or ABO incompatibility (but usually not Rh incompatibility). Neonatal hyperbilirubinemia can be seen in patients with hereditary spherocytosis. The hemolytic manifestations of ABO incompatibility and hereditary spherocytosis are very similar. The blood types of the mother and of the infant should be determined along with the results of a direct Coombs test on the infant and the presence or absence of a family history of hemolytic disease (spherocytosis).

Sickle-cell disease would not be expected to cause problems in newborns because of protection by fetal hemoglobin. Hyperbilirubinemia can be caused by polycythemia, but the spherocytes would be unusual, and the patient in the question had anemia for a newborn. Pyruvate kinase deficiency can cause neonatal hemolytic anemia, but spherocytes are not commonly seen.

406. The answer is a. (Hay et al, pp 837-838. Kliegman et al, pp 2014-2017. McMillan et al, pp 1692-1694. Rudolph et al, pp 1525-1528.) Iron-deficiency anemia is the most common nutritional deficiency in children between 9 and 15 months of age. Low availability of dietary iron, impaired absorption of iron related to frequent infections, high requirements for iron for growth, and, occasionally, blood losses, favor the development of iron deficiency in infants. A history regarding anemia in the family, blood loss, and gestational age and weight can help to establish the cause of an anemia. The strong likelihood is that anemia in a 1-year-old child is nutritional in origin, and its cause will be suggested by a detailed nutritional history.

407. The answer is c. (Hay et al, pp 868-869. Kliegman et al, pp 2080-2081. McMillan et al, pp 1745-1746. Rudolph et al, p 1575.) In disseminated intravascular coagulation (DIC), there is consumption of fibrinogen; factors II, V, and VIII; and platelets. Therefore, there is prolongation of PT, aPTT, and TT and a decrease in factor VIII level and platelet count. In addition, the titer of fibrin split production is usually increased. D-dimer is a fibrin breakdown product and may also be elevated in DIC.

The prolongation of PT, aPTT, and TT excludes the diagnosis of ITP. PT tests principally for factors I, II, V, VII, and X and is not prolonged in hemophilia A (factor VIII deficiency) or hemophilia B (factor IX deficiency). In vitamin K deficiency, there is a decrease in the production of factors II, VII, IX, and X, and PT and aPTT are prolonged. The thrombin time, which tests for conversion of fibrinogen to fibrin, however, should be normal, and the platelet count should also be normal.

408. The answer is d. (Hay et al, p 868. Kliegman et al, pp 2071-2074. McMillan et al, pp 1740-1742. Rudolph et al, p 1573.) Von Willebrand disease is the most common heritable bleeding disorder, with some studies suggesting prevalence of 1% to 2% in the general population. vWF participates in clot formation by adhering to areas of vascular damage and causing platelets to attach and activate. About 85% of cases of vWD are type I, resulting from decreased production of normal vWF. Several variants of type II vWD are described, with abnormal or dysfunctional vWF the etiology. Patients with type III, the most rare, have undetectable levels of vWF. In type I, desmopressin alone can transiently increase the levels of vWF three- to fivefold, so it is frequently used for acute bleeding episodes.

Aminocaproic acid interferes with fibrinolysis and stabilizes a clot (once it is already formed) by inhibiting plasmin, but does not replace desmopressin in treating patients with VWD. vWF and vWF with factor VIII, are used in other types of vWD, but are not usually used first in type I for mild to moderate bleeding. IVIG is not used in vWD.

409. The answer is e. *(Hay et al, pp 797-799, 885-888, 905-906. Kliegman et al, pp 996, 2116-2122, 2147-2148, 2841-2845. McMillan et al, pp 1750-1758, 2497-2499. Rudolph et al, pp 858-859, 904-907, 1594-1604, 1610-1611, 2450-2451.)* The patient in the question likely has osteosarcoma, and the radiograph shows the expected "sunburst" pattern of bone formation. Osteosarcoma occurs most commonly in the second decade of life, and a bit more commonly in boys than in girls. It occurs in all ethnic groups (in contrast, Ewing sarcoma, another bone malignancy, rarely occurs in blacks). The lesion of osteosarcoma is found in the metaphyses of long bones, and usually presents with local pain and swelling. Predisposing factors include a history of retinoblastoma, Li-Fraumeni syndrome, Paget disease, or radiotherapy. Any bone or joint "injury" not responding with conservative therapy within a short period of time should be evaluated.

"Growing pains" are commonly seen in the school-age child. They present with deep, aching pain, usually in the muscles of the leg. They are most common in the evening, gone by the morning, and do not cause joint swelling, redness, heat, or systemic signs or symptoms. The etiology is unknown, but, despite the name, it is not related to growing. Leukemia can present with deep bone pain, but often other signs and symptoms, such as bruising, adenopathy, hepatosplenomegaly, fever, and pallor, will also be seen. Osteomyelitis can present as a localized pain, but systemic signs (such as fever) would also be expected. The radiograph of osteomyelitis would eventually demonstrate a more lytic lesion. Bone fractures can occur in the active child, but the presentation might include a better history of trauma, and the radiograph would demonstrate a fracture or callus formation rather than a sunburst pattern of bone growth.

410. The answer is d. *(Hay et al, pp 896-898. Kliegman et al, pp 2123-2126. McMillan et al, pp 1767-1768. Rudolph et al, pp 1607-1610.)* The patient in this question, especially with the pulmonary findings, may have Hodgkin disease. In underdeveloped countries, the peak incidence of Hodgkin disease is in children under 10 years of age; however, in developed countries, the peak incidence occurs in late adolescence and young adulthood. Systemic symptoms of Hodgkin disease include fever, night sweats, malaise, weight loss, and pruritus. Although a biopsy of the node may prove to be necessary at some point, the first step would involve a radiograph, which may show mediastinal mass suspicious for Hodgkin disease. Depending on the results of the radiograph, a biopsy of a node may be indicated, especially if the question of Hodgkin (or other malignancy) remained high.

A tuberculosis skin test may be indicated, but a trial of antituberculosis drugs without a chest radiograph, a positive purified protein derivative (PPD), or other diagnostic evaluation indicating tuberculosis would be unwise. In Hodgkin disease, the CBC is not diagnostic, but may show nonspecific findings of anemia, neutropenia, or thrombocytopenia; they are useful in the staging process after the diagnosis has been confirmed by biopsy. The presenting complaint with multiple groups of swollen nodes is unlikely to be related to cat-scratch disease.

411. The answer is c. (*Hay et al, pp 838-839. Kliegman et al, pp 2011-2013. McMillan et al, pp 1694-1695. Rudolph et al, pp 1529-1530.*) The finding of hypersegmented neutrophils in the peripheral blood is one of the most useful laboratory aids in making an early diagnosis of folate deficiency. Serum folate levels become low in weeks with an inadequate dietary source. The Pelger-Huët anomaly is an inherited disorder in which neutrophils have no more than two lobes. Neutrophils in severe bacterial infections have toxic granulation, Döhle inclusion bodies, and cytoplasmic vacuoles.

412 to 415. The answers are 412-c, 413-d, 414-a, 415-b. (*Hay et al, pp 840-844, 848, 874. Kliegman et al, pp 2004, 2020-2023, 2032-2037, 2090. McMillan et al, pp 1698, 1699-1703, 2442. Rudolph et al, pp 1531-1534, 1536-1540, 1561.*) Howell-Jolly bodies (slide C) are small, spherical, nuclear remnants seen in the reticulocytes and, rarely, erythrocytes of persons who have no spleen (because of congenital asplenia or splenectomy) or who have a poorly functioning spleen (eg, in hyposplenism associated with sickle-cell disease). Ultrafiltration of blood is a unique function of the spleen that cannot be assumed by other reticuloendothelial organs.

A target cell is an erythrocyte with a membrane that is too large for its hemoglobin content; a thin rim of hemoglobin at the cell's periphery and a small disk in the center give the cell a target-like appearance. Target cells, which are more resistant to osmotic fragility than are other erythrocytes, are seen in children who have α-thalassemia, hemoglobin C disease, or liver disease (eg, obstructive jaundice or cirrhosis). Thalassemia major (slide D) presents in the second 6 months of life with severe anemia requiring transfusion, heart failure, hepatosplenomegaly, and weakness. Later, the typical facial deformities (maxillary hyperplasia and malocclusion) can be seen in a patient inadequately transfused. The diagnosis can be made on peripheral blood smear by the presence of poorly hemoglobinized normoblasts in addition to target cells in the peripheral blood.

Uniformly small microspherocyte (less than 6 μm in diameter) are typical of hereditary spherocytosis (slide A). Because of a decreased surface to volume ratio, these osmotically fragile RBCs have an increased density of hemoglobin. Although spherical RBCs also can appear in other hemolytic states (eg, immune hemolytic anemia, microangiography, ABO incompatibility, and hypersplenism), their cellular volume is only irregularly augmented. Patients with hereditary spherocytosis can present in the newborn period with anemia, hyperbilirubinemia, and reticulocytosis. They may remain asymptomatic until adulthood, when they develop symptoms. After infancy, hepatosplenomegaly and gallstones are common.

Although hemoglobin C disease (slide B) is frequently a mild disorder, target cells constitute a far greater percentage of total RBCs than in thalassemia major. In the heterozygous state, no anemia or disease is noted, but target cells are seen. In the homozygous state, a moderately severe hemolytic anemia, reticulocytosis, and splenomegaly are seen, along with a smear containing a large number of target cells.

Endocrine, Metabolic, and Genetic Disorders

Questions

416. A 6-month-old infant has been exclusively fed a commercially available infant formula. Upon introduction of fruit juices, however, the child develops jaundice, hepatomegaly, vomiting, lethargy, irritability, and seizures. Tests for urine-reducing substances are positive. Which of the following is likely to explain this child's condition?

a. Tyrosinemia
b. Galactosemia
c. Hereditary fructose intolerance
d. α_1-Antitrypsin deficiency
e. Glucose-6-phosphatase deficiency

417. A 12-year-old healthy girl has some dizziness at synagogue. In your office you find her to have a hemoglobin of 8 mg/dL, a white blood cell (WBC) count of 4000/μL, and a platelet count of 98,000/μL. Physical examination reveals an enlarged spleen. An x-ray of the femur is described as "appearing to be an Erlenmeyer flask." Bone marrow examination shows abnormal cells. The diagnosis can be confirmed by measurement of activity of which of the following?

a. Sphingomyelinase activity
b. Hexosamidase A
c. Sulfatase A
d. Glucocerebrosidase
e. Ceramide trihexosidase

418. An infant is born to a woman who has received very little prenatal care. The mother is anxious, complains of heat intolerance and fatigue, and reports that she has not gained much weight despite having an increased appetite. On examination the mother is tachycardic, has a tremor, and has fullness in her neck and in her eyes. The infant is most likely at risk for development of which of the following?

a. Constipation
b. Heart failure
c. Macrocephaly
d. Third-degree heart block
e. Thrombocytosis

419. An otherwise healthy 7-year-old girl is brought to your office by her father because she has some acne, breast development, and fine pubic hair. Which of the following is the most likely etiology for her condition?

a. A feminizing ovarian tumor
b. A gonadotropin-producing tumor
c. A lesion of the central nervous system (CNS)
d. Exogenous estrogens
e. Early onset of "normal" puberty (constitutional)

420. The parents of a 14-year-old boy are concerned about his short stature and lack of sexual development. By history, you learn that his birth weight and length were 3 kg and 50 cm, respectively, and that he had a normal growth pattern, although he was always shorter than children his age. The physical examination is normal and his growth curve is shown on the next page. His upper-to-lower segment ratio is 0.98. A small amount of fine axillary and pubic hair is present. There is no scrotal pigmentation; his testes measure 4.0 cm^3 and his penis is 6 cm in length. In this situation, which of the following is the most appropriate course of action?

a. Measure pituitary gonadotropin
b. Obtain a computed tomographic (CT) scan of the pituitary area
c. Biopsy his testes
d. Measure serum testosterone levels
e. Reassure the parents that the boy is normal

2 to 20 years: Boys
Stature-for-age and Weight-for-age percentiles

NAME _____

RECORD # _____

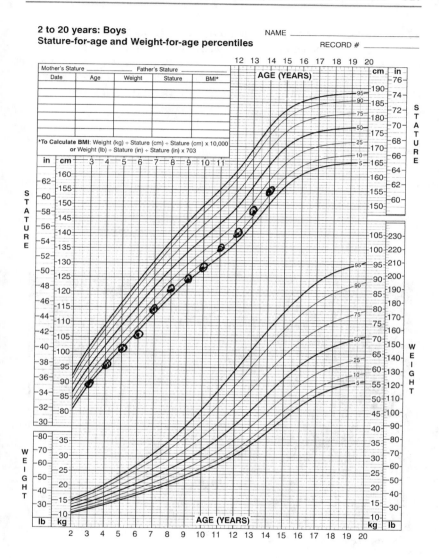

421. Friends are considering adopting a "special needs" child from another country. The family has few details, but the information they have received so far suggests the 4-year-old child has had surgery for an endocardial cushion defect, is short for his age, and had a history of what sounds like surgically repaired duodenal atresia at birth. You are suspicious this child may have which of the following syndromes?

a. Kleinfelter
b. Waardenberg
c. Marfan
d. Down
e. Turner

422. A 13-year-old asymptomatic girl is shown below. She states that the findings demonstrated began more than a year ago. Which of the following is the most likely diagnosis?

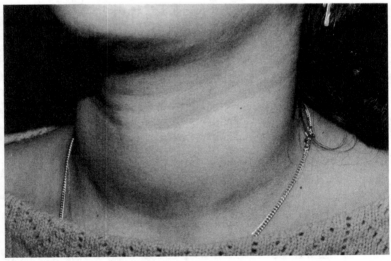

(Courtesy of Adelaide Hebert, MD.)

a. Iodine deficiency
b. Congenital hypothyroidism
c. Graves disease
d. Exogenous ingestion of Synthroid
e. Lymphocytic (Hashimoto) thyroiditis

423. During a routine well-child examination a 10-year-old girl reports that she has occasional headache, "racing heart," abdominal pain, and dizziness. Her mother states that she has witnessed one of the episodes, which occurred during an outing at the mall, and reported the child to be pale and to have sweating as well. Other than some hypertension, she has a normal physical examination. Evaluation of this child is most likely to result in which of the following diagnoses?

a. Hysterical fainting spells
b. Pregnancy
c. Diabetes mellitus
d. Pheochromocytoma
e. Migraine headache

424. A 10-year-old obese child (shown below) has central fat distribution, arrested growth, hypertension, plethora, and osteoporosis. Which of the following disorders is most likely responsible for the clinical picture that this boy presents?

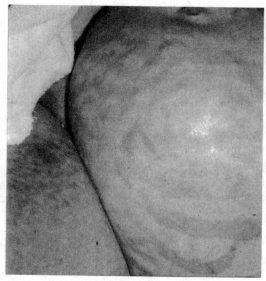

(Courtesy of Adelaide Hebert, MD.)

a. Bilateral adrenal hyperplasia
b. Adrenal adenoma
c. Adrenal carcinoma
d. Craniopharyngioma
e. Ectopic adrenocorticotropin-producing tumor

425. A 6-year-old boy is brought to your practice by his paternal grandmother for his first visit. She has recently received custody of him after his mother entered the penal system in another state; she does not have much information about him. You note that the child is short for his age, has downslanting palpebral fissures, ptosis, low-set and malformed ears, a broad and webbed neck, shield chest, and cryptorchidism. You hear a systolic ejection murmur in the pulmonic region. His grandmother reports that he does well in regular classes, but has been diagnosed with learning disabilities and receives speech therapy for language delay. His constellation of symptoms is suggestive of which of the following?

a. Noonan syndrome
b. Congenital hypothyroidism
c. Turner syndrome
d. Congenital rubella
e. Down syndrome

426. The parents of a 1-month-old infant bring him to the emergency center in your local hospital for emesis and listlessness. Both of his parents wanted a natural birth, so he was born at home and has not yet been to see a physician. On examination, you find a dehydrated, listless, and irritable infant. Although you don't have a birth weight, the parents do not feel that he has gained much weight. He has significant jaundice. His abdominal examination is significant for both hepatomegaly and splenomegaly. Laboratory values include a total bilirubin of 15.8 mg/dL and a direct bilirubin of 5.5 mg/dL. His liver function tests are elevated and his serum glucose is 38 mg/dL. Serum ammonia is normal. A urinalysis is negative for glucose, but it has a "mouse-like" odor. These findings are consistent with which of the following conditions?

a. Homocystinuria
b. Maple syrup urine disease
c. Galactosemia
d. Ornithine transcarbamylase deficiency
e. Phenylketonuria

427. A 2-month-old boy is admitted to the hospital for failure to thrive. You note him to have fatty stools, and consider cystic fibrosis in your differential diagnosis. You order pilocarpine iontophoresis, but the laboratory calls to say they could not collect enough sweat from the infant. Which of the following is another way to make the diagnosis of cystic fibrosis?

a. Quantitative fecal fat
b. Bronchoscopy and bronchoalveolar lavage
c. Pilocarpine iontophoresis for both parents
d. DNA testing for cystic fibrosis transmembrane regulator (CFTR) mutations
e. Pancreatic biopsy

428. An otherwise healthy 7-year-old child is brought to you to be evaluated because he is the shortest child in his class. Careful measurements of his upper and lower body segments demonstrate normal body proportions for his age. Which of the following disorders of growth should remain in your differential?

a. Achondroplasia
b. Morquio disease
c. Hypothyroidism
d. Growth hormone deficiency
e. Marfan syndrome

429. The state laboratory calls your office telling you that a newborn infant, now 8 days old, has an elevated thyroid stimulating hormone (TSH) and low thyroxin (T_4) on his newborn screen. If this condition is left untreated, the infant is likely to demonstrate which of the following in the first few months of life?

a. Hyperreflexia
b. Hyperirritability
c. Diarrhea
d. Prolonged jaundice
e. Hyperphagia

430. A 1-year-old boy presents with the complaint from his parents of "not developing normally." He was the product of an uneventful term pregnancy and delivery, and reportedly was normal at birth. His previous health-care provider noted his developmental delay, and also noted that the child seemed to have an enlarged spleen and liver. On your examination, you confirm the developmental delay and the hepatosplenomegaly, and also notice that the child has short stature, macrocephaly, hirsutism, a coarse facies, and decreased joint mobility. Which of the following is the most likely etiology of his condition?

a. Beckwith-Wiedemann syndrome
b. Crouzon syndrome
c. Trisomy 18 (Edwards syndrome)
d. Jeune syndrome
e. Hurler syndrome

431. A 13-year-old comes to your office expressing concern about his height. He had first seen you a year prior for his routine checkup and a preparticipation sports physical for soccer (see growth curve). Now in the eighth grade, all of his friends are taller than he is, and he is at a disadvantage on the soccer field playing against much larger boys. After obtaining height information from his parents shown here, you order a skeletal bone age radiograph. Which of the following results would allow you to assure him of an excellent prognosis for normal adult height?

a. A bone age of 9 years
b. A bone age of 13 years
c. A bone age of 15 years
d. Being at the 50th percentile for weight
e. Being at the 3rd percentile for weight

2 to 20 years: Boys
Stature-for-age and Weight-for-age percentiles

NAME _____

RECORD # _____

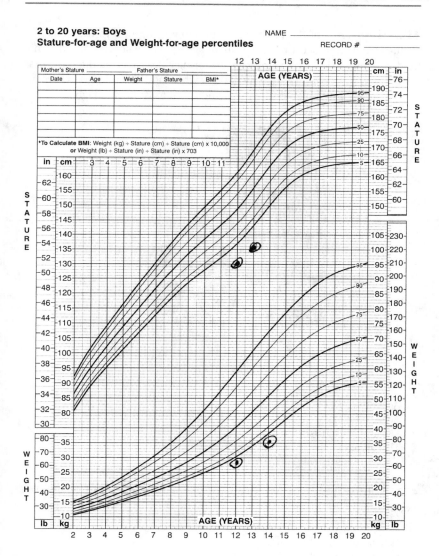

*To Calculate BMI: Weight (kg) ÷ Stature (cm) ÷ Stature (cm) x 10,000
or Weight (lb) ÷ Stature (in) ÷ Stature (in) x 703

432. The parents of the child pictured below bring him to the office for evaluation of short stature. At 5 years of age, he is the shortest child in his kindergarten class. His development is normal, and he is reading on a first grade level. Both parents are of normal height, and this child resembles no one in the family. Which of the following is the most likely diagnosis?

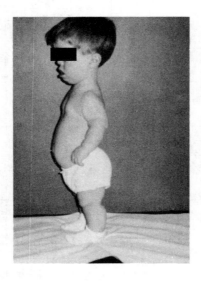

a. Achondrogenesis
b. Achondroplasia
c. Metatropic dysplasia
d. Thanatophoric dwarfism
e. Chondroectodermal dysplasia

433. A 12-year-old girl has a solitary thyroid nodule found on routine examination; she has no symptoms. Which of the following is the most appropriate next step for this patient?

a. Fine needle aspirate
b. CT scan of the neck
c. Serum thyroid function tests
d. Trial of suppressive T_4 treatment to look for nodule shrinkage
e. Excisional biopsy

434. The 16-month-old male infant pictured below was recently brought from a developing country to the United States. The family history reveals that his father had an eye and a leg removed. Which of the following is the most likely diagnosis?

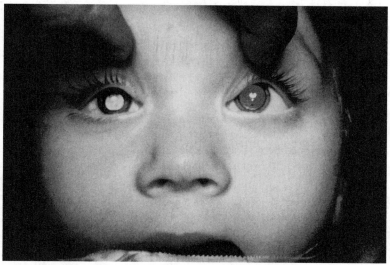

(Courtesy of Kathryn Musgrove, MD.)

a. Coloboma of the choroid
b. Retinal detachment
c. Nematode endophthalmitis
d. Retinoblastoma
e. Persistent hyperplastic primary vitreous

435. A 4-year-old child has mental retardation, shortness of stature, brachydactyly (especially of the fourth and fifth digits), and obesity with round facies and short neck. The child is followed by an ophthalmologist for subcapsular cataracts, and has previously been noted to have cutaneous and subcutaneous calcifications, as well as perivascular calcifications of the basal ganglia. This patient is most likely to have which of the following features?

a. Hypercalcemia
b. Hypophosphatemia
c. Elevated concentrations of parathyroid hormone
d. Advanced height age
e. Decreased bone density, particularly in the skull

436. A 15-year-old boy has been immobilized in a double hip spica cast for 6 weeks after having fractured his femur in a skiing accident. He has become depressed and listless during the past few days and has complained of nausea and constipation. He is found to have microscopic hematuria and a blood pressure of 150/100 mm Hg. Which of the following is the most appropriate course of action?

a. Request a psychiatric evaluation
b. Check blood pressure every 2 hours for 2 days
c. Collect urine for measurement of the calcium to creatinine ratio
d. Order a renal sonogram and intravenous pyelogram (IVP)
e. Measure 24-hour urinary protein

437. An adolescent with type 1 diabetes returns for a follow-up visit after his annual checkup last week. You note that his serum glucose is elevated, and his glycosylated hemoglobin (hemoglobin A_{1C}) is 16.7%. This finding suggests poor control of his diabetes over at least which of the following time periods?

a. 8 hours
b. 1 week
c. 1 month
d. 2 months
e. 6 months

438. A 7-day-old boy is admitted to a hospital for evaluation of vomiting and dehydration. Physical examination is otherwise normal except for minimal hyperpigmentation of the nipples. Serum sodium and potassium concentrations are 120 mEq/L and 9 mEq/L (without hemolysis), respectively; serum glucose is 40 mg/dL. Which of the following is the most likely diagnosis?

a. Pyloric stenosis
b. Congenital adrenal hyperplasia
c. Secondary hypothyroidism
d. Panhypopituitarism
e. Hyperaldosteronism

439. A 14-year-old boy presents with the complaint of "breast swelling." The boy reports that he has been in good health and without other problems, but has noticed over the past month or so that his left breast has been "achy" and that he has now noticed some mild swelling under the nipple. He has never seen discharge; the other breast has not been swelling; and he denies trauma. Your examination demonstrates a quarter-sized area of breast tissue under the left nipple that is not tender and has no discharge. The right breast has no such tissue. He has a normal genitourinary examination, and is Tanner stage 3. Which of the following is the best next course of action?

a. CT scan of the pituitary
b. Measurement of serum luteinizing hormone (LH) and follicle-stimulating hormone (FSH)
c. Measurement of serum testosterone
d. Reassurance of the normalcy of the condition
e. Chromosomes

440. An infant is brought to a hospital because her wet diapers turn black when they are exposed to air. Physical examination is normal. Urine is positive both for reducing substance and when tested with ferric chloride. This disorder is caused by a deficiency of which of the following?

a. Homogentisic acid oxidase
b. Phenylalanine hydroxylase
c. L-histidine ammonia-lyase
d. Ketoacid decarboxylase
e. Isovaleryl-CoA dehydrogenase

441. An 18-year-old girl has hepatosplenomegaly, an intention tremor, dysarthria, dystonia, and deterioration in her school performance. She also developed abnormal urine with excess glucose, protein, and uric acid. She has a several-year history of elevated liver enzymes of unknown etiology. Which of the following best explains her condition?

a. Indian childhood cirrhosis
b. α_1-Antitrypsin deficiency
c. Menkes syndrome
d. Dubin-Johnson syndrome
e. Wilson disease

442. A 3-month-old infant without significant past history was brought to the emergency center by her mother with a generalized tonic-clonic seizure. She is found to have glucose of 5 mg/dL. After correction of her hypoglycemia, she is admitted to your service for further evaluation. Several hours later, her nurse calls to tell you that her bedside glucose check was now 10 mg/dL. You order laboratory work suggested by the pediatric endocrinology team and again correct the infant's hypoglycemia. The results of the laboratory tests you drew include an elevated serum insulin level of 50 μU/mL, and a low IGFBP-1 (plasma insulin-like growth factor binding protein-1). C-peptide levels are not detectable. Which of the following is the likely cause of this child's recurrent hypoglycemia?

a. Nesidioblastosis
b. Pancreatitis
c. Beckwith-Wiedemann syndrome
d. Galactosemia
e. Factitious hypoglycemia

443. An 11-year-old is the tallest child in his sixth grade class. He is thin, has a high arched palate, mild scoliosis, and joint hyperextensibility. He is an honor student, and enjoys basketball but must use prescription sports goggles so he can see the ball on the court. He is likely to have which of the following conditions?

a. Cerebral gigantism (Sotos syndrome)
b. Homocystinuria
c. XXY (Klinefelter syndrome)
d. Marfan syndrome
e. XYY

444. A very upset mother brings her 8-month-old child to the emergency room because he will not move his leg. She reports that when she was carrying him to the car about half an hour ago, she slipped on some ice and fell on top of him. The mother, an 18-year-old African American woman, has been exclusively breast-feeding her child. She has only recently started him on cereals, and has not supplemented his diet with vitamins. A radiograph of the child's leg is shown below. Which of the following laboratory findings would be expected?

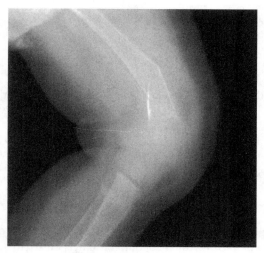

(Courtesy of Susan John, MD.)

a. Hypocalcemia
b. Hypophosphaturia
c. Reduced serum alkaline phosphatase
d. Hypocalciuria
e. Hyperphosphatemia

445. A small-for-gestational-age infant is born at 30 weeks' gestation. At 1 hour of age, his serum glucose is noted to be 20 mg/dL (normally greater than 40 mg/dL). Which of the following is the most likely explanation for hypoglycemia in this infant?

a. Inadequate stores of nutrients
b. Adrenal immaturity
c. Pituitary immaturity
d. Insulin excess
e. Glucagon deficiency

446. A 1-day-old normal-appearing infant develops tetany and convulsions. He was born at 34 weeks' gestation with Apgar scores of 2 and 4 (at 1 and 5 minutes, respectively) to a woman whose pregnancy was complicated by diabetes mellitus and pregnancy-induced hypertension. Which of the following serum chemistry values is likely to be the explanation for his condition?

a. Serum bicarbonate level of 22 mEq/dL
b. Serum calcium of 6.2 mg/dL
c. Serum glucose of 45 mg/dL
d. Serum magnesium level of 5.0 mg/dL
e. Intracranial hemorrhage

Questions 447 to 451

For each of the disorders listed below, select the serum concentration of calcium (Ca_2^+) and phosphate (PO_4) with which it is most likely to be associated. Each lettered option may be used once, more than once, or not at all.

a. Low PO_4, normal Ca
b. Low PO_4, high Ca
c. Normal PO_4, low Ca
d. Normal PO_4, normal Ca
e. High PO_4, low Ca

447. Three boys in a family with hypodense calcification of their bones and a history of fractures; their condition is unresponsive to dietary changes or vitamin supplementation

448. A short, 4-year-old, mentally retarded child with brachydactyly of the fourth and fifth digits; obesity with round facies; short neck; subcapsular cataracts; and cutaneous, subcutaneous, and perivascular calcifications of the basal ganglia

449. A 4-year-old child with blue sclera and a history of multiple fractures with minimal trauma

450. A 6-year-old child who complains of numbness and tingling of the hands, and later develops tonic-clonic seizures

451. An otherwise healthy 18-year-old girl with medullary thyroid carcinoma

Questions 452 to 457

All the syndromes listed below are associated with overweight conditions in children. For each of the other clinical findings that follow, select the syndrome with which it is most likely to be associated. Each lettered option may be used once, more than once, or not at all.

a. Prader-Willi syndrome
b. Laurence-Moon-Biedl syndrome
c. Cushing syndrome
d. Fröhlich syndrome
e. Pseudohypoparathyroidism
f. Polycystic ovary syndrome
g. Type 2 diabetes

452. A 15-year-old defensive lineman for his high school football team whose mother reports that his shoulder pads have permanently stained his neck

453. A 6-day-old infant with severe hypotonia and poor feeding since birth

454. A 5-year-old boy with mental retardation and polydactyly

455. A 5-day-old girl with brachydactyly, round facies, and short neck

456. A 15-year-old girl with menstrual irregularities and hirsutism

457. A 14-year-old boy with hypogonadism and night blindness with retinitis pigmentosa

Questions 458 to 463

For each of the following disorders, select the serum concentrations (mEq/L) of sodium (Na^+) and potassium (K^+) with which it is most likely to be associated in a dehydrated patient. Each lettered option may be used once, more than once, or not at all.

a. Na^+ 118, K^+ 7.5
b. Na^+ 125, K^+ 3.0
c. Na^+ 134, K^+ 6.0
d. Na^+ 144, K^+ 2.9
e. Na^+ 155, K^+ 5.5

458. A 4-month-old boy with salt-losing 21-hydroxylase deficiency (adrenogenital syndrome)

459. An 11-year-old boy with central diabetes insipidus secondary to an automobile accident

460. A 2-year-old girl with nephrogenic diabetes insipidus

461. A 4-year-old boy with hyperaldosteronism

462. An 8-year-old boy with Addison disease (in crisis)

463. A 1-year-old girl with glucose-6-phosphatase deficiency (von Gierke disease)

Questions 464 to 470

Patients with genetic disorders or those affected by specific teratogens *in utero*, typically have certain characteristic dysmorphic features. Match the physical description with the genetic or teratogenic abnormality. Each lettered option may be used once, more than once, or not at all.

a. Trisomy 21 (Down syndrome)
b. Trisomy 18 (Edwards syndrome)
c. Holt-Oram syndrome
d. Diabetic embryopathy
e. Fetal alcohol syndrome
f. Turner syndrome
g. Ehlers-Danlos syndrome

464. A 10-year-old boy with hypermobile joints and poor wound healing.

465. A 6-year-old girl with cognitive delay, a blowing systolic heart murmur, short stature, round face, bilateral transpalmar crease, upslanting palpebral fissures, small ears, and epicanthal folds.

466. A newborn has low sloping shoulders, right hand attached at elbow with agenesis of the forearm, cardiac abnormalities, missing chest wall musculature, and a bifid thumb.

467. A 2-year-old boy, less than the 5% for weight and height, is in early childhood intervention for developmental delay. He has a short nose, thin upper lip with thin vermillion border, a VSD, and short palpebral fissures.

468. A 14-year-old girl with short stature, thick neck, minimal pubertal development, repaired coarctation of the aorta, and normal intelligence.

469. A small newborn with a large ventricular septal defect (VSD), clenched hands, cleft palate, rounded heels, and a horseshoe kidney.

470. A newborn with hypoglycemia, hypocalcemia, and hypoplastic lower extremities.

Questions 471 to 474

New discoveries made possible by advances in molecular genetics have broadened our understanding of nontraditional inheritance. Match the disease with the appropriate genetic mechanism listed below. Each lettered option may be used once, more than once, or not at all.

a. Mitochondrial inheritance
b. Mosaicism
c. Genomic imprinting
d. Sex chromosome imbalance
e. Triplet repeat expansion disorder

471. A 3-year-old boy with myoclonus, ataxia, weakness, and seizures who has cytochrome oxidase-negative ragged red fibers noted on muscle biopsy

472. A mentally retarded 4-year-old boy who was noted to be hypotonic at birth and had failure to thrive in infancy now has a tremendous appetite, obesity, hypogonadism, and small hands and feet

473. A previously normal father of one of your patients, from a family with members known to have fragile X syndrome, develops ataxia and tremor

474. A developmentally delayed 2-year-old has bilateral hypopigmented whorls on the upper extremities

Endocrine, Metabolic, and Genetic Disorders

Answers

416. The answer is c. *(Hay et al, p 993. Kliegman et al, p 611. McMillan et al, pp 2189-2190. Rudolph et al, p 641.)* The patient in the question likely has hereditary fructose intolerance, manifest only when fructose in fruit juice is provided in the diet. Galactosemia, fructosemia, tyrosinosis, and glucose-6-phosphatase deficiency represent diseases in which a congenital deficiency of enzyme causes an interruption of a normal metabolic pathway and an accumulation of metabolic precursors that damage vital organs. Galactose (found in milk) and fructose (found in fruit juices) produce urinary-reducing substances in their respective disorders. The mode of inheritance of galactosemia, fructosemia, and most forms of glucose-6-phosphatase deficiency is autosomal recessive. In galactosemia and fructosemia, errors in carbohydrate metabolism cause the accumulation of toxic metabolites when specific dietary sugars are introduced (lactose in galactosemia; fructose and sucrose in fructosemia). Exclusion of the offending carbohydrate from the diet will prevent liver damage. In tyrosinemia type I, or tyrosinosis, the accumulation of tyrosine and its metabolites is associated with severe involvement of the liver, kidney, and CNS. Manifestations of acute liver failure can appear in infancy. A chronic form of the disorder presents as progressive cirrhosis and leads to liver failure or hepatoma. Dietary management does not prevent liver disease. Glucose-6-phosphatase deficiency often presents at 3 to 4 months of age with failure to thrive, hypoglycemia, hepatomegaly, and acidosis. α_1-Antitrypsin deficiency causes liver disease through accumulation of an abnormal protein, caused by a single amino acid substitution on chromosome 14. It has a variable presentation, but the following are common in infancy: cholestasis; bleeding into the CNS, gastrointestinal (GI) tract, or at the umbilical stump; and elevation of transaminase concentrations. Affected children may have chronic hepatitis with cirrhosis and portal hypertension.

417. The answer is d. *(Hay et al, pp 754-755, 1007. Kliegman et al, pp 595-597. McMillan et al, pp 2208-2209. Rudolph et al, pp 2326-2328.)* Gaucher disease is characterized by β-glucocerebrosidase deficiency, which causes an abnormal accumulation of glucocerebroside in the reticuloendothelial system. Bone marrow aspirate shows the typical Gaucher cells engorged with glucocerebroside. Replacement of marrow with these cells leads to anemia, leukopenia, and thrombocytopenia. The liver and spleen can also be involved. Serum acid phosphatase is elevated. X-ray evaluation demonstrates an Erlenmeyer-flask appearance of the long bones. The diagnosis of Gaucher disease is confirmed by the absence of glucocerebrosidase activity in leukocytes, in cultured skin fibroblasts, and in liver cells. Prenatal diagnosis by enzyme analysis is now possible. In the most common form of Gaucher disease, adult type I, there is no involvement of the CNS. Therefore, magnetic resonance imaging (MRI) of the brain is not indicated.

Sphingomyelinase deficiency causes type A Niemann-Pick disease; hexosaminidase A deficiency causes Sandhoff disease; sulfatase A deficiency causes juvenile metachromatic leukodystrophy; and serum trihexosidase deficiency causes Fabry disease.

418. The answer is b. *(Hay et al, pp 951-952. Kliegman et al, pp 2336-2337. McMillan et al, p 422. Rudolph et al, p 2076.)* The infant is likely at risk for neonatal thyrotoxicosis. Neonatal thyrotoxicosis usually disappears within 2 to 4 months as the concentration of maternally-acquired thyrotropin receptor-stimulating antibody (TRSAb) falls. Unlike TRSAb, TSH does not cross the placenta. All forms of thyrotoxicosis are more common in females, with the exception of neonatal thyrotoxicosis, which has an equal sex distribution. Symptoms include tachycardia and tachypnea, irritability and hyperactivity, low birth weight with microcephaly, severe vomiting and diarrhea, thrombocytopenia, jaundice, hepatosplenomegaly, and heart failure. In severely affected infants, the disease can be fatal if not treated vigorously and promptly. Third-degree heart block is not a feature of this disease, but is sometimes seen in infants born to mothers with systemic lupus erythematosus.

419. The answer is e. *(Hay et al, pp 110-111, 961-964. Kliegman et al, pp 2309-2315. McMillan et al, pp 2080-2082. Rudolph et al, pp 2097-2098.)* The patient in the question appears to have "true sexual precocity," implying that the gonads have matured in response to the secretion of pituitary gonadotropins and have begun secreting sex steroids, causing the development of secondary sexual characteristics. Thus, ovarian tumors and exogenous estrogens, which suppress the function of the pituitary gland, do not cause true precocious puberty; rather, they cause isolated premature telarche and/or vaginal bleeding without pubic hair, body odor, and acne. In girls, the most common form of true precocious puberty is idiopathic and is thought to be caused by early maturation of an otherwise normal hypothalamic-pituitarygonadal feedback system. In boys, true precocious puberty is relatively rare and is more likely to be caused by lesions of the CNS. Hypothalamic hamartomas are a possible cause of precocious puberty in both genders and produce gonadotropin-releasing hormone (GnRH); surgery for these hamartomas is usually not indicated, since GnRH analogs are effective therapy.

420. The answer is e. (*Hay et al, pp 938, 964. Kliegman et al, p 2297. McMillan et al, pp 2085-2090. Rudolph et al, p 2103.*) A record of the sequential pattern of growth in height is very helpful in the differential diagnosis of a child with short stature. A child with constitutionally short stature and delayed puberty will have a consistent rate of growth below, but parallel to, the average for his or her age, whereas patients with organic disease do not follow a given percentile but progressively deviate from their prior growth percentile. Knowledge of the patterns of growth and sexual maturation of family members is helpful, because such patterns are often familial. Reassurance that normal sexual development will occur and that a normal adult height (usually a midparental height) will be attained is frequently the only therapy indicated.

Puberty is said to be delayed in males if physical changes are not apparent by 14 years of age. Identification of the earliest signs of sexual maturation by means of careful physical examination avoids unnecessary workup. In this case, measurement of pituitary gonadotropins is unnecessary because the child already shows evidence of pubertal development (a penile length of more than 2.5 cm and a testicular volume more than 3.0 cm^3). The single most useful laboratory test is the radiographic determination of bone age. In those of constitutionally short stature with delayed pubertal maturation, the bone age is equal to the height age, both of which are behind chronologic age. In familial short stature, bone age is greater than height age and equal to chronologic age. In a child at any age, the administration of human chorionic gonadotropin (hCG) will stimulate interstitial cells of testes to produce testosterone, thereby serving as a method of assessing testicular function. The finding of testicular enlargement is evidence of pituitary secretion of gonadotropins and of testicular responsiveness and obviates the need for administration of hCG. Elevated serum gonadotropins are found in children 12 years of age or older who have primary hypogonadism (Klinefelter syndrome, bilateral gonadal failure from trauma or infection). Because the secretion of gonadotropins is not constant but occurs in spurts, children with constitutional delay of puberty may have normal or low levels of gonadotropins.

421. The answer is d. *(Hay et al, p 1031. Kliegman et al, pp 507-509. McMillan et al, p 2635. Rudolph et al, pp 732-734.)* Down syndrome has many diagnostic features, including short stature, microcephaly, centrally placed hair whorl, small ears, redundant skin on the nape of the neck, upslanting palpebral fissures, epicanthal folds, flat nasal bridge, Brushfield spots, protruding tongue, short and broad hands, simian creases, widely spaced first and second toe, and hypotonia. Cardiac lesions are found in 30% to 50% of children with Down syndrome, including endocardial cushion defect (30%), VSD (30%), and tetralogy of Fallot (about 30%). At birth, duodenal atresia is a common finding. It causes bilious vomiting and a characteristic KUB radiographic findings of a double bubble (dilatation of the stomach and the proximal duodenum).

In Klinefelter syndrome, the testes are smaller than normal for age and feel firm and fibrotic. Physical examination often reveals a eunuchoid body habitus and reduced upper to lower body segment ratio secondary to a long lower segment. Diagnosis is established by means of buccal smear and karyotyping. Levels of luteinizing hormone are elevated after 12 years of age.

Common features of Turner syndrome include female phenotype, short stature, sexual infantilism, streak gonads, broad chest, low hairline, webbed neck, congenital lymphedema of the hands and feet, coarctation of the aorta, and a variety of other anomalies.

Marfan syndrome is a serious disease of connective tissue that is inherited in the autosomal dominant mode. The predominant findings in this condition are bilateral subluxation of the lens, dilatation of the aortic root, and disproportionately long limbs in comparison with the trunk. The decreased upper to lower segment ratio in Marfan syndrome reflects this relative increase in the length of the legs compared with the trunk.

Waardenburg syndrome is the most common of several syndromes that are characterized by both deafness and pigmentary changes. Features of this syndrome, which is inherited as an autosomal dominant disorder, include a distinctive white forelock, heterochromia irides, unilateral or bilateral congenital deafness, and lateral displacement of the inner canthi.

422. The answer is e. *(Hay et al, pp 946, 950. Kliegman et al, pp 2327-2329, 2357. McMillan et al, pp 2128-2129. Rudolph et al, pp 2070-2071.)* The photograph shows thyromegaly. Lymphocytic thyroiditis is a typical organ-specific autoimmune disease characterized by lymphocytic infiltration of the thyroid gland, with or without goiter. It is the most common cause of juvenile hypothyroidism, peaking in adolescence, and affecting as many as 1% of schoolchildren. The condition is 4 to 7 times more prevalent in girls than in boys and may persist for many years without symptoms. Patients are initially euthyroid (with the occasional child having elevated TSH levels), but, with the eventual atrophy of the gland, they become hypothyroid (decreased triiodothyronine [T_3] and T_4, elevated TSH). Spontaneous remission can occur in one-third of the affected adolescents. Hashimoto thyroiditis is not related to endemic goiter caused by iodine deficiency. Autoimmune thyroiditis is associated with many other autoimmune disorders; its association with Addison disease and/or insulin-dependent diabetes mellitus is called type II autoimmune polyglandular syndrome. Family clusters of autoimmune thyroiditis are common; nearly 50% of the patients have siblings with antithyroid antibodies.

423. The answer is d. *(Hay et al, pp 976-977. Kliegman et al, pp 2372-2373. McMillan et al, pp 2144-2145. Rudolph et al, p 2056.)* The child in the question has all of the classic symptoms of childhood pheochromocytoma. In adults, the episodes of hypertension are more paroxysmal than in children, where the hypertension is more sustained. While it is an unusual diagnosis in children, pheochromocytoma must be considered in the evaluation of a patient with hypertension who has intermittent symptoms described. Pheochromocytoma can be associated with tuberous sclerosis, Sturge-Weber syndrome, ataxia-telangiectasia, and it can be inherited as an autosomal dominant trait.

All of the other answers are possibilities in an adolescent-age child, but the concurrent finding of hypertension suggests an alternative diagnosis. Pregnancy would be unusual because of her age, but the diagnosis must be considered for practically all complaints in an adolescent of childbearing age. Migraine headache would be unlikely to produce the cardiac finding of "racing heart" reported in this child. Diabetes can produce a variety of findings, but important clues missing from this case include frequency of urination, weight loss, and other classically seen symptoms. Adolescent fainting spells (vasovagal reaction) are common, and many of the symptoms reported can occur during an episode. They commonly are seen during stressful situations, in groups of adolescents, or sometimes with minor symptoms; hypertension is not one of the features.

424. The answer is a. (*Hay et al, pp 973-974. Kliegman et al, pp 2368-2370. McMillan et al, p 2102. Rudolph et al, pp 2045-2049.*) The photograph shows striae. Although the administration of exogenous adrenocorticotropic hormone or of glucocorticoids is the most common cause of Cushing syndrome, it can also be caused by bilateral adrenal hyperplasia. In the latter case, the concentration of adrenocorticotropic hormone can be normal or high. The basic abnormality, however, is thought to be in the hypothalamic-pituitary axis, not the adrenal gland, because a pituitary adenoma is found in some patients, and those for whom an adenoma is not found, a microadenoma is suspected; many patients who have undergone bilateral adrenalectomy develop Nelson syndrome (invasive pituitary adenoma) despite receiving adequate cortisol replacement. If the patient were an infant, the most likely answer would be an adrenal carcinoma.

425. The answer is a. (*Kliegman et al, p 2380. McMillan et al, p 2650. Rudolph et al, p 2089.*) The constellation of signs described suggest Noonan syndrome. Other features of this syndrome include cubitus valgus, pulmonary stenosis, edema of the dorsum of the hands and feet, hearing loss, pectus excavatum, bleeding diathesis, and mental retardation in about one-fourth of cases. These patients have many features in common with Turner syndrome, and the condition is often referred to as the "male Turner syndrome," although it occurs in both genders. Inheritance is occasionally autosomal dominant, but is more commonly sporadic.

None of the other choices result in a constellation of signs as described. Mental retardation is a prominent feature of untreated congenital hypothyroidism and Down syndrome, and also would be likely in congenital rubella.

426. The answer is c. (*Hay et al, p 992. Kliegman et al, pp 609-610. McMillan et al, pp 2187-2188. Rudolph et al, p 1486.*) The patient has classic findings of galactosemia. Galactose is a component of lactose, found in breast milk and most infant formulas. Symptoms of galactosemia occur in the first weeks of life. While screening for classic galactosemia typically is part of the newborn metabolic panel, patients fitting the clinical presentation as outlined in the question must be evaluated promptly. Signs and symptoms in addition to those presented in the vignette include cataracts and ascites. While three different errors in galactose metabolism are known, most cases result from the deficiency in galactose-1-phosphate uridyl transferase. Urine reducing substances can be positive, but a routine urinalysis will be negative, as the urine strips do not react with galactose. Patients are at increased risk for *E coli* sepsis, and this infection may precede the diagnosis of galactosemia. Prompt removal of galactose from the diet usually reverses the symptoms, including cataracts.

427. The answer is d. (*Hay et al, pp 679-681. Kliegman et al, pp 1803-1816. McMillan et al, pp 1425-1437. Rudolph et al, pp 1967-1979.*) Cystic fibrosis (CF) has an autosomal recessive pattern of inheritance; both parents are usually heterozygous, and the affected child may be a homozygote (two copies of the same mutation) or a compound heterozygote (one copy of each of two different mutations). The ΔF508 mutation, present in about 70% of North American whites, is the most common. In Europe, the incidence of this mutation ranges from 40% to 80% in different population groups. Many other mutations vary in specific ethnic groups.

Identification of a CF mutation in both chromosomes, whether homozygous or compound heterozygous, would be diagnostic in 72%. DNA testing can help predict manifestations of the disease, especially pancreatic involvement. Pancreatic insufficiency is present in 99% of patients who are homozygous for ΔF508, in 72% who are compound homozygous for ΔF508, and in only 32% who do not carry the ΔF508 mutation. DNA analysis for carrier testing is now recommended for relatives of CF patients and for reproductive partners of carriers. Its role in mass population screening is controversial.

The sweat test is diagnostic in virtually all cases of classic CF and is equally useful in all ethnic groups, but it is not useful in detecting heterozygotes. DNA testing is of value for postmortem investigations as well as in sick premature infants and other patients for whom sweat collection is unsuccessful. While genetic testing does not include all of the estimated 1500 defects in the CFTR, it does include 30 to 80 of the most common mutations, representing more than 90% of affected individuals with two CFTR mutations. Sweat testing of asymptomatic parents would not be helpful. While the other studies may indeed be abnormal in a patient with cystic fibrosis, they are not diagnostic.

428. The answer is d. (*Hay et al, pp 938-943. Kliegman et al, pp 2295-2298. McMillan et al, pp 2085-2089. Rudolph et al, pp 2015-2020.*) Alteration of body proportion results from selective regional rates of growth at different stages during the developmental period. At birth, the head is large for the body size, the limbs are short, and the upper to lower segment ratio (crown to pubis/pubis to heel) of 1.7 is high. As the growth of the limbs exceeds that of the trunk from infancy to adolescence, there is a change in body proportions reflected in the upper to lower segment ratios: 1.3 at 3 years, 1.1 at 6 years, and 1.0 at 10 years of age. In achondroplasia, there is a disproportion between the limbs and the trunk; that is, the limbs are relatively short. The head in this condition is also disproportionately large. Achondroplasia is the most common genetic skeletal dysplasia. This disorder has an autosomal dominant mode of inheritance. Marfan syndrome is a serious disease of connective tissue that is inherited in the autosomal dominant mode. The predominant findings in this condition are bilateral subluxation of the lens, dilatation of the aortic root, and disproportionately long limbs in comparison with the trunk. The decreased upper to lower segment ratio in Marfan syndrome reflects this relative increase in the length of the legs compared with the trunk. Morquio syndrome is one of the mucopolysaccharidoses (MPS IV). Abnormal amounts of keratan sulfate accumulate as a result of an enzyme deficiency, and widespread storage of this material in the body results in problems in morphogenesis and function. Skeletal malformations are similar to those seen in osteochondrodysplasias, namely, short trunk with short stature, marked slowing of growth, severe scoliosis, pectus carinatum, and short neck. Thyroid hormone is necessary for physical growth and development and, along with sex hormones, has an essential role in development of bone and linear growth. Thyroid deficiency results in delayed puberty in most cases and in stunting of growth with persistence of immature body proportions; signs and symptoms of hypothyroidism are also frequently seen. In growth hormone deficiency, the upper to lower segment ratio is normal, often without other signs or symptoms.

429. The answer is d. (*Hay et al, pp 947-949. Kliegman et al, pp 2319-2325. McMillan et al, pp 421-422. Rudolph et al, pp 2065-2070.*) Signs of congenital hypothyroidism include constipation, prolonged jaundice, sluggishness, poor feeding, apnea, choking, macroglossia, and excessive sleepiness. The physical examination is usually normal early on except for mild jaundice and a distended abdomen in a sleepy infant. The most appropriate step to manage this condition is to avoid delays and to initiate oral sodium-L-thyroxine, 10 to 15 μg/kg/day. Thyroid dysgenesis is found in 90% of the cases. Neonatal screening for hypothyroidism has allowed for the much earlier diagnosis of hypothyroidism, resulting in an improved prognosis, so that frank cretinism is now quite rare. Most industrialized countries test for phenylketonuria and hypothyroidism; there is variability in testing for other metabolic and genetic diseases.

430. The answer is e. (*Hay et al, pp 1005-1006. Kliegman et al, p 623. McMillan et al, pp 2201-2202. Rudolph et al, pp 657-658.*) Patients born normal who then have progressive developmental delay and hepatosplenomegaly with coarse facial features are likely to have a storage disease. Hurler syndrome, mucopolysaccharidosis type I, is an autosomal condition caused by a deficiency of α-L-iduronidase which causes a deposition of dermatan sulfate and heparan sulfate in the body, and excessive excretion in the urine. Other features of this condition include umbilical hernia, kyphoscoliosis, deafness, cloudy corneas, and claw hand deformity. Death is common in childhood, a result of respiratory or cardiac compromise.

In none of the other choices would one expect to see the development of hepatosplenomegaly or a loss of normal childhood developmental milestones. Jeune syndrome (asphyxiating thoracic dystrophy) is notable for short stature, long and narrow thorax, hypoplastic lungs, fibrotic liver, and short limbs. Death is common, a result of pneumonia or asphyxia because of the abnormally shaped thorax. Crouzon syndrome is an autosomal dominant condition that results in craniosynostosis (usually coronal), proptosis, brachycephaly, hypertelorism and strabismus, "beak" nose, midface hypoplasia, and high and narrow palate. Trisomy 18 (Edwards syndrome) is a condition marked by low birth weight, low-set and malformed ears, micrognathia, clenched hands with overlapping digits, a variety of cardiac defects, and poor subcutaneous fat deposition. About 50% of children with the condition die in the first weeks of life, and less than 10% survive beyond the first year; severe mental retardation is uniform. At birth patients with Beckwith-Wiedemann syndrome are macrosomic with macroglossia, abdominal wall defects, linear ear creases, and organomegaly; they often have hypoglycemia in the newborn period. They have an increased incidence of developing malignancy, especially Wilms tumor, hepatoblastoma, and gonadoblastoma. Intellect is usually normal.

431. The answer is a. (*Hay et al, p 938. Kliegman et al, p 2297. McMillan et al, pp 2084-2092. Rudolph et al, pp 2015-2017, 2094.*) The determination of bone age by the radiographic examination of ossification centers provides a measure of a child's level of growth that is independent of his or her chronologic age. Height age is the age that corresponds to the 50th percentile for a child's height. When bone age and height age are equally retarded several years behind chronologic age, a child is described as having constitutional short stature. Such a child is usually shorter than peers in adolescence because of the delayed growth spurt, but the prognosis for normal adult height is excellent because there is still the potential for growth. Detailed questioning will usually identify other family members with a history of delayed growth and sexual maturation but with ultimately normal stature. Children with genetic or familial short stature grow at an adequate rate, but remain small throughout life; their ultimate height is consistent with predictions based on parental heights. Bone age is within the limits of normal for chronologic age, and puberty occurs at the normal time. In all cases, a thorough history and physical examination are necessary to identify any other cause of growth delay.

432. The answer is b. (*Hay et al, pp 791, 1036. Kliegman et al, pp 2878-2879. McMillan et al, p 2638. Rudolph et al, pp 759-760.*) Achondroplasia, occurring with an incidence of approximately 1 in every 26,000 live births, is the most common genetic form of skeletal dysplasia. Affected persons bear a striking resemblance to one another and are identified by their extremely short extremities; prominent foreheads; short, stubby fingers; and marked lumbar lordosis. Although they go through normal puberty, affected females must have children by cesarean section because of the pelvic deformity. Other complications include hydrocephalus secondary to bony overgrowth at the foramen magnum. Achondroplasia is inherited in an autosomal dominant manner, but most cases represent spontaneous mutations in unaffected parents. Thanatophoric dwarfism has a high incidence of death in the newborn period, as affected patients have a very small thorax and little lung capacity. Chondroectodermal dysplasia, also known as Ellis-van Creveld syndrome, also presents with short limbs but includes dental and nail anomalies, as well as congenital cardiac defects. Patients with metatropic dysplasia also have long torsos and short extremities, but they have progressive kyphoscoliosis and joint restriction; they may also have cervical instability. Achondrogenesis is typically fatal, and involves severe lack of bony development.

433. The answer is c. (*Hay et al, pp 946-953. Kliegman et al, pp 2157-2158, 2338-2339. McMillan et al, pp 2132-2133. Rudolph et al, pp 2077-2078.*) Of the choices, the first step in the management of a pediatric patient with a solitary thyroid nodule is measurement of thyroid function. Decreased incidence of exposure of children to radiation (such as in dental procedures) has resulted in a reduction in the rate of malignancy in the thyroid.

A variety of diagnostic procedures are available to evaluate the patient with a nodule, including measurement of thyroid function, antithyroid antibody determination, ultrasound, and radionuclide uptake and scan. Depending on the results of these tests, a fine needle aspiration may ultimately be required. Trials of T_4 to determine whether the lesion shrinks are not reliable, and excisional surgery would not be indicated unless the mass were rapidly progressing and impinging on a vital structure.

434. The answer is d. (*Hay et al, pp 908-909. Kliegman et al, pp 2151-2152. McMillan et al, pp 1786-1788. Rudolph et al, pp 2395-2396.*) The child pictured is an asymmetric "red" reflex (one eye is lighter than the other). Although all the listed options can produce the symptoms described, the family history supports the diagnosis of retinoblastoma, the most common intraocular tumor in children. Early detection can result in a survival rate of over 90%. The pattern of inheritance of retinoblastoma is complicated: the hereditary form of the disease can be transmitted by means of autosomal dominant inheritance from an affected parent, from an unaffected parent carrying the gene, or from a new germinal mutation. Familial occurrences are usually bilateral. A second primary tumor develops in 15% to 90% of survivors of bilateral retinoblastoma, the most common of which is osteosarcoma, increasing in incidence with time. Retinoblastoma is associated with a mutation or deletion of the long arm of chromosome 13. In addition to specialized ophthalmologic care, management of retinoblastoma includes molecular genetic investigation of the family to identify those who have inherited the tumor-predisposing retinoblastoma gene.

435. The answer is c. (*Hay et al, p 957. Kliegman et al, pp 2344-2345. McMillan et al, p 432. Rudolph et al, p 2151.*) The patient with the features listed likely has pseudohypoparathyroidism (Albright hereditary osteodystrophy). Such patients have chemical findings of hypoparathyroidism (low calcium, high phosphorus), but parathyroid hormone levels are high, indicating resistance to the action of this hormone. Parathyroid hormone infusion does not produce a phosphaturic response. Phenotypically, these patients demonstrate shortness of stature with delayed bone age, mental retardation, increased bone density throughout the body (especially evident in the skull), brachydactyly (especially of the fourth and fifth digits), obesity with round facies and short neck, subcapsular cataracts, cutaneous and subcutaneous calcifications, and perivascular calcifications of the basal ganglia.

436. The answer is c. *(Hay et al, p 960. Kliegman et al, p 2348. McMillan et al, p 2078. Rudolph et al, pp 2154-2155.)* Hypercalcemia can develop in children who are immobilized following the fracture of a weight-bearing bone. Serious complications of immobilization hypercalcemia, and the hypercalciuria that occurs as a result, include nephropathy, nephrocalcinosis, hypertensive encephalopathy, and convulsions. The early symptoms of hypercalcemia—namely, constipation, anorexia, occasional vomiting, polyuria, and lethargy—are nonspecific and may be ascribed to the effects of the injury and hospitalization. Therefore, careful monitoring of these patients with serial measurements of the serum ionized calcium and the urinary calcium to creatinine ratio is critical during their immobilization. A ratio of greater than 0.2 establishes a diagnosis of hypercalciuria. Although complete mobilization is curative, additional measures, such as vigorous intravenous hydration with a balanced salt solution, dietary restrictions of dairy products, and administration of diuretics, can be instituted. For patients who are at risk for symptomatic hypercalcemia, short-term therapy with calcitonin is highly effective in reducing the concentration of serum calcium by inhibiting bone resorption.

437. The answer is d. *(Hay et al, p 982. Kliegman et al, pp 2418-2419. McMillan et al, p 2108. Rudolph et al, p 2111.)* Glucose is nonenzymatically attached to hemoglobin to form glycosylated hemoglobin. The major component of this reaction proceeds very slowly and is irreversible until the hemoglobin is destroyed. The concentration of glycosylated hemoglobin thus reflects glucose concentration over the half-life of the red cell, or about 2 to 3 months. The adolescent in the question may have had poor control of his diabetes for longer than 2 to 3 months, but glycosylated hemoglobin is unable to determine this.

438. The answer is b. *(Hay et al, pp 970-973. Kliegman et al, pp 2360-2364. McMillan et al, pp 2138-2140. Rudolph et al, pp 2038-2042.)* Salt-losing congenital adrenal hyperplasia (adrenogenital syndrome, 21-hydroxylase deficiency) usually manifests during the first 5 to 15 days of life as anorexia, vomiting, diarrhea, and dehydration. Hypoglycemia can also occur. Affected infants can have increased pigmentation, and female infants show evidence of virilization, that is, ambiguous external genitalia. Hyponatremia, hyperkalemia, and urinary sodium wasting are the usual laboratory findings. Death can occur if the diagnosis is missed and appropriate treatment is not instituted.

Although adrenal aplasia, an extremely rare disorder, presents a similar clinical picture, it has an earlier onset than adrenal hyperplasia, and virilization does not occur. In classic 21-hydroxylase deficiency, serum levels of 17-hydroxyprogesterone are markedly elevated beyond 3 days of life (in the first 3 days of life they can normally be high). Blood cortisol levels are usually low in salt-losing forms of the disease.

Pyloric stenosis seems unlikely in this infant in that the vomiting with this disease usually begins after the third week of life. Hypothyroidism would present as a lethargic, poor-feeding infant with delayed reflexes, persistent jaundice, and hypotonia. Hyperaldosteronism would be expected to cause decreased potassium, not increased levels. Panhypopituitarism usually presents with apnea, cyanosis, or severe hypoglycemia.

439. The answer is d. (*Hay et al, pp 125-126. Kliegman et al, pp 2385-2386. McMillan et al, pp 558-559. Rudolph et al, p 248.*) Gynecomastia is a common occurrence in adolescent boys, especially during Tanner stage 2 or 3. It can occur unilaterally or bilaterally, and can affect one breast more significantly than the other. It is thought to be caused by a temporary reduction in the testosterone to estradiol ratio. Spontaneous regression usually occurs; it rarely lasts for more than 2 years. In the child who otherwise has a normal physical examination and no significant past medical history, reassurance of the benign nature of the condition is all that is required for most cases. Rarely, the gynecomastia is significant; antiestrogen agents can be utilized or surgery can be considered. Other, more serious causes for this condition include Klinefelter syndrome, hyperthyroidism, hormone-producing tumors, and drugs (including marijuana). A thorough history and physical examination can help eliminate these relatively unusual causes.

440. The answer is a. (*Kliegman et al, p 534. McMillan et al, pp 2156-2157. Rudolph et al, pp 612-613.*) The infant described in the question has alkaptonuria (alcaptonuria is an alternate spelling), an autosomal recessive disorder caused by a deficiency of homogentisic acid oxidase. The diagnosis is made in infants when their urine turns dark brown or black on exposure to air because of the oxidation of homogentisic acid. Affected children are asymptomatic. In adults, ochronosis—the deposition of a bluish pigment in cartilage and fibrous tissue—develops; symptoms of arthritis may appear later. No specific treatment is available for patients who have alkaptonuria, although supplemental ascorbic acid may delay the onset of the disorder and reduce clinical symptoms. The other deficiencies listed in the question are found in phenylketonuria, histidinemia, maple syrup urine disease, and isovaleric acidemia, respectively.

441. The answer is e. *(Hay et al, pp 661-663. Kliegman et al, pp 1677-1678. McMillan et al, pp 2021-2022. Rudolph et al, pp 1491-1492.)* Wilson disease is an autosomal recessive disorder characterized by liver disease (usually seen in childhood), neurologic and behavioral disturbances (seen by adolescence), renal tubular dysfunction (Fanconi syndrome), and eye findings (Kayser-Fleischer rings). Its multisystem manifestations are caused by the deposition of copper in various tissues (resulting in low serum levels), and therapy is aimed at the prevention of accumulation of copper. Defective metabolism of the copper-binding protein ceruloplasmin (usually reduced) has been demonstrated by some.

Indian childhood cirrhosis is a nontreatable, fatal condition found in rural India, affecting children aged 1 to 3 years with hepatomegaly, fever, anorexia, and jaundice. It rapidly progresses to cirrhosis and liver failure. Serum immunoglobulin levels and hepatic copper concentrations are elevated. α_1-Antitrypsin deficiency, which causes liver disease through accumulation of an abnormal protein, is caused by a single amino acid substitution on chromosome 14. It has a variable presentation, but in infancy the following are common: cholestasis; bleeding into the CNS, GI tract, or at the umbilical stump; and elevation of transaminase concentrations. In childhood, a picture of chronic hepatitis with cirrhosis and portal hypertension is seen, but the neurologic and behavior changes typical of Wilson disease are not seen. Menkes syndrome presents in the first months of life and includes hypothermia, hypotonia, and myoclonic seizures. These children have chubby, rosy cheeks and kinky, colorless, and friable hair. Severe mental retardation is always seen. Low serum copper and ceruloplasmin levels are found, with a copper absorption/transport problem being the cause. Dubin-Johnson syndrome is inherited as an autosomal recessive condition with patients being unable to excrete conjugated bilirubin. Such patients present during adolescence or early adulthood, sometimes earlier. Morbidity owing to this condition is unusual.

442. The answer is e. *(Kliegman et al, p 659. McMillan et al, p 2354. Rudolph et al, p 2110.)* Hypoglycemia with hyperinsulinemia but without evidence of C-peptide suggests that the insulin is exogenous; these findings occurring while the patient is in the hospital would suggest that the current caretaker is injecting insulin into the baby causing hypoglycemia. The caretaker (more commonly the mother) may be suffering from Munchausen by proxy (MPB) syndrome, a disorder in which a parent induces illness in the child or reports symptoms repeatedly to represent the child as ill. There is usually no obvious secondary gain for the parent, as there is with the diagnosis of malingering. Protective services should always be notified about suspected MBP cases, as there are sometimes fatalities.

Nesidioblastosis, Beckwith-Wiedemann, and galactosemia can all cause hypoglycemia, but do not fir the story and the laboratory values. Pancreatitis can cause hyperglycemia.

443. The answer is d. *(Hay et al, pp 1035-1036. Kliegman et al, pp 2890-2893. McMillan et al, pp 2230-2233. Rudolph et al, pp 762-764.)* Marfan syndrome is a genetic disorder transmitted as an autosomal dominant trait with variable expression. People with this disorder typically have tall stature, arachnodactyly, subluxation of the lens, dilatation of the aorta, and dissecting aneurysm. Mental retardation is not a part of this syndrome. Vascular complications can be serious if not identified early; aortic dissection can lead to sudden death. Patients with any of the other syndromes listed have tall stature and are more likely to have varying degrees of mental retardation or behavioral problems among their clinical findings.

444. The answer is d. *(Hay et al, pp 294-295. Kliegman et al, pp 253-258. McMillan et al, p 113. Rudolph et al, pp 2156-2160.)* The x-ray demonstrates a fracture of the femur, and also a significant decreased bone mineralization. The child in the question (exclusively breast-fed, no vitamin D supplementation, northern climate with limited sun exposure, African American mother) is at risk for simple (nutritional) rickets. Nutritional rickets is caused by a dietary deficiency of vitamin D and lack of exposure to sunlight.

Intestinal absorption of calcium and phosphorus is diminished in vitamin D deficiency. Transient hypocalcemia stimulates the secretion of parathyroid hormone and the mobilization of calcium and phosphorus from bone; enhanced parathyroid hormone activity leads to phosphaturia and diminished excretion of calcium. In children with nutritional rickets, the concentration of serum calcium usually is normal and the phosphate level is low. Increased serum alkaline phosphatase is a common finding. The excretion of calcium in the urine is increased only after therapy with vitamin D has been instituted.

445. The answer is a. *(Hay et al, pp 17-19. Kliegman et al, pp 655-658. McMillan et al, pp 411-413. Rudolph et al, pp 155-159.)* Glycogen and fat stores are diminished in premature infants and those who are small for gestational age. Energy stores are inadequate to meet the energy demands after the maternal supply of glucose is interrupted at birth, and hypoglycemia ensues. Deficiency of cortisol or growth hormone is a rare cause of neonatal hypoglycemia.

Insulin excess, common in infants of diabetic mothers, is unusual in other infants. Hypoglycemia associated with a deficiency of glucagon has been reported but is very rare.

446. The answer is b. *(Hay et al, pp 953-957. Kliegman et al, pp 259, 778. McMillan et al, pp 2075-2076. Rudolph et al, pp 2149-2152, 2268-2269.)* Hypocalcemia of newborn infants can be divided into two groups: early (during the first approximately 72 hours of life) and late (after approximately 72 hours). The most common type of early neonatal hypocalcemia is the so-called idiopathic hypocalcemia.

Other causes early on include maternal illness (diabetes, toxemia, and hyperparathyroidism), neonatal respiratory distress (perinatal asphyxia) or sepsis, low birth weight because of prematurity, or hypomagnesemia. Transient or permanent hypoparathyroidism and high phosphate intake are the most common factors associated with late hypocalcemia. The bicarbonate and glucose levels in the question are normal, while the elevated magnesium level may cause sedation and apnea but not tetany and seizures. Intracranial hemorrhages are less common in an infant of this gestational age, and usually do not present with tetany.

447 to 451. The answers are 447-a, 448-e, 449-d, 450-e, 451-d. *(Hay et al, pp 953, 955-958, 1036. Kliegman et al, pp 259-260, 2339-2340, 2342-2345, 2887-2890. McMillan et al, pp 432, 1898-1900, 2075-2076, 2133, 2236-2237. Rudolph et al, pp 163-164, 761-762, 2057-2059, 2151, 2156-2160.)* The boys in the first question have rickets unresponsive to vitamin supplementation; vitamin D–resistant rickets is caused by a genetic abnormality in the renal tubular reabsorption of phosphate with resultant hyperphosphaturia and hypophosphatemia and also in the conversion of 25-hydroxyvitamin D to 1,25-dihydroxyvitamin D. The intestinal absorption of phosphate is also abnormal, and calcium absorption from the gut can be secondarily affected. Calcium concentration is usually normal. The disorder is usually transmitted as an X-linked dominant trait.

The patient in the second question has a form of pseudohypoparathyroidism (Albright hereditary osteodystrophy). Patients with pseudohypoparathyroidism have the same chemical abnormality (low Ca, high PO_4) as those with hypoparathyroidism. They are distinguished from the latter group by the phenotypic features demonstrated by the girl in the question (Albright hereditary osteodystrophy) and high serum concentration of parathyroid hormone. The basic abnormality in these patients is the unresponsiveness of the renal tubules to parathyroid hormone. They are classified into two groups, depending on the site of the defect. Type I patients have failure to generate cyclic adenosine monophosphate (AMP) and do not have an increase in urinary concentration of cyclic AMP or phosphate in response to parathyroid hormone. Type II patients have a defect in the renal tubules that causes failure to respond to high concentrations of cyclic AMP. These patients, if given parathyroid hormone, have increased urinary excretion of cyclic AMP but not of phosphate.

Osteogenesis imperfecta (blue sclera, easily broken bones with minimal trauma) is transmitted as an autosomal recessive (severe form) or, more commonly, autosomal dominant (milder form) disorder. The basic defect is an abnormality in the production and composition of the matrix of bone. Serum calcium and phosphate concentrations are normal.

Hypoparathyroidism is unusual in children outside the newborn period, usually presenting with neuromuscular instability such as seizures, with numbness and tingling possibly preceding the seizures, like those in the patient in the question, who had numbness and tingling of the hands and who later developed seizures. In response to low concentrations of parathyroid hormone, there is reduced bone resorption. In the kidney, there is reduced excretion of phosphate and reduced formation of 1,25-dihydroxyvitamin D. The reduced 1,25-dihydroxyvitamin D formation in turn reduces the absorption of calcium and, secondarily, of phosphorus from the gut. The net effect is hypocalcemia and hyperphosphatemia.

Medullary carcinoma of thyroid arises from the C cells of the thyroid. These tumors secrete excessive amounts of calcitonin, and, accordingly, the concentration of this hormone in the blood is increased. Despite elevated levels of calcitonin, the serum concentrations of calcium and phosphorus are usually normal unless the patient has associated hyperparathyroidism (multiple endocrine adenomatosis, type II).

452 to 457. The answers are 452-g, 453-a, 454-b, 455-e, 456-f, 457-b. (*Hay et al, pp 130-132, 957-958, 966, 973-974, 978-985, 1039-1040. Kliegman et al, pp 233, 2282-2283, 2344-2345, 2368-2370, 2379, 2425-2427. McMillan et al, pp 432, 562, 2102, 2115-2122, 2640-2641, 2653. Rudolph et al, pp 249, 1708, 2045-2049, 2134-2136, 2152, 2303.*) Patients with type 2 diabetes mellitus have insulin resistance in their skeletal muscles, increased hepatic glucose production, and decreased insulin secretion in response to elevated levels of glucose. They also develop hyperlipidemia and many complications of chronic hyperglycemia. Acanthosis nigricans, as described in the question, is a common finding in type 2 diabetes.

The Prader-Willi syndrome is a disorder consisting of hypotonia, hypogonadism, hyperphagia after the newborn period, hypomentia, and obesity. A deletion of a portion of chromosome 15 has been found in approximately 70% of patients. Children affected by this syndrome exhibit little movement *in utero* and are hypotonic during the neonatal period. Feeding difficulties and failure to thrive can be the presenting complaints in the first year; later, obesity becomes the most common presenting complaint. The enormous food intake of affected children is thought to be caused by a defect in the satiety center in the hypothalamus. Stringent caloric restriction is the only known treatment.

Laurence-Moon-Biedl (Bardet-Biedl) syndrome is transmitted as an autosomal recessive trait. Obesity, mental retardation, hypogonadism, polydactyly, and retinitis pigmentosa with night blindness are the principal findings in affected children. There is no known effective treatment.

Fröhlich syndrome, also known as adiposogenital dystrophy, is a rare cause of childhood obesity associated with a hypothalamic tumor.

Pseudohypoparathyroidism is a collective term for a variety of diseases. Affected patients have biochemical findings (low serum calcium and high serum phosphorus levels) similar to those associated with hypoparathyroidism, but they also have high levels of endogenous parathyroid hormone; in addition, exogenous parathyroid hormone fails to increase their phosphate excretion or raise their serum calcium level. The defects in these patients appear to be at the hormone receptor site or in the adenylate cyclase-cyclic AMP system. The symptoms of pseudohypoparathyroidism are caused by hypocalcemia. Affected children are short, round-faced, and mildly retarded. Metacarpals and metatarsals are shortened, and subcutaneous and basal ganglia calcifications as well as cataracts can be present. The current treatment consists of large doses of vitamin D and reduction of the phosphate load.

Polycystic ovary disease classically presents at or shortly after puberty with obesity, hirsutism, and secondary amenorrhea. Later, these women have anovulatory infertility. The cause of this condition is not entirely clear.

The initial complaint in Cushing syndrome may be obesity. Accumulation of fat in the face, neck, and trunk causes the characteristic "buffalo hump" and "moon" facies. Characteristic features include growth failure, muscle wasting, thinning of the skin, plethora, and hypertension. The bone age of affected patients is retarded, and osteoporosis can be present. The disorder results from an excess of glucocorticoids that may be caused by a primary adrenal abnormality (adenoma or carcinoma) or secondary hypercortisolism, which may be owing to excess adrenocorticotropin. Exogenous glucocorticoids administered in supraphysiologic doses for a prolonged period of time will produce a similar picture in normal subjects.

458 to 463. The answers are 458-a, 459-e, 460-e, 461-d, 462-a, 463-b.
(Hay et al, pp 703-704, 945-946, 968-974, 991-992. Kliegman et al, pp 602-604, 2300-2301, 2355-2356, 2367-2368. McMillan et al, pp 1901-1904, 2138-2141, 2143, 2183-2185, 2303. Rudolph et al, pp 634-636, 1651, 1714, 2026-2028, 2038-2044, 2245.) In the salt-losing variety of 21-hydroxylase deficiency, the synthesis of both mineralocorticoids (eg, aldosterone) and cortisol is impaired. Aldosterone deficiency impairs the exchange of potassium for sodium in the distal renal tubule. Affected patients have hyponatremia and hyperkalemia. Dehydration, hypotension, and shock may be present.

In the absence of vasopressin (central diabetes insipidus), renal collecting tubules are impermeable to water, resulting in the excretion of hypotonic urine. Patients with diabetes insipidus present with polyuria and polydipsia. Net loss of water leads to dehydration and hemoconcentration and, therefore, to relatively high serum concentrations of sodium and potassium. Patients with nephrogenic diabetes insipidus have similar laboratory findings. This genetic disorder is unresponsive to antidiuretic hormone (ADH). These patients are unable to concentrate their urine and present in the neonatal period with hypernatremic dehydration.

In hyperaldosteronism, renal tubular sodium–potassium exchange is enhanced. Hypokalemia, hypernatremia, hyperchloremia, and alkalosis are the usual findings. Primary hyperaldosteronism (Conn syndrome) is very rare in children.

Addison disease is associated with a combined deficiency of glucocorticoids and mineralocorticoids. Resorption of sodium and excretion of potassium and hydrogen ions are impaired at the level of the distal renal tubules. Sodium loss results in loss of water and depletion of blood volume. Persons with compensated Addison disease can have relatively normal physical and laboratory findings; Addisonian crisis, however, characteristically produces hyponatremia, hyperkalemia, and shock. The pathophysiology of the serum electrolyte abnormalities in this disorder is the same as in the salt-losing variety of adrenogenital syndrome.

Patients with a deficiency of glucose-6-phosphatase (von Gierke disease) are, as a rule, hyperlipidemic. Increased triglyceride concentration in the serum decreases the volume of the aqueous compartment. Because electrolytes are present only in the aqueous compartment of the serum but are expressed in milliequivalents per liter of serum as a whole, the concentrations of sodium and potassium can be factitiously low in these patients.

464 to 470. The answers are 464-g, 465-a, 466-c, 467-e, 468-f, 469-b, 470-d. *(Hay et al, pp 17-18, 99-100, 555, 871-872, 1031-1032. Kliegman et al, pp 507-509, 780-781, 783-785, 1883, 2386-2389, 2717-2718. McMillan et al, pp 2630-2634. Rudolph et al, pp 124-126, 731-734, 744, 764-768, 775, 2087-2089.)* Ehlers-Danlos syndrome is characterized by thin fragile skin, easy bruising, and joint hypermobility. Mitral valve prolapse has been reported. There are several different variants. One of these variants, the vascular form (type 3), can result in rupture of the aorta.

Trisomy 21, also known as Down syndrome, is easily recognized in older children and adults, but may be more difficult to diagnose in infancy. Characteristics include upslanting palpebral fissures with epicanthal folds, hypotonia, small ears, and a single transverse palmar crease. About half of patients with Down syndrome will have some type of cardiac abnormality.

Holt-Oram syndrome is characterized by abnormalities in the upper extremities, hypoplastic radii, thumb abnormalities, and cardiac anomalies. Occasionally the pectoralis major muscle is missing in Holt-Oram, and as such it needs to be considered when discussing Poland syndrome.

Mothers who consume alcohol during pregnancy put their infant at risk of fetal alcohol syndrome. Key features include growth retardation, short palpebral features, short nose, thin upper lip, mental retardation, heart defects, and behavioral abnormalities.

Turner syndrome (XO) is characterized by short stature, low ears, a wide chest with widely spaced nipples, broad based neck, low hairline, extremity edema, and congenital heart defects (typically coarctation or bicuspid aortic valve). Intelligence is normal.

Trisomy 18 (Edwards syndrome) babies are small with low-set ears, a prominent occiput, a short sternum, a closed hand with overlapping fingers, cardiac defects, rocker-bottom (rounded) feet, cleft lip and/or palate, and renal and genital abnormalities. Mortality is 50% in the first week and 90% in the first year.

Infants born to diabetic mothers are frequently macrosomic and may become hypoglycemic. However, they can have many other problems as well, including cardiac septal hypertrophy, congenital heart disease, caudal regression, vertebral defects, and a single umbilical artery.

471 to 474. The answers are 471-a, 472-c, 473-e, 474-b. (*Hay et al, pp 1025-1026. Kliegman et al, pp 495-502, 515. McMillan et al, pp 89-90. Rudolph et al, pp 649-650, 717-720, 2303.*) The mitochondrial genome originates only from the ovum and is therefore transmitted by the mother to her offspring of both genders. Mitochondrial disease involves mainly brain and muscle. Ragged red fibers seen on muscle biopsy are present in several inherited enzyme defects. Examples of mitochondrial inheritance include myoclonic epilepsy and ragged red fibers (MERF); mitochondrial myopathy, encephalopathy, lactic acidosis, and strokelike episodes (MELAS); and Leber hereditary optic neuropathy (LHON), a condition not associated with myopathy.

Prader-Willi syndrome, which is characterized by hypotonia, obesity, hypogonadism, mental retardation, and characteristic hands, feet, and facies, is caused by a chromosomal deletion of 15q11-13 when the chromosome is of paternal origin. In some syndromes, such as Angelman syndrome, chromosomal deletion of maternal origin results in a syndrome characterized by a specific facies, happy disposition, mental retardation, bizarre movements, and seizures. More recently, cases of Prader-Willi syndrome have been found wherein there is no DNA deletion but both copies of chromosome 15 have been inherited from the mother; similarly, some cases of Angelman syndrome have been shown to have two copies of paternally derived chromosome 15. This suggests that it is the lack of part of paternal chromosome 15 that causes Prader-Willi syndrome and the lack of part of maternal chromosome 15 that causes Angelman syndrome.

Some conditions have a more dynamic mutation that can continue to expand with errors in replication. These are called triplet repeat expansion disorders, and include fragile X syndrome, Huntington disease, and myotonic dystrophy. As the gene is further replicated and expanded, protein production ceases and clinical symptoms are expressed.

Hypomelanosis of Ito is not thought to be inherited, but does display mosaicism in that about half of affected patients have two distinct cell lines of skin fibroblasts. Other examples of inherited mosaicism include higher functioning patients with trisomy 21, who may display some physical findings consistent with the syndrome but may not have as severe cognitive delay, as some cells have trisomy 21 and others do not.

The Adolescent

Questions

475. A 15-year-old female presents to your office with secondary amenorrhea. As part of your evaluation, you find that she is pregnant. After informing her of the pregnancy, you continue to explain that young mothers have a higher risk of several pregnancy-related complications, including which of the following?

a. Twin gestation
b. Low-birthweight infants
c. Hypotension
d. Excessive weight gain
e. Infants with genetic defects

476. A 12-year-old boy has scant, long, slightly pigmented pubic hairs; slight enlargement of his penis, and a pink, textured, and enlarged scrotum. He is most likely at which sexual maturation rating (SMR, also called Tanner) stage?

a. SMR 1
b. SMR 2
c. SMR 3
d. SMR 4
e. SMR 5

477. A 16-year-old boy who is the backup quarterback for the local high school team is in your office complaining of worsening acne. For the last few months he has noted more acne and more oily hair. On his examination, you note gynecomastia and small testicular volume. He is SMR 5. Which of the following drugs of abuse is the likely explanation for all of his findings?

a. Cocaine
b. Oxandrolone
c. Marijuana
d. Toluene
e. Methylenedioxymethamphetamine

478. A 15-year-old girl is brought to the pediatric emergency room by the lunchroom teacher, who observed her sitting alone and crying. On questioning, the teacher learned that the girl had taken five unidentified tablets after having had an argument with her mother about a boyfriend of whom the mother disapproved. Toxicology studies are negative, and physical examination is normal. Which of the following is the most appropriate course of action?

a. Hospitalize the teenager on the adolescent ward.
b. Get a psychiatry consultation.
c. Get a social service consultation.
d. Arrange a family conference that includes the boyfriend.
e. Prescribe an antidepressant and arrange for a prompt clinic appointment.

479. A 15-year-old girl is seen in your clinic with a sprained ankle, which occurred the previous day while she was exercising in her room. You realize that you have not seen her for quite some time, and begin to expand your examination beyond the ankle. You find relatively minimal swelling on her right ankle. She has dental decay, especially of anterior teeth and a swollen, reddened, irritated uvula. She seems to be somewhat hirsute on her arms and legs, but has thinning of her hair of the head. She has a resting heart rate of 60 beats per minute, and her oral temperature is 35.5°C (96°F). Further questioning suggests that she has developed secondary amenorrhea. Which of the following is the most appropriate next step in the management of this girl?

a. Human immunodeficiency virus (HIV) testing
b. Radiograph of ankle
c. Thyroid function panel
d. Comparison of current and past weights
e. Pregnancy testing

480. A 17-year-old sexually active girl comes to your office complaining of acne that is unresponsive to the usual treatment regimen. Physical examination reveals severe nodulocystic acne of her face, upper chest, and back. You consider prescribing isotretinoin (Accutane), but you are concerned about side effects. Reviewing the literature, you find which of the following to be true about isotretinoin?

a. Its efficacy can be profound and permanent.
b. It is not known to be a teratogen.
c. Most patients experience excessive tearing and salivation.
d. Severe arthritis necessitating cessation of the drug occurs in about 15% of patients.
e. Significant decrease in serum triglyceride levels are noted in 25% of patients.

481. A 15-year-old presents with the complaint of a rash, as pictured below. Which of the following statements is correct concerning the management of this common condition?

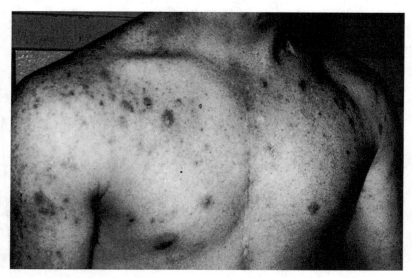

(Courtesy of Adelaide Hebert, MD.)

a. Fried foods must be avoided.
b. Frequent scrubbing of the affected areas is key.
c. Topical antibiotics are of no value.
d. Topical benzoyl peroxide is the mainstay of treatment.
e. This rash is solely a disease of the adolescent.

482. A 15-year-old athlete is in your office for his annual physical examination before the start of football season. He has no complaints, has suffered no injuries, and appears to be physically fit. On his heart examination, you note a heart rate of 100 beats per minute, and a diffuse point of maximal impulse (PMI) with a prominent ventricular lift. He has a normal S_1 and S_2, with an S_4 gallop. He has no murmur sitting, but when he stands you clearly hear a systolic ejection murmur along the lower left sternal edge and the apex. For which of the following conditions is this examination most consistent?

a. Wolff-Parkinson-White syndrome
b. Valvular aortic stenosis
c. Valvular pulmonic stenosis
d. Myocarditis
e. Hypertrophic cardiomyopathy

483. You are the sideline physician for a local high school football team. During a district playoff game, the starting quarterback is sacked for a loss on third down. As the punter heads out onto the field, the quarterback is slow to come to the sidelines. He seems confused and dazed. Aside from his confusion, his examination is normal. After 10 minutes, he is lucid and wants to get back into the game. Based on published guidelines, which of the following is your correct course of action?

a. Allow the player back in the game
b. Hold the player out for at least 30 minutes
c. Hold the player out for the rest of the game
d. Hold the player out for this game and the next game
e. Send the player to a hospital for evaluation

484. A 16-year-old girl, accompanied by her mother, is in your office for a well-adolescent visit. The mother asks about drug and alcohol abuse. You explain that the warning signs of abuse include which of the following?

a. Excessive concern for weight and body configuration
b. Improved school performance
c. Recent changes from age-appropriate, acceptable friends to younger associates
d. Deterioration in personal habits, hygiene, dress, grooming, speech patterns, and fluency of expression
e. Improvement in relationships with adults, siblings, and authority figures

485. The recent suicide of a well-known high school cheerleader in your community has generated an enormous amount of community concern and media coverage. A girl who was close friends with the deceased makes an appointment and comes in to your office to discuss the event with you. You ask, and she denies suicidal ideation, but she has many questions about suicide. Correct statements about adolescent suicide include which of the following?

a. Girls tend to use more lethal means.
b. The number of attempted suicides is much higher among boys.
c. Those who are successful have a history of a prior attempt or prior serious suicidal ideation.
d. Inquiry by pediatricians, high school teachers, parents, or friends about suicidal thoughts typically precipitates the act.
e. The number of suicides in adolescents 10 to 19 years of age has decreased significantly since the 1950s.

486. A 16-year-old girl is in your office for a preparticipation sports examination. She plans to play soccer in the fall, and needs her form filled out. Which of the following history or physical examination findings is usually considered a contraindication to playing contact sports?

a. Congenital heart disease, repaired
b. Obesity
c. Absence of a single ovary
d. Absence of a single eye
e. Diabetes mellitus

487. A 15-year-old boy is in the office for a preparticipation sports physical examination before he begins playing with the varsity football team at his school. Although he is a skilled receiver, he will be one of the smallest players on the field and is concerned about the potential for injury. He asks how to bulk up. Appropriate advice to increase muscle mass includes which of the following?

a. Taking extra vitamins
b. Doubling protein intake
c. Using anabolic steroids
d. Increasing muscle work
e. Taking ergogenic medication

488. An 18-year-old male college student is seen in the student health clinic for urinary frequency, dysuria, and urethral discharge. Which of the following is likely to explain his condition?

a. Herpes simplex
b. *Escherichia coli* urinary tract infection
c. Chlamydial urethritis
d. Syphilis
e. HIV infection

489. A 19-year-old male college student returns from spring break in Fort Lauderdale, Florida, with complaints of acute pain and swelling of the scrotum. Physical examination reveals an exquisitely tender, swollen right testis that is rather hard to examine. The cremasteric reflex is absent, but there is no swelling in the inguinal area. The rest of his genitourinary examination appears to be normal. A urine dip is negative for red and white blood cells. Which of the following is the appropriate next step in management?

a. Administration of antibiotics after culture of urethra for *Chlamydia* and gonorrhea
b. Reassurance
c. Intravenous fluid administration, pain medications, and straining of all voids
d. Ultrasound of the scrotum
e. Laparoscopic exploration of both inguinal regions

490. A 16-year-old girl presents with lower abdominal pain and fever. On physical examination, a tender adnexal mass is felt. Further questioning in private reveals the following: she has a new sexual partner; her periods are irregular; she has a vaginal discharge. Which of the following is the most likely diagnosis?

a. Appendiceal abscess
b. Tubo-ovarian abscess
c. Ovarian cyst
d. Renal cyst
e. Ectopic pregnancy

491. The parents of a 16-year-old girl complain that she does not get enough sleep. They recently discovered that she stays awake most nights until 1:00 AM reading and text messaging her friends. She wakes at 6:30 AM for school, and complains of sleepiness during the day. On weekends she sleeps until noon. Her parents have tried taking away her computer and phone, but she still would go to bed at the same time. The parents are looking for advice in dealing with their "night owl" daughter. Which of the following is appropriate advice for this family?

a. Teens need less sleep than adults.
b. Effects of puberty on melatonin cause a phase delay with later sleep onset.
c. Most teens get an adequate number of hours of sleep each night.
d. Daytime sleepiness is a clear manifestation of an inadequate number of hours of sleep.
e. Sleeping in on weekends should repay the "sleep debt".

Questions 492 to 495

Listed below are diagnostic tests for various types of genital ulcers. Match each with the appropriate vignette. Each lettered option may be used once, more than once, or not at all.

a. Dark-field microscopic examination
b. Special chocolate agar culture
c. Bordet-Gengou medium culture
d. Tzanck preparation for multinucleated giant cells
e. *Chlamydia* culture
f. Loeffler medium culture

492. A 16-year-old female has a positive rapid plasma reagin (RPR) of 1:64 and an ulcer on her labia.

493. A 19-year-old male has recurrent episodes of painful, erythematous, small vesicles, and ulcers on his glans penis.

494. A 15-year-old male had a painless papule on his genitals that resolved, but he has now developed a unilateral draining inguinal lymphadenitis.

495. A 19-year-old female has a few small papules on her labia and perineum. The papules become pustular, eroded, and ulcerated over the next few days; at the same time, the patient develops painful, tender inguinal lymphadenopathy.

Questions 496 to 500

Listed below are common adolescent activities that may result in injury. Match each with the injury with which the activity is most commonly associated. Each lettered option may be used once, more than once, or not at all.

a. A 15-year-old competitive swimmer
b. A 17-year-old high school quarterback
c. A 17-year-old starting center for a high school basketball team
d. A 14-year-old long-distance runner
e. An 11-year-old ballerina
f. A 16-year-old high school wrestling champion
g. A 14-year-old snow skier
h. An 18-year-old college hockey star

496. Patellar tendinitis and Osgood-Schlatter disease

497. Injuries almost exclusively related to the shoulder, including rotator cuff tendinitis

498. Delayed menarche and eating disorder

499. Hyperextension of the thumb and sprains of the anterior cruciate ligament

500. Shoulder subluxation, knee injuries, and dermatologic problems such as herpes simplex, impetigo, and staphylococcal furunculosis or folliculitis

The Adolescent

Answers

475. The answer is b. *(Hay et al, pp 140-141. Kliegman et al, pp 850-852. McMillan et al, pp 566-567. Rudolph et al, pp 254-255.)* Adolescents are typically healthy and do not have chronic disease. However, several pregnancy complications occur more frequently in teens, including poor weight gain in the mother, premature delivery, low birth weight, and an increased risk of pregnancy-induced hypertension. The risk of violence is also elevated for teen mothers. As both parents age, the risk of genetic defects in their infant increases. Teen mothers have a lower risk of twin gestation.

476. The answer is b. *(Hay et al, pp 112-113. Kliegman et al, pp 60-62. McMillan et al, pp 531-536. Rudolph et al, pp 224-226.)* Normal sexual maturation during puberty follows a consistent pattern. The first sign of puberty in boys is scrotal and testicular growth; penis growth usually occurs about a year after. Pubic hair growth is more variable. In girls, the first sign of puberty is the development of breast buds. The SMRs are not synchronized, in that a girl with SMR 3 pubic hair doesn't always have SMR 3 breasts.

The description in the question is typical of SMR 2 in males: sparse, thin, and long pubic hair with slight penile enlargement. In SMR 3, pubic hair becomes darker and begins to curl, and the penis lengthens. In SMR 4 it is starting to resemble adult pubic hair but without complete coverage, and the penis continues to grow. At SMR 5, pubic hair extends to the inner thigh and is in the typical adult configuration.

Females have sparse pubic hair to start SMR 2 as well, and progress over time to full pubic coverage with medial thigh extension in SMR 5. Breasts start with buds in SMR 2, and progress to larger breasts and areola without a separate areolar contour in SMR 3. Breasts at SMR 4 will have elevation of the areola, but by SMR 5 the areola is part of the general breast contour.

477. The answer is b. *(Hay et al, pp 144-162. Kliegman et al, pp 824-834. McMillan et al, pp 579-584. Rudolph et al, pp 376-378.)* Substance abuse in adolescence is a common concern, and rightly so: 75% of high school students have tried an alcoholic drink, with 25% trying alcohol before they were 13; and more than 40% of seniors have tried marijuana. The average starting age of smokers is 12 years. Inhalants of volatile organic compounds, such as gasoline, glue, refrigerant, and paint thinner are frequently used earlier, as they are easier to obtain. Although many children see inhalants as "safe" drugs, they are anything but, as acute use can result in arrhythmia and death, and chronic use can result in brain damage, peripheral neuropathies, and spasticity. Cocaine abuse leads to euphoria, increased motor activity, tachycardia, and dizziness, Marijuana cause elation and euphoria, short-term memory impairment, distorted time perception, and flashbacks. Methylenedioxymethamphetamine (more commonly known as MDMA, or even more commonly Ecstasy) is a "club drug" for all-night parties, and typically causes euphoria and increased energy. Of the list, only anabolic steroids have been associated with increased hirsutism, acne, and breast development with testicular wasting.

478. The answer is a. (*Hay et al, pp 192-194. Kliegman et al, pp 124-125. McMillan et al, pp 648-650. Rudolph et al, pp 501-503.*) The adolescent who has attempted suicide should be hospitalized so that a complete medical, psychological, and social evaluation can be performed and an appropriate treatment plan developed. Hospitalization also emphasizes the seriousness of the adolescent's action to her and to her family and the importance of cooperation in carrying out the recommendations for ongoing future therapy. The treatment plan may include continued counseling or supportive therapy with a pediatrician, outpatient psychotherapy with a psychiatrist or other mental health worker, or family therapy.

479. The answer is d. (*Hay et al, pp 163-174. Kliegman et al, pp 127-130. McMillan et al, pp 655-661. Rudolph et al, pp 231-233.*) The young lady in the question could have any number of problems, and all of the answers could ultimately prove to be helpful. As a first step, however, a close look at her weight in comparison to previous ones is in order; she has some physical examination findings seen with bulimia (dental decay, irritated uvula), and others seen with anorexia nervosa (lanugo, thinning hair, low resting heart rate, hypothermia, secondary amenorrhea).

Eating disorders have become increasingly prevalent in recent years. Symptoms of finicky appetite, progressively restricted food intake, distress at looking fat, and compulsively pursuing thinness can appear after puberty. Parents may not appreciate the magnitude of weight loss until it reaches 10% or more of body weight, because those girls will not undress in their parents' presence and because the facial contours are the last parts to be affected. Bulimia usually appears in mid adolescence rather than early adolescence and is characterized by sessions of gorging, often in secret and often involving a single favored snack food such as ice cream, cake, or candy, although it may also be manifested as immoderate eating at mealtimes. This gorging is followed by secret bouts of self-induced vomiting. Some bulimics also use laxatives and purgatives. Physical consequences of bulimia include esophageal varices and hemorrhage; dental decay, especially of anterior teeth (because of exposure of enamel to gastric HCl); and a swollen, reddened, irritated uvula (also from chronic HCl exposure). Physical consequences of anorexia include profound weight loss (25%-30% or more of body weight), dehydration, facial and arm hirsutism, loss of hair of the head, bradycardia, cardiac conduction problems, reduced cardiac output, hypothermia, impaired renal function, multiple malnutrition effects (including avitaminoses), a primary or secondary amenorrhea, and osteoporosis. Significant mortality in treatment-resistant cases is seen. The psychologic component of these disorders is not a unitary one. Some anorexic patients have an underlying obsessive-compulsive or narcissistic personality disorder, some are borderline psychotic, and some are depressed. Bulimic patients have a significant underlying depression. Patients with eating disorders have exceedingly ambivalent feelings toward parents, especially mothers, and in turn evoke great ambivalence on the part of parents. Therapy includes behavior modification to deal with eating behavior per se, family therapy, and individual or group therapy. Imipramine, when used appropriately, is a useful adjunct treatment for this condition. In cases of life-threatening degrees of weight loss or vomiting, hospitalization to limit freedom, restore physiologic equilibrium, and provide a controlled eating environment can be indicated.

480. The answer is a. *(Hay et al, pp 406-409. Kliegman et al, pp 2759-2762. McMillan et al, pp 875-877. Rudolph et al, pp 1208-1210.)* Isotretinoin (13-cis-retinoic acid; Accutane) has proved to be very effective in the treatment of refractory nodulocystic acne. The effects of treatment appear to be long-lasting. Precautions regarding its use, however, are essential. Because of its teratogenic effects (isotretinoin syndrome), the drug is contraindicated during pregnancy and within 1 month of becoming pregnant. Dry skin, eyes, and mucous membranes are the most frequent complications of therapy. Other associated problems include musculoskeletal pain and hyperostosis, inflammatory bowel disease, pseudotumor cerebri, and corneal opacities. Patients on isotretinoin therapy can often develop abnormal liver function tests, elevated triglyceride and cholesterol levels, and lowered levels of high-density lipoproteins. Some have suggested that an increased risk of suicide is related to its use, although this link is less well established.

481. The answer is d. *(Hay et al, pp 406-409. Kliegman et al, pp 2759-2762. McMillan et al, pp 875-877. Rudolph et al, pp 1208-1210.)* Acne is a skin disorder that affects virtually all adolescents and is seen less commonly in older patients. There is a wide spectrum of clinical findings, ranging from a few papules and comedones to a disfiguring nodulocystic disease of the face and trunk. The goals of therapy are to prevent scarring and disfigurement and to avoid loss of self-esteem. The chief benefit of benzoyl peroxide is derived from its antibacterial activity, but it also functions as an exfoliant and comedolytic. A combination of benzoyl peroxide and retinoic acid is particularly effective in sloughing the epithelium, and statics, such as oral tetracycline, and the use of topical antibiotics can be necessary to control the inflammatory component of acne. Studies have failed to demonstrate adverse effects of any particular foods on disease activity. Vigorous facial or body scrubbing can traumatize the skin and aggravate the problem.

482. The answer is e. *(Hay et al, pp 585-586. Kliegman et al, pp 1967-1969. McMillan et al, pp 1638-1641. Rudolph et al, pp 1805, 1862.)* Hypertrophic cardiomyopathy (HCM) should be a significant concern to anyone caring for young athletes. Although uncommon (one study of asymptomatic young adults found echocardiographic evidence of HCM in 2 of 1000 patients), the sudden death of an athlete on the playing field generates significant public awareness of the condition. Unfortunately, youth afflicted with HCM are frequently asymptomatic. The first hint of the condition may be when the athlete collapses during a practice or game. Thus, potential warning signs are extremely important and should not be missed. A family history of sudden death or early myocardial infraction (MI), a past history of syncope during exercise, or the physical examination described in the question above should prompt further evaluation with an echocardiograph.

Wolff-Parkinson-White (WPW) is a reentrant tachycardia with abrupt onset and termination. WPW has been associated with HCM, but would not present by itself as the above vignette. Valvular aortic stenosis presents with and left ventricular thrust, a systolic thrill, a prominent aortic ejection click between S_1 and S_2, and a loud rough systolic ejection murmur is heard in the first and second intercostal spaces. Valvular pulmonic stenosis presents with a right ventricular heave and systolic thrill and a prominent ejection click best heard in the left third intercostal space that is more easily identified during expiration. Myocarditis can be acute or chronic, and should display some elements of heart failure.

483. The answer is a. *(Hay et al, p 815. Kliegman et al, pp 2862-2863. McMillan et al, pp 741-742. Rudolph et al, p 2244.)* Return to Play guidelines were published in 1997 by the American Academy of Neurology. The guidelines divide concussions into three categories. Grade 1 (mild) concussions have no loss of consciousness and a return to baseline in less than 15 minutes. Grade 2 (moderate) concussions also have no loss of consciousness, but include confusion lasting longer than 15 minutes. Grade 3 (severe) concussions include any loss of consciousness. The player in the vignette had a grade 1 concussion with no other sign of injury, and as such may be allowed back into the game. If, later in the game, he were to have a second grade 1 concussion, he should be removed from the game and held out of play for a week. A player with a grade 2 concussion may not return to the game and must remain out for at least a week; he should be evaluated in a hospital if symptoms last for more than an hour. A player with a grade 3 concussion should be evaluated immediately at the hospital.

484. The answer is d. *(Hay et al, pp 144-162. Kliegman et al, pp 824-834. McMillan et al, pp 579-584. Rudolph et al, pp 226-230.)* When an adolescent shows evidence of declining school performance or truancy, a change for the worse in personal habits and grooming, exaggerated mood swings, change in friends to an older and unacceptable group, and frequent hostile reactions in relationships with others, the possibility that he or she is abusing drugs or alcohol, or both, should be considered strongly. Dependence on drugs is a progressive disorder; therefore, prompt identification and intervention are required if serious complications are to be avoided. Routine health assessment of adolescents should include inquiry about the use of cigarettes, alcohol, and other drugs, and about school performance and family and peer relationships.

485. The answer is c. *(Hay et al, pp 192-194. Kliegman et al, pp 124-126. McMillan et al, pp 648-650. Rudolph et al, pp 37, 501-503.)* Suicide among teenagers has increased steadily since 1950 and is now the third leading cause of adolescent death, following accidents and homicides. Suicide attempts occur more often in girls, but in all age groups males outnumber females in completed suicides because boys tend to use more lethal means, such as firearms, hanging, jumping, and inhalation of carbon monoxide. Most suicide attempters and completers (where history can be established) have a history of a prior attempt or prior serious suicidal ideation. Therefore, direct questioning of the adolescent about feelings of sadness, hopelessness, concerns about death, and thoughts of committing suicide is important, and suicidal ideation must be taken seriously. There are no data to indicate that such inquiry precipitates suicidal behavior.

486. The answer is d. *(Hay et al, p 811. Kliegman et al, p 2849.)* The preparticipation sports physical examination is important in that it allows the physician to screen patients for potential risks associated with the sport they intend to play. That said, there are few real contraindications to sports participation. Having one eye is typically seen as a contraindication to playing contact sports like football or soccer. There are eye shields available, but in general these children are advised to avoid contact sports. Stable, repaired congenital heart disease; obesity; girls with a single ovary; and controlled diabetics are routinely allowed to participate. Other reasons to recommend against contact sports participation include hemophilia, single kidney, and unexplained syncope (until evaluated).

487. The answer is d. *(Hay et al, pp 151-152. Kliegman et al, pp 833-834. McMillan et al, p 884.)* Increased muscle work (along with increased calories) is the only appropriate way to increase muscle mass. Measurements of skinfold thickness, performed serially, are a useful way to detect changes in the amount of body fat, so that obesity can be avoided. Protein loading or using drugs, hormones, and vitamins will not be helpful and may be harmful.

488. The answer is c. *(Hay et al, pp 1255-1256, 1264. Kliegman et al, pp 1285-1286. McMillan et al, pp 585-586. Rudolph et al, pp 261-266.)* Urethritis in an adolescent male is almost always a sexually transmitted disease (STD), either gonococcal or nongonococcal urethritis (NGU). *Chlamydia trachomatis* is usually the causative agent in NGU. Less frequently, NGU can be caused by *Ureaplasma urealyticum, Trichomonas vaginalis,* and yeast. Herpes simplex can cause an NGU, but it is considerably less likely than *C trachomatis.* Gonococcal culture and Gram stain are easily available; chlamydial culture may not be. Direct monoclonal antibody tests as well as enzyme immunoassay and molecular probe tests are alternative methods for *Chlamydia* identification, although they are less sensitive and less specific than chlamydial culture. Urine ligase testing for *Chlamydia* and gonococcus is available. Serologic testing for syphilis should always be done, but in none of its normal presentations is urethral discharge common. Testing for HIV should be offered and safe sexual practices encouraged; HIV does not cause urethral discharge. Urinary tract infection is not associated with a urethral discharge.

489. The answer is d. (*Hay et al, p 1265. Kliegman et al, pp 856-857, 2262. McMillan et al, pp 1832-1833. Rudolph et al, pp 260-270.*) The patient in the question may have a torsion of his testis that requires immediate attention. Another possibility would be epididymitis, especially if there is a possible antecedent history of sexual activity or urinary tract infection. Prehn sign, although not totally reliable, is elicited by gently lifting the scrotum toward the symphysis. Relief of the pain points to epididymitis; it's worsening, to torsion. Doppler ultrasound (or surgical consultation) is a logical first step in this man's evaluation, demonstrating absence of flow in torsion and increased flow in epididymitis. Alternatively, a radionuclide scan will show diminished uptake in torsion and increased uptake in epididymitis.

Treatment for torsion is surgical exploration and detorsion and scrotal orchiopexy. Causative organisms for epididymitis include *Neisseria gonorrhoeae, C trachomatis,* and other bacteria. Treatment with appropriate antibiotics and rest is indicated. However, treating this patient with antibiotics without first excluding testicular torsion is ill-advised; loss of the testis can be expected after 4 to 6 hours of absent blood flow if the testis has torsioned. Strangulated hernia is associated with evidence of intestinal obstruction.

490. The answer is b. (*Hay et al, pp 1262-1264. Kliegman et al, pp 857-858, 861. McMillan et al, p 587. Rudolph et al, pp 268-269.*) Pelvic inflammatory disease (PID) refers to sexually transmitted infections of the female upper genital tract including tubo-ovarian abscess, endometritis, salpingitis, and pelvic peritonitis. Each year, a diagnosis of PID is made in more than 1 million women. Sexually active teenagers are at great risk of acquiring PID because of their high-risk behavior, exposure to multiple partners, and failure to use contraceptives. The strong likelihood of PID in the patient presented should not preclude consideration of serious conditions requiring surgical intervention, such as appendiceal abscess, ectopic pregnancy, and ovarian cyst. Renal cyst does not present in the manner described. An episode of PID raises the risk of ectopic pregnancy, and about 20% of women become infertile following one episode of PID. Other sequelae include dyspareunia, pyosalpinx, tubo-ovarian abscess, and pelvic adhesions. Endometriosis is not related to PID.

491. The answer is b. (*Hay et al, pp 88-90. Kliegman et al, pp 91-93. McMillan et al, p 665.*) Adolescents typically require about 9 hours of sleep a night, but on average get about 7 hours. Changes due to puberty cause a phase delay in the normal sleep-wake cycle, meaning teens will almost universally prefer to stay up late. Left to their own devices, they would choose to sleep later into the morning as well, but most high schools start early in the morning, forcing adolescents to wake early and not get adequate sleep. Sleeping late on the weekends does not reverse the symptoms of chronic sleep deprivation, which include daytime sleepiness, inattention, and emotional lability. However, sleepiness during the day does not always mean the patient is getting insufficient number of hours of sleep; medical conditions, such as obstructive sleep apnea, can cause sleep fragmentation and daytime sleepiness, and should be considered in any sleep evaluation.

492 to 495. The answers are 492-a, 493-d, 494-e, 495-b. (*Hay et al, pp 1115-1116, 1206, 1269. Kliegman et al, pp 1177-1178, 1266-1267, 1287, 1363-1364. McMillan et al, pp 983, 1139-1140, 1255-1256. Rudolph et al, pp 928-929, 1002-1005, 1168, 1173.*) In the first patient, syphilis is likely. A scraping from a genital ulcer could be examined under dark-field microscopy for *Treponema pallidum*. A serologic test for syphilis is indicated for every sexually active patient recently infected with a STD. In the event of a negative serologic test result, consideration should be given to repeating this test at a later date, because serologic tests performed too early in the disease may not be reliable.

Herpes should be suspected in a patient with recurrent shallow, painful ulcers of the genitourinary tract. A herpes simplex ulcer can be either a primary or a secondary infection (as in the case presented). Examination of a Tzanck preparation of scraping from the ulcer reveals multinucleated giant cells and intranuclear inclusions. Herpes simplex virus is readily cultured. In addition, rapid diagnostic tests using immunofluorescence or enzyme-linked immunosorbent assay (ELISA) are available, as is a herpes simplex virus polymerase chain reaction (HSV PCR) assay.

Lymphogranuloma venereum (LGV) is caused by serotypes of *C trachomatis,* which can be cultured. Serial serologic testing for chlamydial antibodies can be of diagnostic value retrospectively.

Chancroid caused by *Haemophilus ducreyi* is difficult to culture. Special chocolate agar medium is only 65% sensitive. Indirect immunofluorescence using monoclonal antibodies or PCR is more commonly used. Inguinal adenopathy that suppurates and causes chronic draining of sinuses is commonly seen in chancroid and can be confused with LGV. Typically, the inguinal adenopathy of chancroid occurs at the same time as the genital ulcer, while the adenopathy in LGV occurs after the ulcer has healed.

496 to 500. The answers are 496-c, 497-a, 498-e, 499-g, 500-f. *(Hay et al, pp 814-821. Kliegman et al, pp 2848-2869. McMillan et al, pp 884-899. Rudolph et al, pp 2432, 2448, 2449-2451.)* A wide variety of injuries occur in adolescents who participate in sports. Some injuries, however, are more common in certain sports than in others.

For swimmers, shoulder injuries are the most common type of problem seen. Rotator cuff tendinitis of the biceps and/or the supraspinatus muscles presents as shoulder pain and tenderness.

In football, head and neck injuries are not uncommon, but, fortunately, serious injuries are rare. Knee injuries such as anterior cruciate, posterior cruciate, and collateral ligament tears do occur. In addition, turf toe, injury to the first metatarsophalangeal joint, is seen when play is on artificial turf.

Basketball and volleyball tend to produce lower extremity problems, including those of the knee, with such injuries as Osgood-Schlatter disease and sprains to the ligaments of the knee. Ankle injuries, too, are quite common in these sports.

Injuries caused by running are frequently muscle strains in the hamstrings, adductors, soleus, and gastrocnemius muscles. *Runner's knee,* anterior knee pain because of patellofemoral stress, is also seen.

Ballet can be associated with delayed menarche and eating disorders (more commonly in the female dancers). In addition, a variety of mostly lower extremity problems can be seen, ranging from bunions to knee and ankle problems from serious overuse.

Injuries in wrestlers are frequently seen in the upper extremities, especially shoulder subluxation, and in the knees, usually prepatellar bursitis from traumatic impact to the floor. Additionally, a variety of skin conditions are common, ranging from contact dermatitis and superficial fungal infections to herpes simplex (herpes gladiatorum), impetigo, and staphylococcus furunculosis or folliculitis.

Availability of better equipment has resulted in a decrease in the number of serious skiing injuries. Thumb injuries during a fall, *skier's thumb* (abduction and hyperextension of the thumb, causing a sprain of the ulnar collateral ligament), remains the most common injury seen.

Hockey injuries range from mild contusions to significant lacerations. No particular type of injury (with the exception of, perhaps, loss of teeth) is characteristic of this sport.

Bibliography

Hay WW, Levin MJ, Sondheimer JM, Deterding RR, eds. *Current Diagnosis and Treatment in Pediatrics*. 18th ed. New York, NY: McGraw-Hill; 2007.

Kliegman RM, Behrman RE, Jenson HB, Stanton BF, eds. *Nelson Textbook of Pediatrics*. 18th ed. Philadelphia, PA: WB Saunders Co.; 2007.

McMillan JA, Feigin RD, DeAngelis CD, Jones MD, eds. *Oski's Pediatrics*. 4th ed. Philadelphia, PA: Lippincott Williams & Wilkins; 2006.

Rudolph CD, Rudolph AM, Hostetter MK, Lister G, Siegel NJ, eds. *Rudolph's Pediatrics*. 21st ed. New York, NY: McGraw-Hill; 2003.

Index

Notes